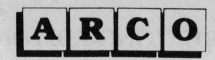

NURSING SCHOOL ENTRANCE EXAMINATIONS

CANCELLED

Marion F. Gooding, R.N., Ph. D.
Professor of Nursing
North Carolina Central University

Prentice Hall
New York • London • Toronto • Sydney • Tokyo • Singapore

CONTRIBUTING EDITORS

Mattie Moss, Ed.D.
Associate Professor of Mathematics
North Carolina Central Univerity
Durham, North Carolina

John C. Clamp, Ph.D.
Associate Professor of Biology
North Carolina Central University
Durham, North Carolina

Louise Gooch, R.N., Ed.D.
Director, Practical Nurse Program
Durham Technical Community College
Durham, North Carolina

Doris E. Wilson, B.A.
Language Arts Instructor
Sampson G. Smith School
Somerset, New Jersey

12th Edition

Prentice Hall General Reference
15 Columbus Circle
New York, NY 10023

Library of Congress Cataloging-in-Publication Data

Gooding, Marion F.
    Nursing school entrance examinations.—12th ed. / Marion F. Gooding.
    p. cm.
    ISBN 0-671-86750-4
    1. Nursing schools—United States—Entrance examinations—
Study guides. I. Title.
    [DNLM: 1. Nursing—examination questions. 2. Educational
Measurement. WY 18 G652n 1993]
RT79.G66   1993
610.73'076—dc20
DNLM/DLC
for Library of Congress   93-22714
                                           CIP

Manufactured in the United States of America

1 2 3 4 5 6 7 8 9 10

CONTENTS

Part Three: Practice for Practical Nursing School Entrance Examinations

PREFACE

If you are planning to apply to a nursing program, you will probably be required to take an entrance examination. These examinations are designed to measure your abilities in subject areas pertinent to nursing. Since nursing is an art as well as a science, it takes creativity, a trained intellect, and a noble spirit to develop the skills of a competent practitioner. Therefore, it is important for persons desiring to enter the field to be able to think quantitatively and qualitatively, to communicate effectively, and to be able to conceptualize—put terms, concepts, facts, and principles together in a meaningful way. The entrance examinations include mathematics, science, reading comprehension and verbal ability, all of which are directly related to nursing competencies.

The results of the entrance examinations are used for selection of students, for placement within nursing programs, or for guidance to students who have academic deficiencies and need remedial work. Each nursing program establishes procedures for using the test results.

This book is specifically designed to prepare you for the Psychological Corporation Entrance Examinations and the National League for Nursing Prenursing and Guidance Examination. The Psychological Corporation has one Entrance Examination for schools of Nursing and one Entrance Examination for schools for Practical/Vocational Nursing. The National League for Nursing also has two separate examinations, one for entrance into registered-nurse programs, and one for entrance into licensed practical-nurse programs.

This book also provides preparation for the Allied Health Admissions Test offered by Psychological Corporation for persons entering a variety of programs, such as dental hygiene, respiratory therapy, physical therapy, surgical technology, medical technology, dietetics and nutrition, environmental health, physician's assistant, and several other occupations and professions. The Psychological Services Bureau's Entrance Examination for practical nursing, registered nursing, and health occupations includes a battery of tests similar to the tests mentioned above.

The areas covered include verbal ability, mathematics, health sciences, and reading comprehension. This is the only review book with comprehensive preparation for entrance examinations for nursing and allied health occupations and professions. If you use this book as directed, you should be prepared to take the entrance examinations successfully.

Part One

INFORMATION ABOUT THE NURSING PROFESSION AND NURSING SCHOOL ENTRANCE EXAMINATIONS

ABOUT THE NURSING PROFESSION

SELECTING A NURSING CAREER

Regardless of which kind of nursing program you choose to enter, you will have opportunities to provide an important service to humanity. You may enter nursing at one level and expand your skills through practice and additional education. Advancement within the nursing profession comes about in several ways. A practical nurse may decide to become a registered nurse, an upward move. A registered nurse may decide to move from the hospital setting into community-based care, a horizontal move that expands the types of services a nurse can provide. A registered nurse who does not have a baccalaureate degree may decide to earn one in order to step up to a management position.

There are four kinds of programs that prepare for entrance into nursing:

The practical-nurse programs are usually offered in vocational schools, hospitals, and community colleges. The program varies from 9–18 months. The courses include the basic sciences and medical–surgical, pediatric, and obstetrical nursing. Some mental-health concepts are included. The major focus is on technical skills. A practical nurse works under the supervision of a registered nurse (RN).

The associate-degree nurse is a graduate of a two-year college program that is designed with a balance between clinical nursing courses (medical, surgical, psychiatric, obstetrical, and pediatric nursing) and general-education courses (biological and physical sciences, behavioral sciences, humanities, and electives) to provide a background for making important judgments about patient care. The graduate is prepared for technical expertise in the assessment, planning, and delivery of direct patient care in the hospital setting.

The graduate of the hospital-based diploma program functions on the nursing team in the same manner as the associate-degree nurse. Most diploma programs are 24–30 months in length, and the non-nursing courses may be offered through a college.

The baccalaureate nursing program is four years in length and is offered in senior colleges and universities. The required courses in the biological, physical, and behavioral sciences are both basic and advanced. These general-education requirements, along with courses that provide a broad liberal-arts background, are taken during the first two years. The major clinical courses are offered in the third and fourth years and include the five clinical areas identified above, with an emphasis on community-health nursing and the role of the professional nurse as a manager. Most nursing programs offering the professional baccalaureate degree admit graduates from the diploma and associate degree programs with varying degrees of advanced standing.

The graduates of all four programs take a licensing examination. At the present time, there are two kinds of licenses: the practical-nurse license and the registered-nurse license for graduates of the diploma, associate degree, and baccalaureate degree programs.

A nurse may continue studies to receive a master's degree and a doctorate with a major in clinical specialties, teaching, administration, or research, depending on his or her career choice. There is a great demand for nurses in hospitals, schools, clinics, public-health agencies, and many other settings throughout the world. Nurses may become anesthetists, enter the military, or become writers, consultants, or private practitioners. Nursing provides a basis for many careers and, more importantly, a personally and financially satisfying experience.

SELECTING A NURSING PROGRAM

The first factor you should take into consideration is your career goal. Do you plan to work in hospitals as a member of the health team? Is your ultimate goal to function as a manager or an administrator? Are you primarily interested in teaching? Do you want to specialize in a specific clinical area? Are you planning to work in a community setting providing services to families? Is your ultimate goal to become an entrepreneur?

The rapidly moving trend in nursing today is to license two levels of nursing for entry into the professional services. The assistant level will be represented by graduates of the associate degree nursing programs; the professional level, by graduates of the baccalaureate nursing programs. Baccalaureate education in nursing forms the foundation for graduate education in nursing, where specialization as a clinical practitioner, administrator, and teacher occurs. Other types of graduates (practical nurse and diploma) will achieve these credentials through career mobility programs.

A second factor to consider is costs. The demands for full-time study and the length of the program may necessitate resigning from your job.

A third factor is whether you qualify for admission. As the levels of performance increase, so do the academic requirements. In some cases, a student may enter at the associate degree level and upon graduating and receiving a license (RN), enter the baccalaureate program because the requirements are different for the RNs.

Once you have matched your career with a program, you should use the guidelines listed below to make your final choice.

1. Is the program approved by the state regulating body (most often the Board of Nursing)?
2. Is the program accredited by a voluntary agency (National League for Nursing)?
3. What is the program's reputation in terms of graduate performance?
4. How does the social and academic environment meet your needs?

FINANCIAL AID SOURCES

With the increasing costs of education, and the decreasing federal sources for financial aid, the competition for funds is increasing. It is therefore important to know what the sources are, the eligibility requirements, and how to apply. It is equally important to apply as early as possible to a variety of programs.

To initiate the application process, get a financial aid form from your local high school counseling office, or directly from the school to which you are seeking admission. This form must be completed and mailed to the *College*

Scholarship Service (address is on the form). In approximately six weeks, a report is sent back that identifies whether you are eligible for financial aid. This report must be sent to the school of your selection so that the amount you are eligible for and amount you will have to pay can be determined.

The amount of money a recipient can receive is dependent on the need analysis derived from the financial aid form and the financial aid program in which the nursing school, college, or university is participating. The school usually prepares a financial aid package that is a combination of financial sources to make up for the difference between the amount the student is able to contribute and the total costs for the nursing program.

Some financial aid programs are loans, which must be paid back at a low interest rate over a prolonged period of time. Other sources are grants and scholarships, which do not have to be paid back. The obligation for debt payment requires serious thought on the part of the student since a default can affect his or her credit ranking.

When shopping for financial aid, check the accreditation status of the nursing program and the institution's eligibility for such aid. All nursing programs accredited by the National League for Nursing are eligible for federal funding, but some institutions have limited federal sources due to high default rates.

Federal Sources of Financial Aid

All federal funds are based on need. The United States Department of Education currently offers five programs that are described below.

Pell Grant (Basic Education Opportunity Grant [BEOG]). This award is based on a formula that considers family income, which must be documented by IRS statements. The maximum award per student is $2,200 per year and may not exceed half the total cost of a year's study. If need is documented, the student may receive additional moneys from other sources. There is no repayment.

Supplemental Education Opportunity Grant (SEOG). The student must demonstrate exceptional need. Awards may be up to $4,000 per year and must not exceed one-half of the total financial package. There is no repayment.

College Work Study (WS). The student is given a work assignment on or off campus. The maximum workload is twenty hours per week. The recipient is paid a salary that must meet the minimum wage. The government provides the award moneys to the school for tuition. Depending on the institutional policies, the student's salary may be credited to his or her account, or the salary may be paid directly to the student.

Stafford Loan (Formerly Guaranteed Student Loan). The moneys are secured through a lender, such as a bank or credit union or other commercial lender, at a low interest rate. The amount of the loan varies. The repayment starts after graduation or termination of studies at an interest rate fixed at the time the loan is granted. Additional funds are available through *PLUS Loans.*

Other Sources of Financial Aid

Because of the nursing shortage, the financial aid sources for nursing education have greatly expanded. Some of these awards are not based on financial need. Some are aimed at recruitment into a specialty, such as geriatric nursing.

At the federal and state levels, there are nursing student loan programs for full- or part-time study, ranging from $2500 up to $10,000. Many of these loans are repayable through employment.

In your state, you will find many health-care agencies that provide scholarships or tuition reimbursement plans. Individual nursing programs have additional scholarship and or loan monies.

Some of the community-based sources might be the state nurses association, the state constituent of the National League for Nursing (NLN), religious organizations, fraternal organizations, and civic and corporate organizations. Some of the nationally known sources include:

- American Association of Critical Care Nurse Scholarships

- American Cancer Society

- American Nurse Association Ethnic/Racial Minority Fellowships

- Association of Operating Room Nurses

- Eight and Forty American Legion

- National Student Nurse Association

- International Council of Nurses

Interested persons should purchase *Scholarships and Loans for Nursing*, published by the National League for Nursing; Scholarships and Loans, 350 Hudson Street, New York, NY 10014 (212) 989-9393.

SPECIAL FEATURES OF THIS BOOK

Simulated Tests

By studying the more than 1300 test questions in this book, which are similar to the items included in the entrance examinations, you will review material already learned, gain new knowledge, and become familiar with the format of timed tests. The sections for the registered-nurse and practical-nurse examinations are separated; however, the entire book may be used to prepare for all examinations.

Test-Taking Skills

By following the guidelines presented on test-taking skills, you will be able to increase your chances for success by using the "educated guess" technique.

Presentation of Basic Concepts

The verbal ability, mathematics, and science sections include a summary of basic facts, principles, and concepts related to the content area. This provides a study guide and helps you select correct answers.

Explanatory Answers

For selected tests, explanations of the correct answers are given. This provides another opportunity to reinforce principles which apply to the test items.

ABOUT THE EXAMINATIONS

How to Apply for an Entrance Examination

The procedures for applying for the Psychological Corporation, National League for Nursing, or other entrance examination will be provided by the specific school that you have selected to study nursing. It will notify you which examination it requires, where the local testing centers are located, and the specific time you are scheduled to take the examination. An application card must be completed and submitted with a test fee. You must follow all instructions given by the specific program for which you are applying. All applications and test results are handled through the specific schools.

Administration of the Examinations

The examinations are administered by qualified persons, usually in a testing center. You will be scheduled to take the tests along with other candidates. Specific directions for taking the examinations will be given by the person proctoring the examination. All tests are timed. The proctor will tell you when to begin and when to stop.

All answers are placed on a separate answer sheet so that your results can be analyzed by computer. The computerized answer sheets are similar to the answer sheets in this book.

The National League for Nursing examination for entrance into registered-nurse programs takes approximately four hours, and the practical-nurse entrance exam takes three and one-half hours. The Psychological Corporation examination takes approximately two and one-half hours. The proctor arranges for a break between test portions of each exam.

Answer sheets are sent to the respective testing centers for analysis. A computerized report is sent to the program from which the application was obtained, and the person taking the examination can also receive a report. The average time for receiving the test results is three weeks.

The tests are developed from a blueprint that identifies the number and type of items. There are several forms for each examination. If the blueprint calls for ten items related to understanding electrolytes, each form will have ten such items, but the specific test items may differ. That is why this book provides a variety of test items along with basic guidelines for answering similar questions.

HOW TO INTERPRET TEST SCORES

Simulated Report of Performance

NLN PRENURSING AND GUIDANCE EXAMINATION

Applicant	Identification No.	Test Date
Mary Brown 100 Oaks Road Clearview, OK 74835	6-5081-599	04/11/90

Test	Score	Percentile Norms*		
		DI	AD	ALL
Verbal Ability	026	22	20	21
Mathematics	013	20	29	24
Science	024	20	18	18
Composite	082	17	20	19

* Percentile Norms Are Based on Performance of:

	INDIV.	PROG.	STATES	PERIOD
Applicants to Diploma Programs	995	61	20	1990
Applicants to Associate Degree Programs	1449	43	20	1990
All Applicants to Basic Nursing Programs	2756	114	27	1990

Norms not available for applicants to baccalaureate degree programs.

Report Date	Program Code	Head
05/13/90	99-999	Department of Nursing Centerville State Community College P.O. Box 341 Centerville, OK 74830

The sample on page 8 represents a test report. Notice that it is an individual report with the examinee name and identification number. This sample is for the NLN Prenursing and Guidance Examination.

The scores represent the candidate's achievement on each one of the subtests on the examination:

1. *Verbal ability*—Word knowledge, vocabulary, reading.

2. *Mathematics*—Proportions, fractions, ratios, decimals, basic algebra.

3. *Science*—Biology, chemistry, physics, general science.

The score for each test represents the number of correct items. The composite score (a standard score) reflects the score achieved in relation to the group average, with a composite of 100 being the mean or midpoint. The candidate above scored well below the group mean. The scores are then compared with all of the examinees who took the test in 1990. See the lower portion of sample, which gives an indication of how the candidate's achievement on this examination compares with other examinees on a nationwide basis. The information is reported in percentiles, that is, the percentage of individuals who took the test and scored lower than this candidate did. Therefore, the 50th percentile represents a midpoint. Percentiles above 50 are considered above average and percentiles below 50 are considered below average. A percentile of 74 would be interpreted as the examinee did as well as or better than 74 percent of the group.

There are two groups (norms); those who apply to diploma programs (DI) and those applying to associate-degree programs (AD). The third percentile, ALL, describes performance in relation to both groups. In the example on page 8, the individual scored below the 50th percentile in all subtests. This level of performance is reflected in the composite scores for DI, AD, and ALL.

The Psychological Corporation also offers a standardized admissions test for applicants to registered-nurse programs and practical-nurse programs. The content on the Registered Nurse Entrance Examination includes:

1. *Verbal Ability*—Identifying synonyms and antonyms to measure vocabulary.

2. *Numerical Ability*—Emphasizing arithmetic operations, word problems, algebra, and geometry.

3. *Life Sciences*—Focusing on principles and concepts of the biological sciences specifically related to body structure and functions, heredity and development, microorganisms and health.

4. *Physical Sciences*—Measuring understanding of principles and concepts of chemistry and physics which includes the nature of matter, changes, and energy.

5. *Reading Skill*—Drawing inferences, interpreting, and evaluating reading passages from natural and social sciences.

The Practical Nurse Entrance Examination includes four content areas: verbal ability, numerical ability, science, and reading skill. The reporting and interpretation of test results on both the registered- and practical-nurse entrance examinations are similar to the NLN tests that were previously explained. There are subtest scores representing the content and a percentile rank.

The Allied Health Admissions Test and the Psychological Services Bureau's Entrance Examinations have similar test reports in verbal ability, numerical or quantitative ability, sciences, and reading comprehension.

Each program determines how these scores will be used in the admission process. It is, therefore, advisable to seek this information directly from the program to which you are applying.

PREPARING FOR THE EXAMINATIONS

Reducing Test Anxiety

Most people become very anxious about taking an examination because they feel threatened by the possibility of doing poorly. So the first step in preparing is to reduce your anxiety by increasing the possibility of doing well. You can do this by using effective study techniques and developing test-taking skills.

For each section, we recommend that you first study the section overview, which outlines the major concepts, principles, and important facts. If you have completed several courses in the basic sciences, the overview should be a "brush-up." However, if your previous science background has been limited, the "overview" might be a completely new course. The overview explains basic facts, principles, and concepts so that you can answer questions requiring knowledge and understanding.

Answering Test Items

After completing the overview of a section, answer the sample tests. Please note that many items are multiple-choice. This type of item requires knowing the answer or making an educated guess. (You are not penalized for guessing wrong on these examinations.) Therefore, you should go through the entire test, answering all the questions that you know, and then go back to the items you are not sure about to make an educated guess. This is how it's done.

1. *Carefully* read the question (the *stem*). Look for clues or the main ideas in the stem that will lead you to the correct answer.

2. Go through the entire examination, answering all questions that you feel sure about. This will give you an overall idea of what the test is about and lessen the time pressure, and you may run across related items that will help you to answer those you aren't sure about.

3. Now go back to those items you didn't answer and use the test-taking techniques. First, look for the key word(s) or clue(s) in the stem. Keeping that in mind, try to eliminate those options that do not relate to the clue. Look at the remaining options to identify similarities and differ-

ences. Compare the difference with the clue to see if you can eliminate another option. Select the remaining option.

Example:

Which of the following may be an indication of high blood pressure?

(A) flushed skin

(B) pale skin

(C) cold skin

(D) weak pulse

What is the *clue*?
Answer: high pressure
Can I eliminate any options?
Answer: Yes. There is a direct relationship between pressure and force; therefore, (D) cannot be the correct answer.
What are the similarities and differences among options (A), (B), and (C)?
Answer: They all relate to changes in skin characteristics. However, items (B) and (C) are alike. As a matter of fact, if (B) were correct, (C) would also be correct.
The selected answer, then, is (A).
Now, let's assume that the following question is also on the test.

Why do some people with high blood pressure have flushed skin?

(A) The pulse weakens, and blood pools in the skin.

(B) The skin temperature lowers, and the skin blood vessels dilate.

(C) The increased pressure increases the volume of blood to the arteries.

(D) The increased pressure forces the arteries to dilate.

Based on your experience with the previous item, you would immediately eliminate options (A) and (B). Looking at (C) and (D), you might think that both would cause reddened skin. However, you would either eliminate (D) because it contradicts the relationship between pressure and volume, or you would select (C) because it supports the relationship between pressure and volume.

PLEASE PRACTICE THIS TECHNIQUE WITH THE SAMPLE ITEMS!

A summary of the steps for preparing to take a nursing-school entrance examination is presented below:

1. Study the concepts and principles presented in each section so that you will have a good base of knowledge.

2. Study one section at a time over a period of time—whatever is reasonable for your learning style. Do not cram!

3. Take the tests related to each section immediately after studying the explanatory materials.

4. Follow all directions for each test carefully.

5. Utilize the guidelines for test-taking as presented in this section.

6. Check your answers in order to diagnose your strengths and weaknesses.

7. Seek additional information from reliable resources in the areas in which you are weak.

Part Two

PRACTICE FOR REGISTERED NURSING SCHOOL ENTRANCE EXAMINATIONS

UNIT 1   VERBAL ABILITY

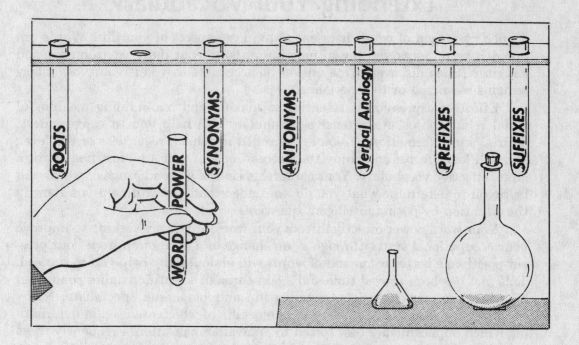

WHAT VERBAL ABILITY IS AND HOW IT IS MEASURED

Verbal ability may be defined as skill with word usage and comprehension. It is often evaluated in the form of written vocabulary tests. These vocabulary tests measure the test taker's ability to recall and produce *lexical units*. A lexical unit is a word or group of words possessing a specific meaning. A single word can have a variety of meanings in different contexts (that is, phrases or sentences). For this reason, a single word may represent several lexical units. Consider the following example:

> Her answer to the question was *right*.
> She handed the paper to the person on her *right*.
> She has a *right* to know the results of the test.
> She felt compelled to help *right* the wrong that was done.

The vocabulary test usually includes words from your *active* vocabulary—those words that you see, hear, and use frequently—and words from your *passive* vocabulary—words that you have heard and seen, and might comprehend, but that you rarely if ever use. It also includes words that may be common in written language but are not often used in spoken expression, and vice versa.

Measurement of verbal skill encompasses many elements. Although vocabulary test items may or may not appear on your test, it is advisable to study and practice with the kind of material presented in this verbal ability section. Words and their meanings are vital for good scores on tests of reading comprehension, effective writing, and current usage. Expanding your vocabulary will result in a marked improvement in your scores in these and similar subjects.

Extending Your Vocabulary

A good command of words is essential to most aspects of your life. Words can broaden your vistas and reveal new interests in your daily environment and activities. Such discoveries may never be accessible to you if your vocabulary remains restricted or too specialized.

Effective expression is essential to making and maintaining meaningful social relationships. An extensive vocabulary will help you to convey ideas, desires, and information. If you are enrolled in school, regardless of the level, you will learn faster and enjoy the process more if you are "fortified" with a large, effective vocabulary. Your comprehension of a broad range of words will help you to determine what you do *not* understand and will help you remedy the situation by posing intelligent questions.

Your word power directly affects your work. If you are seeking to improve your occupational status through a job change or a promotion from your present position, a better command of words will undoubtedly help you to succeed. This fact has been proved time and again through scientific studies conducted by educators, psychologists, sociologists, and personnel specialists. Many employers require a battery of tests, the results of which are used in determining which applicants are best suited to an available position. Frequently these tests incorporate a number of items designed to measure verbal ability.

Attaining a leadership role depends on, among other things, the extent of your vocabulary. Leadership tasks demand that you get your ideas across, that you speak and are heard. You will need to use all your expressive powers to voice your opinion with conviction. Articulation can furnish you with an astonishing amount of persuasive power.

A larger vocabulary will help you feel secure and competent in every undertaking. Let's explore the means by which this vocabulary may be acquired.

The following strategies are designed to increase your vocabulary and help you achieve word mastery. Word mastery implies reaching a level of verbal ability at which you can both recognize and comprehend words—and use them frequently and properly.

1. Read as much as you can, taking care not to confine yourself to one kind of reading material. Seek variety in what you read—periodicals, newspapers, nonfiction, novels and other fiction, poetry, prose, essays, etc. Reading from a broad range of material will accelerate your vocabulary growth. You will learn the meaning of words by context. This means that at times you will not know the definition of an isolated word, but the words or phrase with which this word appears will be familiar and therefore provide a clue to its meaning.

2. Take vocabulary tests. There are many practice books containing word tests; we recommend *Webster's New World Power Vocabulary*. These tests are challenging and make an enjoyable leisure-time activity. More important, they are fast vocabulary builders.

3. Listen to lectures, discussion, and talks given by people who speak well. TV and radio are excellent means of learning new terminology coming into common usage in the English language. A word of caution: you cannot always rely on a speaker's pronunciation. Always check your dictionary for proper pronunciation.

4. Use a dictionary when you are not certain of a word's meaning. If you do not have access to a dictionary when you encounter the word, make a note of it (and its context) and research it at your earliest convenience. Find out how it is pronounced, what words are related to it, and its finer shades of meaning and correct usage. A good dictionary is a must! Any one of the following is highly recommended:

   Funk and Wagnall's Standard College Dictionary
   Webster's New World Dictionary®
   Random House College Dictionary

   Also, use of the following is encouraged: *Roget's International Thesaurus; Webster's New World Dictionary® of Synonyms;* and *Harper Dictionary of Contemporary Usage.*

5. Word games, such as Scrabble® and Boggle®, are an effective and pleasurable means of encountering new words. Crossword puzzles, anagrams, and similar word games provide a relaxing method of acquiring new vocabulary. Most of these puzzles are published in varying degrees of difficulty. Start with the easy level and progress to the expert. You will find it a challenging learning experience.

6. Review the etymological charts and diagrams in this book, which explain word derivations. A knowledge of roots, or stems, of words will enable you to infer the meaning of new words having roots similar to words you already know.

7. Study words by central ideas. It is difficult to study and retain isolated words. Even context clues sometimes are not enough to help you remember a word, its meaning, or its appropriate use. Studying vocabulary by central idea encourages you to consider groups of related words. As you learn each term, you associate it with some other word. For example: the words *ingest, devour, consume, voracious, edible, delectable,* and *palatable* are all tied to the principle idea of eating. The central idea strategy of studying words will not only provide you with a basis for remembering the word but will also motivate you to use the word in your everyday oral and written expression. Frequent use of the word will in turn ensure your ability to recall its meaning in a testing situation. This word study method also fosters comprehension of jargon or word usage peculiar to specific fields. A number of workbooks and study materials present words according to a central idea and feature exercises formatted to this method. Such books may be found in the "study aids" section of most bookstores.

   Be sure to record all new words in a notebook dedicated to that purpose. Make notes alongside each entry that include a simple definition or synonym, finer shades of meaning, related forms, and sample sentences of the word in context. Finally, make these words your own. Use them in your writing and speaking. Remember—verbal ability is a skill you can improve at any age.
   The purpose of this section is to provide you with practice exercises representative of the three most common kinds of verbal-ability test items—syno-

nyms, antonyms, and verbal analogies. This section covers these question types in three separate subsections.

An explanation of each kind of test item, helpful study hints, and test-taking strategies precede each subsection. Subsections also include a 75-question, multiple-choice test. An answer key follows each sample test to help you evaluate your performance immediately and to help you determine areas of weakness. You may wish to use these answer keys to compile a word study list.

ETYMOLOGY—KEY TO WORD RECOGNITION

Etymology is the study of the history and origin of words. It explains how a word came into being, the place of its beginning, and how it has been used through the ages. The etymology of a word also outlines alterations in its meaning, usage, and spelling through the years.

Although the term "etymology" sounds somewhat complex and weighty, the science itself is not difficult to understand. Etymologies may be simple and concise or lengthy and intricate. To find them, you should use your dictionary. Etymologies are usually found at the beginning of a definition of a principal entry (the word you are looking up, usually printed in heavy type), enclosed in brackets and placed directly before the definition.

> **arris** \'ar əs\ *n, pl* **arris** or **arrises** [probably modif. of MF *areste*, lit., fishbone, fr LL *arista*, ear of grain]: the sharp edge or salient angle formed by the meeting of two surfaces, esp. in moldings.

You probably should familiarize yourself with the abbreviations used to denote the origin of words. Consult the front pages of your dictionary where you will find a guide to the use of that particular publication. Look for a heading that refers to etymologies or abbreviations and symbols used in etymologies. These keys will help you interpret a word's entry. For instance, the entry printed above uses the abbreviations MF and LL indicating that the entry *arris* is derived from Middle French or Late Latin.

Many English words have their origin in Greek and Roman myths and legends. If you are well-read, you may already have an edge in using the etymological method of determining word meaning. For instance, if you have read the story of the mythical king Tantalus, you would understand the derivation of the verb *tantalize*. King Tantalus, after his death, was punished for his wickedness by being placed in water up to his chin. When he stooped to drink, the water would recede. Above his head, branches laden with fruit bobbed out of his reach. So from the name Tantalus came the word *tantalize,* meaning "to tease."

A great many of the words we use daily came into our language from the Latin and Greek. Approximately half the words in the dictionary are derived from Latin. Many Latin words and phrases have been borrowed and adopted by other languages. European languages such as French and Spanish came directly from Latin and are known as Romance languages. Consequently, if you are or have been a student of Latin, you will find it easier to build your vocabulary.

Many foreign terms were absorbed into English as parts of several different words related in meaning to each other. These parts of words fall into three groups.

Roots (or stems)—These carry the basic meaning and are combined with each other and with prefixes and suffixes to create other words with related meanings.

Prefixes—Letter combinations with their own particular meaning that appear at the beginning of a word.

Suffixes—Letter combinations with their own particular meaning that appear at the end of a word.

The lists of roots, prefixes, and suffixes in this section are accompanied by words in which the letter combinations appear. Use the dictionary to look up any words that are not clear in your mind.

Remember that this section is not meant for easy reading. It is a guide to a program of study that will prove invaluable if you do your part. Do not try to absorb too much at one time. If you can put in a half-hour every day, your study will yield better results.

After you have done your preliminary work and have formed a better idea of how words are formed in English, schedule the various vocabulary tests we have provided. They cover a wide variety of the vocabulary questions commonly encountered on examinations. These lengthy tests are not meant to be taken all at one time. Space them out. Adhere closely to the directions, which differ for the different kinds of tests. Keep an honest record of your scores. Study your corrected mistakes and look them up in your dictionary. Concentrate closely on each sample test . . . and watch your scores improve.

KNOW YOUR ROOTS

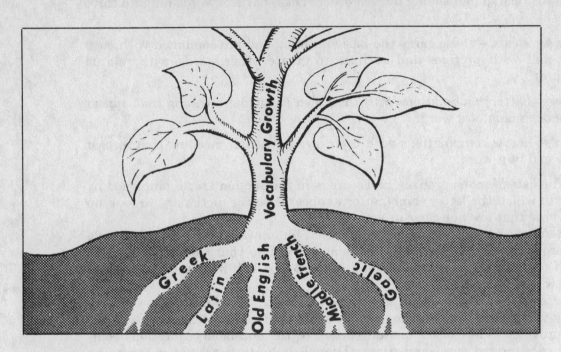

Roots or Stems

The root or stem is that part of the word that conveys the basic meaning of the word. For example, in the word *introduction, duct* is the root. It means "lead." *Intro-* means *within, into,* and *-tion* is a noun ending. Hence, the meaning of introduction—a "leading into."

Below is a chart of common stems. See how well you "know your roots."

STEMS

Stem	Meaning	Example
ag, ac	do	agenda, action
agri	farm	agriculture
aqua	water	aquatic
auto	self	automatic
biblio	book	bibliography
bio	life	biography
cad, cas	fall	cadence, casual
cap, cep, cept	take	captive, accept
capit	head	capital, decapitate
ced, cede, ceed, cess	go	intercede
celer	speed	accelerate
chrom	color	monochromatic
chron	time	chronological
cide, cis	cut	incision
clude, clud, clus	close, close in	include, cluster
cog, cogn	knowledge of	recognize

Stem	Meaning	Example
cur, curs	run	recur, cursive
ded	give	dedicate
dent, dont	tooth	dental
duce, duct	lead	induce, deduct
fact, fect, fict	make, do	perfect, fiction, factory
fer, late	carry	refer, dilate, transfer, translate
flect, flex	bend, turn	reflect
fring, fract	break	infringe, refract
graph, gram	picture, writing	graphic, telegram
greg	group, gather	gregarious, congregation
gress, grad	step, walk	progress, degrade
hydr	water	hydrate
ject	throw	inject
jud	right	judicial
junct	join	conjunction
juris	law, justice	jurist
lect, leg	read, choose	collect, legible
logue	speech, speaking	dialogue
logy	study of	psychology
loq, loc	speak	elocution
lude, lus	play, perform	elude, ludicrous
manu	by hand	manuscript
mand	order	remand
mar	sea	maritime
med	middle	intermediate
ment, mem	mind, memory	mention
meter	measure	thermometer
micro	small	microscope
min	lessen	miniature
mis, miss, mit	send	remit, dismiss
mot, mov	move	remote, remove
mute	change	commute, mutation
naut	sailor, sail	nautical
nounce, nunci	declare, state	announce, enunciate
ped, pod	foot	pedal
pel, pulse	drive, push	dispel, impulse
pend, pense	hang	depend, dispenser
plac	please	placate
plic	fold	implicate
port	carry	portable
pose, pone	put, place	depose, component
reg, rect	rule	regulate, direct
rupt	break	disruption
sec, sect	cut	bisect
sed	remain	sedentary

Stem	Meaning	Example
sert	weave, bind	insert
serve	keep, save	preserve
scend, scent	climb	ascent
scribe, script	write	describe, transcript
sist	stand, set	insist
spect	look	inspect
spire, spirat	breath, breathe	perspire
strict	tighten	restrict
tain	hold	detain
term	end	terminate
tract	draw, drag	detract
tort	twist	distort
vene, vent	come	intervene, invent
vict	overcome, conquer	evict
volve, volu	roll, turn	evolve, evolution

PREFIXES AND SUFFIXES

Down to the Letter

Prefixes and suffixes are the "beginning and end!" We will begin by reviewing the term *prefix*. A prefix is a letter-combination attached to the beginning of a word; it usually carries a meaning independent of the word to which it is attached. For example, the prefix *semi* means "half." It can be added to many words—*semicircle, semilunar, semiprofessional, semiformal*. Attaching a prefix sometimes requires the placement of a hyphen between the prefix and the root word. A hyphen is used when the prefix is attached to a proper noun: *all-American, pro-British, anti-Fascist, un-Christian*.

A *suffix* is a combination of letters attached to the end of a word and usually possessing a meaning separate from the word to which it is affixed, for example: *-less* (without)—*careless, hopeless, meaningless*. Usually, affixing a suffix to a word changes its part of speech, for example: *Assert* (verb)—*assertion* (noun); *beautiful* (adjective)—*beautifully* (adverb).

Study the following prefix and suffix charts to increase your understanding of related words and inflected (changed) forms.

Prefixes

Prefix	Meaning	Example
a	not	amoral
ab, a	away from	absent
ad, ac, ag, at	to	advent, accrue, attract, aggressive
an	without	anarchy
ante	before	antedate
anti	against	antipathy

Prefix	Meaning	Example
aud, audit	hear	auditor
bene	well	beneficent
bi	two	bicameral
cap, capt, cept	take, seize, hold	capture
ced, cess	go, yield	rescind, recess
circum	around	circumspect
com, con, col	together	commit, confound, collate
contra	against	contraband
cred, credit	believe	credible
de	from, down	descend
dic, dict	say	dictionary
dis, di	apart	distract, divert
dom	home, rule	domicile, dominate
duc, duct	lead	induce
ex, e	out	exit, emit
extra	beyond	extracurricular
fac, fact	make	facsimile
in, im, ir, il, un	not	inept, irregular, illegal
in, im	in, into	interest, imbibe
inter	between	interscholastic
intra, intro	within	intramural
mal	bad	malcontent
mis	wrong	misnomer
non	not	nonentity
ob	against	obstacle
omni	all	omnivorous
per	through	permeate
peri	around	periscope
poly	many	polytheism
post	after	postmortem
pre	before	premonition
pro	forward	propose
re	again	review
se	apart	seduce
semi	half	semicircle
sub	under	subvert
sui	self	suicide
super	above	superimpose
sur	on, upon	surcharge
trans	across	transpose
un	not	unwelcome
vice	instead of	vice-president

Suffixes

Suffix	Meaning	Example
able, ible	capable of being	capable, reversible
age	state of	storage
al	pertaining to	instructional

Suffix	Meaning	Example
ance	relating to	reliance
ary	relating to	dictionary
ate	act	confiscate
ation	action	radiation
cy	quality	democracy
ed	past action	subsided
ence	relating to	confidence
er, or	one who	adviser, actor
ic	pertaining to	democratic
ing	present action	surmising
ious	full of	rebellious
ish	like, as	childish
ive	having the quality of	creative
ize	to make like	harmonize
less	without	hopeless
ly	the quality of	carefully
ment	result	amusement
ness	the quality of being	selfishness
ty	condition	sanity

Increased Word Power From Beginning to End

Using the etymological approach can simplify the process by which you attack the monumental feat of learning medical terminology. By knowing that the suffix *itis* implies inflammation and *ectomy* means "the cutting out or removal of," you can easily deduce that the term *appendicitis* means "inflammation of the appendix" and *appendectomy* means "the cutting out or removal of the appendix."

Now that you have studied the various letter combinations or word components, see if you can make an educated guess at the meanings of the terms listed below. Start with the root or stem. Next, add the suffix and/or prefix to the interpretation in the order that provides a clear definition. The result will be increased word power from "beginning to end!" It's as challenging as a jig-saw puzzle! Be sure to compare your definitions with those in the dictionary.

decapitate

emissary

incursion

involuted

convocation

colloquy

aggregation

retractable

implacable

celerity

SYNONYMS

The Name's the Same

Synonyms are words that share meanings. The English language abounds in synonyms. In your effort to acquire word mastery, you must learn to express your ideas without redundancy and constant use of overworked words. Effective writing and speaking may be achieved through the precise use of synonyms.

Words such as *brave* and *courageous,* which may allude to an identical quality, can be used interchangeably. Some synonyms, however, differ in definition or usage. For example, *fewer* refers to number, while *less* refers to quantity: John has *fewer* books and *less* money than his brother. These words are indeed similar in meaning, but one cannot be substituted for the other.

The adjectives *beautiful* and *handsome* both describe someone or something attractive or pleasing to the eye. Nevertheless, you would not usually speak of a "beautiful man" or a "handsome young lady." In our society, common usage would cause one to reverse these expressions to "beautiful young lady" and "handsome man."

A study of the finer shades of meaning of synonyms will help you be more precise when you convey your exact feelings or mental picture of an object or scene. For instance, if you were to say, "The *bottom* of the lamp is made of Indian brass and features intricate carvings," one might simply envision the underside of the lamp. However, if you were to substitute *base* for the word *bottom,* one would instead get a visual image of something highly decorative that supports the upper structure of the lamp. So even though the "name" appears to be the same, an investigation into various shades of definition will assist you in distinguishing variations in usage.

If you wish to expand your vocabulary of synonyms and familiarize yourself with their correct use, you will find the following reference books helpful:

Webster's Dictionary of Synonyms
Crabb's English Synonyms
Roget's International Thesaurus
Harper Dictionary of Contemporary Usage

Familiar Surroundings?

The most common way of testing vocabulary on a standardized test is in context, that is, to present the items in a sentence or phrase so that you can see how a word is used. You can then determine whether the word is used as a noun, a verb, an adjective, etc. The test, therefore, is designed to encourage the extraction of word meaning from context; however the context will not be so explicit that you can easily infer the meaning of a word.

More specifically, the synonym test item is usually a multiple-choice item that appears in one of three formats:

Type A—Given an underlined or italicized word in a complete sentence, the test-taker is required to identify which of the four other words is a synonym for the underlined or italicized word.

Example: The disinterested witness was able to give a *candid* account of the incident.

(A) complete
(B) impartial
(C) biased
(D) candescent

Type B—Given an underlined or italicized word in a phrase, the test-taker is required to identify which of the four other words is a synonym for the underlined or italicized word.

Example: The *emaciated* patient

(A) discharged
(B) emancipated
(C) emotional
(D) shriveled

Type C—Given a sentence with a missing word, the test-taker is required to identify which of the four other words best completes the sentence.

Example: An *apology* is appropriate when a person feels

(A) sorry
(B) apathetic
(C) rejected
(D) elated

OR

Example: He is a *staunch* supporter of the presidential candidate. Staunch means

(A) stubborn
(B) faithful
(C) inflexible
(D) hopeful

In completing a synonym test item, remember to look for a word which means the same, or almost the same, as the target word in the item (the underlined or italicized word). Do not be distracted by a word that is a look-alike, that is, one that looks similar or begins with the same three or four letters but is unrelated in meaning. When possible, apply the etymological approach of interpreting roots, prefixes, and suffixes. Now try completing the sample synonym test. There is a total of 75 items. An answer key appears on page 35.

Answer Sheet
Synonyms

1. Ⓐ Ⓑ Ⓒ Ⓓ   20. Ⓐ Ⓑ Ⓒ Ⓓ   39. Ⓐ Ⓑ Ⓒ Ⓓ   58. Ⓐ Ⓑ Ⓒ Ⓓ

2. Ⓐ Ⓑ Ⓒ Ⓓ   21. Ⓐ Ⓑ Ⓒ Ⓓ   40. Ⓐ Ⓑ Ⓒ Ⓓ   59. Ⓐ Ⓑ Ⓒ Ⓓ

3. Ⓐ Ⓑ Ⓒ Ⓓ   22. Ⓐ Ⓑ Ⓒ Ⓓ   41. Ⓐ Ⓑ Ⓒ Ⓓ   60. Ⓐ Ⓑ Ⓒ Ⓓ

4. Ⓐ Ⓑ Ⓒ Ⓓ   23. Ⓐ Ⓑ Ⓒ Ⓓ   42. Ⓐ Ⓑ Ⓒ Ⓓ   61. Ⓐ Ⓑ Ⓒ Ⓓ

5. Ⓐ Ⓑ Ⓒ Ⓓ   24. Ⓐ Ⓑ Ⓒ Ⓓ   43. Ⓐ Ⓑ Ⓒ Ⓓ   62. Ⓐ Ⓑ Ⓒ Ⓓ

6. Ⓐ Ⓑ Ⓒ Ⓓ   25. Ⓐ Ⓑ Ⓒ Ⓓ   44. Ⓐ Ⓑ Ⓒ Ⓓ   63. Ⓐ Ⓑ Ⓒ Ⓓ

7. Ⓐ Ⓑ Ⓒ Ⓓ   26. Ⓐ Ⓑ Ⓒ Ⓓ   45. Ⓐ Ⓑ Ⓒ Ⓓ   64. Ⓐ Ⓑ Ⓒ Ⓓ

8. Ⓐ Ⓑ Ⓒ Ⓓ   27. Ⓐ Ⓑ Ⓒ Ⓓ   46. Ⓐ Ⓑ Ⓒ Ⓓ   65. Ⓐ Ⓑ Ⓒ Ⓓ

9. Ⓐ Ⓑ Ⓒ Ⓓ   28. Ⓐ Ⓑ Ⓒ Ⓓ   47. Ⓐ Ⓑ Ⓒ Ⓓ   66. Ⓐ Ⓑ Ⓒ Ⓓ

10. Ⓐ Ⓑ Ⓒ Ⓓ   29. Ⓐ Ⓑ Ⓒ Ⓓ   48. Ⓐ Ⓑ Ⓒ Ⓓ   67. Ⓐ Ⓑ Ⓒ Ⓓ

11. Ⓐ Ⓑ Ⓒ Ⓓ   30. Ⓐ Ⓑ Ⓒ Ⓓ   49. Ⓐ Ⓑ Ⓒ Ⓓ   68. Ⓐ Ⓑ Ⓒ Ⓓ

12. Ⓐ Ⓑ Ⓒ Ⓓ   31. Ⓐ Ⓑ Ⓒ Ⓓ   50. Ⓐ Ⓑ Ⓒ Ⓓ   69. Ⓐ Ⓑ Ⓒ Ⓓ

13. Ⓐ Ⓑ Ⓒ Ⓓ   32. Ⓐ Ⓑ Ⓒ Ⓓ   51. Ⓐ Ⓑ Ⓒ Ⓓ   70. Ⓐ Ⓑ Ⓒ Ⓓ

14. Ⓐ Ⓑ Ⓒ Ⓓ   33. Ⓐ Ⓑ Ⓒ Ⓓ   52. Ⓐ Ⓑ Ⓒ Ⓓ   71. Ⓐ Ⓑ Ⓒ Ⓓ

15. Ⓐ Ⓑ Ⓒ Ⓓ   34. Ⓐ Ⓑ Ⓒ Ⓓ   53. Ⓐ Ⓑ Ⓒ Ⓓ   72. Ⓐ Ⓑ Ⓒ Ⓓ

16. Ⓐ Ⓑ Ⓒ Ⓓ   35. Ⓐ Ⓑ Ⓒ Ⓓ   54. Ⓐ Ⓑ Ⓒ Ⓓ   73. Ⓐ Ⓑ Ⓒ Ⓓ

17. Ⓐ Ⓑ Ⓒ Ⓓ   36. Ⓐ Ⓑ Ⓒ Ⓓ   55. Ⓐ Ⓑ Ⓒ Ⓓ   74. Ⓐ Ⓑ Ⓒ Ⓓ

18. Ⓐ Ⓑ Ⓒ Ⓓ   37. Ⓐ Ⓑ Ⓒ Ⓓ   56. Ⓐ Ⓑ Ⓒ Ⓓ   75. Ⓐ Ⓑ Ⓒ Ⓓ

19. Ⓐ Ⓑ Ⓒ Ⓓ   38. Ⓐ Ⓑ Ⓒ Ⓓ   57. Ⓐ Ⓑ Ⓒ Ⓓ

SYNONYM TEST

30 Minutes   **75 Questions**

Directions: *In each of the sentences below, one word is italicized. Following each sentence are four words or phrases. For each sentence, choose the word or phrase that most nearly corresponds in meaning with the italicized word.*

1. The *diction* acceptable in speech is usually more informal than that required in writing.

   (A) conviction
   (B) language
   (C) discourse
   (D) decrement

2. It is apparent that Mr. Smith is the most *sedulous* and active member of the group.

   (A) hideous
   (B) generous
   (C) infirm
   (D) industrious

3. During the hockey game several *altercations* took place.

   (A) fracases
   (B) substitutions
   (C) alterations
   (D) plays

4. The carrot is a perfect illustration of a *biennial*.

   (A) occurring quarterly
   (B) occurring once in two years
   (C) perennial
   (D) bisection

5. She has run the *gamut* of clerical jobs in this office.

   (A) periphery
   (B) margin
   (C) range
   (D) imperception

6. His deeds amounted to nothing more than those of a *sanctimonious* hypocrite.

   (A) parsimonious
   (B) perpetual
   (C) intrinsic
   (D) affectedly pious

7. He displayed the manners of an *urbane* gentleman.

   (A) suave
   (B) poignant
   (C) spasmodic
   (D) pensive

8. The *slogan* is appropriate for both the product and its service.

   (A) catchword
   (B) sample
   (C) design
   (D) passage

9. We do not wish to *pursue* the discussion.

   (A) conclude
   (B) interrupt
   (C) continue
   (D) influence

10. He was determined to *foil* the scheme of his opponent.

    (A) heighten
    (B) secure
    (C) disencumber
    (D) thwart

11. The examiner *purported* to be an official representative.

    (A) addressed
    (B) claimed
    (C) propitiated
    (D) conciliated

12. The ship carried refugees of every *persuasion*.

    (A) mediocrity
    (B) sort
    (C) prospectus
    (D) compendium

13. The child could not *recollect* the incident.

    (A) remember
    (B) dubitate
    (C) interrogate
    (D) illumine

14. The Supreme Court *rescinded* the law.

    (A) complicated
    (B) inveigled
    (C) revoked
    (D) accepted

15. The implementation of the plan was given *scant* consideration.

    (A) audacious
    (B) fervid
    (C) little
    (D) clothed

16. The key speaker in his lengthy presentation *scoffed at* religion.

    (A) exonerated
    (B) amplified
    (C) confuted
    (D) mocked

17. She completed the *sprint* with a sudden surge of energy.

    (A) relaxation
    (B) adventure
    (C) run
    (D) convergence

18. The content of the message was *urgent*.

    (A) privileged
    (B) amendable
    (C) pressing
    (D) absolved

19. A *simulated* rescue mission was conducted by the forest rangers.

    (A) pretended
    (B) superficial
    (C) stimulated
    (D) simultaneous

20. He spoke the language with native *fluency*.

    (A) meritoriousness
    (B) variety
    (C) ephemera
    (D) ease

21. Her quickening gait seemed regulated by the *pulse* of the big city.

    (A) utility
    (B) pace
    (C) reverence
    (D) solace

22. The language of the publication is *unsophisticated* but informative.

    (A) ponderous
    (B) elaborate
    (C) simple
    (D) superficial

23. All the evidence presented pointed to *willful* execution of a crime.

    (A) deliberate
    (B) eminent
    (C) amicable
    (D) remorseful

24. There is no *provision* for deadlines in the contract.

    (A) improvement
    (B) convenience
    (C) aggregation
    (D) stipulation

25. The furnishings *impart* an air of elegance to the room.

    (A) communicate
    (B) indemnify
    (C) reinforce
    (D) disguise

26. She exhibited great *valor* in handling the emergency. If the woman exhibited great valor, she demonstrated

    (A) ingeniousness
    (B) courage
    (C) discretion
    (D) optimism

27. Various courses were *fused* in the revision of the curriculum.

    (A) required
    (B) implicated
    (C) combined
    (D) involved

28. A *document* was presented as proof of citizenship.

    (A) notification
    (B) an official paper
    (C) memorandum
    (D) coalition

29. The task of choosing one from so many qualified applicants *bewildered* the employer.

    (A) perplexed
    (B) aggravated
    (C) subdued
    (D) infuriated

30. The revision of the city plan incorporated adjustments in the projected *modes* of transportation.

    (A) increments
    (B) expenditures
    (C) means
    (D) modifications

31. The politician sought to *aggrandize* himself at the expense of the people.

    (A) exhaust
    (B) subjugate
    (C) sacrifice
    (D) exalt

32. The newcomer made an effort to *mingle* with the crowd.

    (A) argue
    (B) mix
    (C) disrupt
    (D) flout

33. If an organization's programs were described as *philanthropic,* the programs would be

    (A) primitive
    (B) deleterious
    (C) extraneous
    (D) benevolent

34. If the traits of a nation's leader *were covetous,* they were

    (A) greedy
    (B) exemplary
    (C) disparate
    (D) adventitious

35. Rabbits *breed* offspring rapidly.

    (A) raise
    (B) gather
    (C) propagate
    (D) destroy

36. It was necessary to *iterate* one procedure of the experiment.

    (A) adjust
    (B) defend
    (C) ferment
    (D) repeat

37. A shadow of a man *loomed* ominously in the dimly lit corridor.

    (A) asserted
    (B) yielded
    (C) appeared
    (D) rebuffed

38. Alcohol consumption often exerts a *malign* influence on an individual.

    (A) ecstatic
    (B) injurious
    (C) luminous
    (D) gloomy

39. The girl is reported to have left of her own *volition.*

    (A) flight
    (B) will
    (C) repudiation
    (D) recognizance

40. Cultural differences caused him not to understand the *significance* of the ceremony.

    (A) meaning
    (B) ritual
    (C) scheme
    (D) loquacity

41. The *similitude* between the original painting and the reproduction is remarkable.

    (A) incongruity
    (B) connection
    (C) resemblance
    (D) relationship

42. A *prudent* individual will save some portion of his or her wage.

    (A) judicious
    (B) terse
    (C) audacious
    (D) laconic

43. His decision to return home was *instinctive*.

    (A) spontaneous
    (B) turbid
    (C) premeditated
    (D) irrelevant

44. The mountain *torrent* flowed over the rocks.

    (A) slide
    (B) avalanche
    (C) deluge
    (D) air

45. The book was written to *embody* all aspects of life science.

    (A) combat
    (B) eliminate
    (C) abjure
    (D) incorporate

46. Her sudden decision is typical of her *impetuous* behavior.

    (A) contemptible
    (B) sophisticated
    (C) impulsive
    (D) fallacious

47. It is fitting that we *eulogize* one who has contributed so greatly to our society.

    (A) promulgate
    (B) praise
    (C) denigrate
    (D) append

48. The convention hall swelled with the *vociferation* of various campaign groups.

    (A) clamor
    (B) taciturnity
    (C) oblivion
    (D) discernment

49. The blackmailer has placed her in a *precarious* position.

    (A) mellifluous
    (B) intrusive
    (C) unusual
    (D) unstable

50. Her display of so much fine china was too *ostentatious*.

    (A) pretentious
    (B) inconspicuous
    (C) ascribable
    (D) candid

51. To *manifest* interest

    (A) conceal
    (B) diminish
    (C) augment
    (D) display

52. *Banter* and laughter

    (A) discourse
    (B) singing
    (C) toasting
    (D) raillery

53. *Aesthetic* value

    (A) practical
    (B) artistic
    (C) monetary
    (D) intrinsic

54. Confirmed his *apostasy*

    (A) defiance
    (B) defection
    (C) belief
    (D) inference

55. The *cryptic* message

    (A) cynical
    (B) mysterious
    (C) critical
    (D) censorious

56. New witnesses *emerged*

    (A) deviated
    (B) divested
    (C) declined
    (D) appeared

57. The *contumacious* youngster

    (A) exuberant
    (B) rebellious
    (C) awkward
    (D) mischievous

58. *Cognizant* of the ill will

    (A) ignorant
    (B) aware
    (C) insensitive
    (D) remorseful

59. *Glacial* region

    (A) glass-like
    (B) illiberal
    (C) frigid
    (D) reticent

60. *Instigated* the rebellion

    (A) quelled
    (B) incited
    (C) assisted
    (D) depressed

61. A fight *ensued*

    (A) followed
    (B) terminated
    (C) was avoided
    (D) culminated

62. *Retrospect* of events

    (A) review
    (B) concept
    (C) knowledge
    (D) awareness

63. *Malice* toward my friend

    (A) adoration
    (B) sympathy
    (C) ill will
    (D) apathy

64. *Saturated* with moisture

    (A) void of
    (B) mixed with
    (C) full of
    (D) replaced with

65. *Debilitating* to people

    (A) invigorating
    (B) stimulating
    (C) tolerable
    (D) weakening

66. Ten years' *servitude*

    (A) freedom
    (B) lethargy
    (C) vicissitude
    (D) bondage

67. *Relish* the thought

    (A) enjoy
    (B) dread
    (C) spread
    (D) implant

68. A *lackadaisical* attitude

    (A) enthusiastic
    (B) complacent
    (C) profound
    (D) indifferent

69. To *hoist* the sails

    (A) cast
    (B) raise
    (C) prepare
    (D) repair

70. *Asperse* the family's good name

    (A) slander
    (B) fathom
    (C) extol
    (D) palliate

71. *Sordid* details

    (A) bizarre
    (B) wretched
    (C) primordial
    (D) exaggerated

72. Sudden *alienation*

    (A) agitation
    (B) inception
    (C) subsidence
    (D) isolation

73. *Sauntered* into the room

    (A) ambled
    (B) slithered
    (C) danced
    (D) dragged

74. *Accede* to the request

    (A) attend
    (B) refer
    (C) adjust
    (D) agree

75. The *proximity* of the lake

    (A) worthlessness
    (B) nearness
    (C) level
    (D) ebullition

Answer Key

1.	**B**	26.	**B**	51.	**D**
2.	**D**	27.	**C**	52.	**D**
3.	**A**	28.	**B**	53.	**B**
4.	**B**	29.	**A**	54.	**B**
5.	**C**	30.	**C**	55.	**B**
6.	**D**	31.	**D**	56.	**D**
7.	**A**	32.	**B**	57.	**B**
8.	**A**	33.	**D**	58.	**B**
9.	**C**	34.	**A**	59.	**C**
10.	**D**	35.	**C**	60.	**B**
11.	**B**	36.	**D**	61.	**A**
12.	**B**	37.	**C**	62.	**A**
13.	**A**	38.	**B**	63.	**C**
14.	**C**	39.	**B**	64.	**C**
15.	**C**	40.	**A**	65.	**D**
16.	**D**	41.	**C**	66.	**D**
17.	**C**	42.	**A**	67.	**A**
18.	**C**	43.	**A**	68.	**D**
19.	**A**	44.	**C**	69.	**B**
20.	**D**	45.	**D**	70.	**A**
21.	**B**	46.	**C**	71.	**B**
22.	**C**	47.	**B**	72.	**D**
23.	**A**	48.	**A**	73.	**A**
24.	**D**	49.	**D**	74.	**D**
25.	**A**	50.	**A**	75.	**B**

ANTONYMS

The Turnabout

In the preceding part of this section, emphasis was placed on synonyms or words with similar or identical meanings. You are now ready to make a "turnabout" and embark upon increasing your word power from a contrasting point of view. *Antonyms* are words that are opposite in meaning. Some very explicit and simple samples are: *hot/cold, strong/weak, sit/stand, night/day*, and *lazy/industrious*.

Antonyms are extremely useful to express contrast. The use of certain antonyms can result in the verbal creation of a universal portrait or concept. For instance, everyone associates the name "Scrooge" with *penny-pinching or miserly* traits. The Dickens character was anything but philanthropic, a term that characterizes people or agencies who devote themselves to helping and giving to humanity. Therefore, if you read that "a former Scrooge has transformed himself into a philanthropist" you would surmise that the person being described has had a complete change of heart. The term *philanthropist* has been contrasted with a symbol of *miserly and penny-pinching* traits.

In taking a test measuring your comprehension of verbal contrasts, be certain to select a response that is the same part of speech as the term in question. Although *discourtesy* and *insolent* share the same shade of meaning, one could not be substituted for the other—the former is a noun and the latter an adjective. Therefore, they could not play identical roles in a sentence.

If you are stumped by any one test item, move on quickly to the next. When you have completed the test, and if time permits, return to any test item(s) you have skipped. Mentally put the various word choices, including the test item, in a sentence. Then remove the test item again.

Example:
Polite

(A) desperate
(B) discourtesy
(C) insolent
(D) discriminate

For the above example, make up a sentence using the word *polite* and then substitute the options in its place, such as "The boy is *discourtesy*." *The boy is insolent*." Obviously, *insolent* is the correct response, as it is the word opposite in meaning to *polite* and best fits the sentence pattern "The boy is...."

USING PREFIXES

Another helpful technique in taking antonym tests is the close examination of prefixes. Review the etymological information before attempting the sample antonym test, and pay special attention to prefixes. Prefixes can often be the key to contrast in meaning. For example, the prefixes *un, im*, and *in* frequently denote the opposite meaning of the word to which they are affixed: *happy/unhappy*; *adequate/inadequate*; *polite/impolite*. These examples make it apparent that the actual meaning of the prefixes is "not." The prefixes *in* and *ex* are opposite in meaning. *In* means, "in", "into," "inside;" and *ex* means "out," "outside of." If the target word is *internal*, which of the following words would you select as its antonym?

(A) interior
(B) ephermeral
(C) illegal
(D) external

Of course, *external* is the correct response. Study the list of contrasting prefixes below. Then try your hand at making the "turnabout!"

CONTRASTING PREFIXES

ad, ac, ag, at (to)   *ab, a* (away from)
ante (before)   *post* (after)
anti, contra (against)   *pro* (for)
bene (well, good)   *mal* (bad)
com, con, col (together)   *dis, di* (apart)
con, com (with)   *an* (without)
eu (good)   *dys* (bad)
in, im (in)   *e, ex* (out)
hypo (under)   *hyper* (over)
pro (forward)   *retro* (backward)
sub (under)   *super, sur* (above)

Answer Sheet Antonyms

1. Ⓐ Ⓑ Ⓒ Ⓓ	16. Ⓐ Ⓑ Ⓒ Ⓓ	31. Ⓐ Ⓑ Ⓒ Ⓓ	46. Ⓐ Ⓑ Ⓒ Ⓓ	61. Ⓐ Ⓑ Ⓒ Ⓓ
2. Ⓐ Ⓑ Ⓒ Ⓓ	17. Ⓐ Ⓑ Ⓒ Ⓓ	32. Ⓐ Ⓑ Ⓒ Ⓓ	47. Ⓐ Ⓑ Ⓒ Ⓓ	62. Ⓐ Ⓑ Ⓒ Ⓓ
3. Ⓐ Ⓑ Ⓒ Ⓓ	18. Ⓐ Ⓑ Ⓒ Ⓓ	33. Ⓐ Ⓑ Ⓒ Ⓓ	48. Ⓐ Ⓑ Ⓒ Ⓓ	63. Ⓐ Ⓑ Ⓒ Ⓓ
4. Ⓐ Ⓑ Ⓒ Ⓓ	19. Ⓐ Ⓑ Ⓒ Ⓓ	34. Ⓐ Ⓑ Ⓒ Ⓓ	49. Ⓐ Ⓑ Ⓒ Ⓓ	64. Ⓐ Ⓑ Ⓒ Ⓓ
5. Ⓐ Ⓑ Ⓒ Ⓓ	20. Ⓐ Ⓑ Ⓒ Ⓓ	35. Ⓐ Ⓑ Ⓒ Ⓓ	50. Ⓐ Ⓑ Ⓒ Ⓓ	65. Ⓐ Ⓑ Ⓒ Ⓓ
6. Ⓐ Ⓑ Ⓒ Ⓓ	21. Ⓐ Ⓑ Ⓒ Ⓓ	36. Ⓐ Ⓑ Ⓒ Ⓓ	51. Ⓐ Ⓑ Ⓒ Ⓓ	66. Ⓐ Ⓑ Ⓒ Ⓓ
7. Ⓐ Ⓑ Ⓒ Ⓓ	22. Ⓐ Ⓑ Ⓒ Ⓓ	37. Ⓐ Ⓑ Ⓒ Ⓓ	52. Ⓐ Ⓑ Ⓒ Ⓓ	67. Ⓐ Ⓑ Ⓒ Ⓓ
8. Ⓐ Ⓑ Ⓒ Ⓓ	23. Ⓐ Ⓑ Ⓒ Ⓓ	38. Ⓐ Ⓑ Ⓒ Ⓓ	53. Ⓐ Ⓑ Ⓒ Ⓓ	68. Ⓐ Ⓑ Ⓒ Ⓓ
9. Ⓐ Ⓑ Ⓒ Ⓓ	24. Ⓐ Ⓑ Ⓒ Ⓓ	39. Ⓐ Ⓑ Ⓒ Ⓓ	54. Ⓐ Ⓑ Ⓒ Ⓓ	69. Ⓐ Ⓑ Ⓒ Ⓓ
10. Ⓐ Ⓑ Ⓒ Ⓓ	25. Ⓐ Ⓑ Ⓒ Ⓓ	40. Ⓐ Ⓑ Ⓒ Ⓓ	55. Ⓐ Ⓑ Ⓒ Ⓓ	70. Ⓐ Ⓑ Ⓒ Ⓓ
11. Ⓐ Ⓑ Ⓒ Ⓓ	26. Ⓐ Ⓑ Ⓒ Ⓓ	41. Ⓐ Ⓑ Ⓒ Ⓓ	56. Ⓐ Ⓑ Ⓒ Ⓓ	71. Ⓐ Ⓑ Ⓒ Ⓓ
12. Ⓐ Ⓑ Ⓒ Ⓓ	27. Ⓐ Ⓑ Ⓒ Ⓓ	42. Ⓐ Ⓑ Ⓒ Ⓓ	57. Ⓐ Ⓑ Ⓒ Ⓓ	72. Ⓐ Ⓑ Ⓒ Ⓓ
13. Ⓐ Ⓑ Ⓒ Ⓓ	28. Ⓐ Ⓑ Ⓒ Ⓓ	43. Ⓐ Ⓑ Ⓒ Ⓓ	58. Ⓐ Ⓑ Ⓒ Ⓓ	73. Ⓐ Ⓑ Ⓒ Ⓓ
14. Ⓐ Ⓑ Ⓒ Ⓓ	29. Ⓐ Ⓑ Ⓒ Ⓓ	44. Ⓐ Ⓑ Ⓒ Ⓓ	59. Ⓐ Ⓑ Ⓒ Ⓓ	74. Ⓐ Ⓑ Ⓒ Ⓓ
15. Ⓐ Ⓑ Ⓒ Ⓓ	30. Ⓐ Ⓑ Ⓒ Ⓓ	45. Ⓐ Ⓑ Ⓒ Ⓓ	60. Ⓐ Ⓑ Ⓒ Ⓓ	75. Ⓐ Ⓑ Ⓒ Ⓓ

ANTONYM TEST

Directions: *For each of the following questions, select the word opposite in meaning to the word printed in capital letters.*

1. DEFACE

   (A) defame
   (B) embellish
   (C) vilify
   (D) disfigure

2. SUPERFLUOUS

   (A) coarse
   (B) transient
   (C) insufficient
   (D) abundant

3. ASSUAGE

   (A) presume
   (B) agitate
   (C) alleviate
   (D) absorb

4. AUGURY

   (A) gentility
   (B) relentlessness
   (C) supremacy
   (D) science

5. TERMINATE

   (A) withhold
   (B) construe
   (C) repel
   (D) initiate

6. VITIATE

   (A) liquidate
   (B) revive
   (C) validate
   (D) slander

7. JUBILANT

   (A) lugubrious
   (B) irrepressible
   (C) discernible
   (D) jocular

8. HOSTILE

   (A) affable
   (B) awkward
   (C) judicious
   (D) coxcombical

9. TACITURN

   (A) tactful
   (B) talkative
   (C) crucial
   (D) impetuous

10. LAGGARDLY

    (A) laboriously
    (B) languidly
    (C) briskly
    (D) cowardly

11. PHLEGMATIC

    (A) vital
    (B) apparent
    (C) conversant
    (D) apprehensive

12. LOATHSOME

    (A) alluring
    (B) mournful
    (C) indifferent
    (D) preposterous

13. EXALT

    (A) degrade
    (B) gratify
    (C) expose
    (D) desiderate

14. PACIFY

    (A) conciliate
    (B) palliate
    (C) quell
    (D) exasperate

15. SUBSEQUENT

   (A) worthless
   (B) inactive
   (C) preceding
   (D) demeaning

16. ULTIMATE

   (A) initial
   (B) equitable
   (C) irrefutable
   (D) turbid

17. LEEWAY

   (A) relevance
   (B) restriction
   (C) protection
   (D) satisfaction

18. PRETENTIOUS

   (A) flagrant
   (B) diabolical
   (C) officious
   (D) modest

19. QUANDARY

   (A) certainty
   (B) mediocrity
   (C) ruthlessness
   (D) criterion

20. SAGACIOUS

   (A) obtuse
   (B) scurrilous
   (C) indulgent
   (D) impertinent

21. SAVANT

   (A) savage
   (B) master
   (C) neophyte
   (D) constituent

22. SQUALID

   (A) staunch
   (B) stately
   (C) avaricious
   (D) equivocal

23. EXQUISITE

   (A) exorbitant
   (B) inobscure
   (C) extraneous
   (D) ordinary

24. FACILITATE

   (A) falsify
   (B) delude
   (C) hinder
   (D) assimilate

25. FLAWLESS

   (A) pertinent
   (B) conventional
   (C) defective
   (D) complacent

26. RECOMPENSE

   (A) renovate
   (B) misrequite
   (C) miscompute
   (D) sanction

27. FERVENT

   (A) nonchalant
   (B) lenient
   (C) meager
   (D) liable

28. AVERT

   (A) pursue
   (B) forestall
   (C) reject
   (D) relinquish

29. ARID

   (A) fragrant
   (B) moist
   (C) parched
   (D) odoriferous

30. IMPERATIVE

   (A) conceptive
   (B) illustrative
   (C) speculative
   (D) optional

31. SUCCINCT

    (A) corporeal
    (B) graphic
    (C) princely
    (D) loquacious

32. JEOPARDY

    (A) security
    (B) discernment
    (C) curiosity
    (D) tedium

33. SOMBER

    (A) insipid
    (B) congruous
    (C) festive
    (D) voluminous

34. EXOTIC

    (A) diachronic
    (B) erotic
    (C) common
    (D) harmonious

35. AFFILIATE

    (A) annihilate
    (B) disassociate
    (C) proffer
    (D) disparage

36. SINISTER

    (A) auspicious
    (B) immaculate
    (C) fanatical
    (D) transitory

37. INEXTRICABLE

    (A) intricate
    (B) judicious
    (C) disentangled
    (D) desperate

38. PROFLIGATE

    (A) insolvent
    (B) virtuous
    (C) redundant
    (D) incessant

39. TURBULENT

    (A) diaphanous
    (B) tranquil
    (C) formidable
    (D) diffident

40. UNWARRANTED

    (A) justifiable
    (B) baneful
    (C) depleted
    (D) contemplated

41. PLAINTIVE

    (A) embellished
    (B) peccant
    (C) rational
    (D) gleeful

42. ORNATE

    (A) unadorned
    (B) deft
    (C) subtle
    (D) conspicuous

43. ABROGATE

    (A) ratify
    (B) reconcile
    (C) abridge
    (D) alleviate

44. ABASE

    (A) cede
    (B) dignify
    (C) repudiate
    (D) engulf

45. RENOUNCE

    (A) claim
    (B) deride
    (C) conceive
    (D) alienate

46. SABOTAGE

    (A) compensate
    (B) reinforce
    (C) restrain
    (D) release

47. OBLIVIOUS

    (A) latent
    (B) integrant
    (C) repugnant
    (D) cognizant

48. SUBMISSIVE

    (A) offensive
    (B) tactless
    (C) incompliant
    (D) manifest

49. NURTURE

    (A) distinguish
    (B) impart
    (C) neglect
    (D) disclose

50. PRUDENCE

    (A) compunction
    (B) dilemma
    (C) anticipation
    (D) recklessness

51. LAMENT

    (A) rejoice
    (B) acclaim
    (C) surmise
    (D) deceive

52. GRUELING

    (A) relaxing
    (B) satisfying
    (C) taming
    (D) suppressing

53. TRIVIAL

    (A) nugatory
    (B) ungainly
    (C) critical
    (D) solicitous

54. ZENITH

    (A) vitality
    (B) rage
    (C) reverence
    (D) nadir

55. UNOBTRUSIVE

    (A) resonant
    (B) interfering
    (C) controlled
    (D) subjective

56. REFRACTIVE

    (A) cryptic
    (B) interruptive
    (C) applicable
    (D) direct

57. REBUFF

    (A) exclusion
    (B) disturbance
    (C) recall
    (D) encouragement

58. ADVERSARY

    (A) opponent
    (B) administrator
    (C) accomplice
    (D) enemy

59. ANTAGONIST

    (A) rival
    (B) protagonist
    (C) analyst
    (D) pessimist

60. ALIEN

    (A) native
    (B) anonymous
    (C) verified
    (D) copious

61. ERUDITE

    (A) contagious
    (B) inadvertent
    (C) benevolent
    (D) ignorant

62. PARAMOUNT

    (A) admissible
    (B) inconsequential
    (C) tolerable
    (D) supreme

63. SURREPTITIOUS

    (A) authoritative
    (B) candid
    (C) vulnerable
    (D) subjugated

64. MENDACIOUS

    (A) meddlesome
    (B) incomparable
    (C) malicious
    (D) creditable

65. UNCTUOUS

    (A) awkward
    (B) dubious
    (C) furtive
    (D) disputable

66. IMPETUOUS

    (A) subdued
    (B) unmitigated
    (C) substantial
    (D) egregious

67. PENURIOUS

    (A) frugal
    (B) extravagant
    (C) plausible
    (D) absurb

68. ODIOUS

    (A) attentive
    (B) considerate
    (C) acceptable
    (D) unascertained

69. OSTENSIBLE

    (A) hidden
    (B) preliminary
    (C) authentic
    (D) unsuitable

70. DELETERIOUS

    (A) distressing
    (B) beneficial
    (C) grievous
    (D) delirious

71. IGNOMINY

    (A) honor
    (B) aversion
    (C) perplexity
    (D) remoteness

72. COMPATIBLE

    (A) dexterous
    (B) repugnant
    (C) incongruous
    (D) captivating

73. PREMEDITATED

    (A) devoted
    (B) condescending
    (C) improvised
    (D) supposed

74. PERNICIOUS

    (A) restorative
    (B) conclusive
    (C) tractable
    (D) capricious

75. UMBRAGE

    (A) pique
    (B) monstrous
    (C) reliance
    (D) amity

Answer Key

1.	**B**	26.	**B**	51.	**A**
2.	**C**	27.	**A**	52.	**A**
3.	**B**	28.	**A**	53.	**C**
4.	**D**	29.	**B**	54.	**D**
5.	**D**	30.	**D**	55.	**B**
6.	**C**	31.	**D**	56.	**D**
7.	**A**	32.	**A**	57.	**D**
8.	**A**	33.	**C**	58.	**C**
9.	**B**	34.	**C**	59.	**B**
10.	**C**	35.	**B**	60.	**A**
11.	**A**	36.	**A**	61.	**D**
12.	**A**	37.	**C**	62.	**B**
13.	**A**	38.	**B**	63.	**B**
14.	**D**	39.	**B**	64.	**D**
15.	**C**	40.	**A**	65.	**A**
16.	**A**	41.	**D**	66.	**A**
17.	**B**	42.	**A**	67.	**B**
18.	**D**	43.	**A**	68.	**C**
19.	**A**	44.	**B**	69.	**A**
20.	**A**	45.	**A**	70.	**B**
21.	**C**	46.	**B**	71.	**A**
22.	**B**	47.	**D**	72.	**C**
23.	**D**	48.	**C**	73.	**C**
24.	**C**	49.	**C**	74.	**A**
25.	**C**	50.	**D**	75.	**D**

SKILL WITH VERBAL ANALOGIES

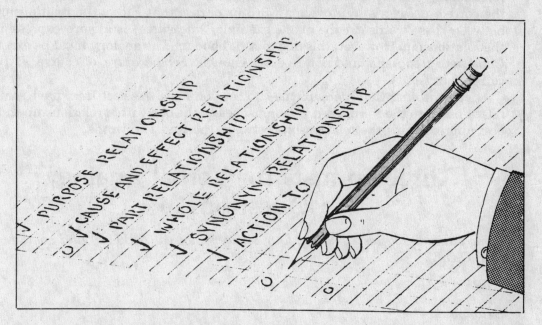

The verbal analogy is one variation of the vocabulary question often encountered on nursing school tests. It tests your understanding of word meanings *and* your ability to grasp relationships between words and ideas. This practice in mental agility will help you do better with all the other questions on the test.

In addition to their simple meanings, words carry subtle shades of implication that depend in some degree upon the relationship they bear to other words. There are various classifications of relationship, such as similarity (synonyms) and opposition (antonyms). Careful students will try to examine each shade of meaning they encounter.

The ability to detect the exact nature of the relationship between words is a function of your intelligence. In a sense, the verbal analogy test is a vocabulary test. But it is also a test of your ability to analyze meanings, think things out, and see the relationships between ideas and words. In mathematics, this kind of situation is expressed as a proportion problem: $3 : 5 :: 6 : X$. Sometimes, verbal analogies are written in this mathematical form:

CLOCK : TIME :: THERMOMETER :

(A) hour
(B) degrees
(C) climate
(D) temperature

Or the question may be put:

CLOCK is to TIME as THERMOMETER is to

(A) hour
(B) degrees
(C) climate
(D) temperature

The problem is to determine which of the lettered words has the same relationship to *thermometer* as *time* has to *clock*. The best way of determining the correct answer is to provide a word or phrase that shows the relationship between these words. In the above example, "measures" is a word expressing the relationship. However, this may not be enough. The analogy must be exact. *Climate* or *weather* would not be exact enough. *Temperature,* of course, is the correct answer.

You will find that many of the choices you have to select from have some relationship to the third word. You must select the one with a relationship that *best* approximates the relationship between the first two words.

Three Formats for Verbal Analogy Questions

Some standarized tests provide four answer choices (A,B,C,D) and some five (A,B,C,D,E).

TYPE 1

Example:

From the four pairs of words that follow, you are to select the pair related in the same way as are the words of the first pair.

SPELLING : PUNCTUATION ::

(A) pajamas : fatigue
(B) powder : shaving
(C) bandage: cut
(D) biology : physics

Spelling and *Punctuation* are elements of the mechanics of English; *Biology* and *Physics* are two of the subjects that make up the field of science. The other choices do not possess this part : part relationship. Therefore, (D) is the correct choice.

TYPE 2

Example:

Another popular format gives two words followed by a third word. The latter is related to one word in a group of choices in the same way that the first two words are related.

WINTER : SUMMER :: COLD :

(A) wet
(B) future
(C) hot
(D) freezing

Winter and *Summer* bear an opposite relationship. *Cold* and *hot* have the same kind of opposite relationship. Therefore, (C) is the correct answer.

TYPE 3

Example:

Still another analogy format has a variable construction. Any four relationship elements may not be specified. From choices offered—regardless of position— you are to select the one choice that completes the relationship with the other three items. In this example the third element is not specified.

SUBMARINE : FISH :: _____ : BIRD

(A) kite
(B) limousine
(C) feather
(D) chirp

Both a *submarine* and a *fish* are usually found in the water; both a *kite* and a *bird* are customarily seen in the air. (A), consequently, is the correct answer.

This third type is used in the Miller Analogy Test, considered one of the most reliable and valid tests for selection of graduate students for universities and high level personnel for government, industry, and business.

Categorizing the Kinds of Analogy Relationships

1. Purpose Relationship
   GLOVE : BALL ::
   (A) hook : fish
   (B) winter : weather
   (C) game : pennant
   (D) stadium : seats

   (Answer: A)

2. Cause-and-Effect Relationship
   RACE : FATIGUE ::
   (A) track : athlete
   (B) ant: bug
   (C) fast : hunger
   (D) walking : running

   (Answer: C)

3. Part : Whole Relationship
   SNAKE : REPTILE ::
   (A) patch : thread
   (B) removal : snow
   (C) struggle : wrestle
   (D) hand : clock

   (Answer: D)

4. Part : Part Relationship
   GILL : FIN ::
   (A) tube : antenna
   (B) instrument : violin
   (C) sea : fish
   (D) salad : supper

   (Answer: A)

5. Action : Object Relationship
   KICK : FOOTBALL ::
   (A) kill : bomb
   (B) break : pieces
   (C) question : team
   (D) smoke : pipe

   (Answer: D)

6. Object : Action Relationship
   STEAK : BROIL ::
   (A) bread : bake
   (B) food : eat
   (C) wine : pour
   (D) sugar : spill

   (Answer: A)

7. Synonym Relationship
ENORMOUS : HUGE ::
(A) rogue : rock
(B) muddy : unclear
(C) purse : kitchen
(D) black : white

(Answer: B)

8. Antonym Relationship
PURITY : EVIL ::
(A) suavity : bluntness
(B) north : climate
(C) angel : horns
(D) boldness : victory

(Answer: A)

9. Place Relationship
MIAMI : FLORIDA ::
(A) Chicago : United States
(B) New York : Albany
(C) United States : Chicago
(D) Albany : New York

(Answer: D)

10. Degree Relationship
WARM : HOT ::
(A) glue : paste
(B) climate : weather
(C) fried egg : boiled egg
(D) bright : genius

(Answer: D)

11. Characteristic Relationship
IGNORANCE : POVERTY ::
(A) blood : wound
(B) money : dollar
(C) schools : elevators
(D) education : stupidity

(Answer: A)

12. Sequence Relationship
SPRING : SUMMER ::
(A) Thursday : Wednesday
(B) Wednesday : Monday
(C) Monday : Sunday
(D) Wednesday : Thursday

(Answer: D)

13. Grammatical Relationship
RESTORE : CLIMB ::
(A) segregation : seem
(B) into : nymph
(C) tearoom : although
(D) overpower : seethe

(Answer: D)

14. Association Relationship
DEVIL : WRONG ::
(A) color : sidewalk
(B) slipper : state
(C) ink : writing
(D) picture : bed

(Answer: C)

15. Numerical Relationship
4 : 12 ::
(A) 10 : 16
(B) 9 : 27
(C) 3 : 4
(D) 12 : 6

(Answer: B)

Points to Remember

In many analogy questions, the incorrect choices may be related in some way to the first two words. Don't let this association mislead you. For example, in number 4 (part : part relationship,) the correct answer is (A), *tube : antenna.* Choice (C), *sea : fish,* is incorrect, although these two latter words are associated in a general sense with the first two words (*gill : fin*).

Often, the relationship of the first two words may apply to *more than one* of the choices given. In such a case, you must narrow down the initial relationship in order to get the correct choice. For example, in number 6 (object : action relationship), a *steak* is something that you *broil.* Now let us consider the choices: *bread* is something that you *bake; food* is something that you *eat; wine* is something that you *pour* and *sugar* is something that you (can) *spill.* Thus far, each choice seems correct. Let us now narrow down the relationship: a *steak* is something that you *broil* with *heat.* The only choice that fulfills this *complete* relationship is (A), *bread*—something that you *bake* with *heat.* It follows that (A) is the correct choice.

Remember that the keys to analogy success are:

Step One determine the relationship between the first two words.

Step Two find the same relationship among the choices that follow the first two words.

Answer Sheet Verbal Analogies

PART A

1. Ⓐ Ⓑ Ⓒ Ⓓ	6. Ⓐ Ⓑ Ⓒ Ⓓ	11. Ⓐ Ⓑ Ⓒ Ⓓ	16. Ⓐ Ⓑ Ⓒ Ⓓ	21. Ⓐ Ⓑ Ⓒ Ⓓ
2. Ⓐ Ⓑ Ⓒ Ⓓ	7. Ⓐ Ⓑ Ⓒ Ⓓ	12. Ⓐ Ⓑ Ⓒ Ⓓ	17. Ⓐ Ⓑ Ⓒ Ⓓ	22. Ⓐ Ⓑ Ⓒ Ⓓ
3. Ⓐ Ⓑ Ⓒ Ⓓ	8. Ⓐ Ⓑ Ⓒ Ⓓ	13. Ⓐ Ⓑ Ⓒ Ⓓ	18. Ⓐ Ⓑ Ⓒ Ⓓ	23. Ⓐ Ⓑ Ⓒ Ⓓ
4. Ⓐ Ⓑ Ⓒ Ⓓ	9. Ⓐ Ⓑ Ⓒ Ⓓ	14. Ⓐ Ⓑ Ⓒ Ⓓ	19. Ⓐ Ⓑ Ⓒ Ⓓ	24. Ⓐ Ⓑ Ⓒ Ⓓ
5. Ⓐ Ⓑ Ⓒ Ⓓ	10. Ⓐ Ⓑ Ⓒ Ⓓ	15. Ⓐ Ⓑ Ⓒ Ⓓ	20. Ⓐ Ⓑ Ⓒ Ⓓ	25. Ⓐ Ⓑ Ⓒ Ⓓ

PART B

1. Ⓐ Ⓑ Ⓒ Ⓓ Ⓔ	6. Ⓐ Ⓑ Ⓒ Ⓓ Ⓔ	11. Ⓐ Ⓑ Ⓒ Ⓓ Ⓔ	16. Ⓐ Ⓑ Ⓒ Ⓓ Ⓔ	21. Ⓐ Ⓑ Ⓒ Ⓓ Ⓔ
2. Ⓐ Ⓑ Ⓒ Ⓓ Ⓔ	7. Ⓐ Ⓑ Ⓒ Ⓓ Ⓔ	12. Ⓐ Ⓑ Ⓒ Ⓓ Ⓔ	17. Ⓐ Ⓑ Ⓒ Ⓓ Ⓔ	22. Ⓐ Ⓑ Ⓒ Ⓓ Ⓔ
3. Ⓐ Ⓑ Ⓒ Ⓓ Ⓔ	8. Ⓐ Ⓑ Ⓒ Ⓓ Ⓔ	13. Ⓐ Ⓑ Ⓒ Ⓓ Ⓔ	18. Ⓐ Ⓑ Ⓒ Ⓓ Ⓔ	23. Ⓐ Ⓑ Ⓒ Ⓓ Ⓔ
4. Ⓐ Ⓑ Ⓒ Ⓓ Ⓔ	9. Ⓐ Ⓑ Ⓒ Ⓓ Ⓔ	14. Ⓐ Ⓑ Ⓒ Ⓓ Ⓔ	19. Ⓐ Ⓑ Ⓒ Ⓓ Ⓔ	24. Ⓐ Ⓑ Ⓒ Ⓓ Ⓔ
5. Ⓐ Ⓑ Ⓒ Ⓓ Ⓔ	10. Ⓐ Ⓑ Ⓒ Ⓓ Ⓔ	15. Ⓐ Ⓑ Ⓒ Ⓓ Ⓔ	20. Ⓐ Ⓑ Ⓒ Ⓓ Ⓔ	25. Ⓐ Ⓑ Ⓒ Ⓓ Ⓔ

PART C

1. Ⓐ Ⓑ Ⓒ Ⓓ Ⓔ	6. Ⓐ Ⓑ Ⓒ Ⓓ Ⓔ	11. Ⓐ Ⓑ Ⓒ Ⓓ Ⓔ	16. Ⓐ Ⓑ Ⓒ Ⓓ Ⓔ	21. Ⓐ Ⓑ Ⓒ Ⓓ Ⓔ
2. Ⓐ Ⓑ Ⓒ Ⓓ Ⓔ	7. Ⓐ Ⓑ Ⓒ Ⓓ Ⓔ	12. Ⓐ Ⓑ Ⓒ Ⓓ Ⓔ	17. Ⓐ Ⓑ Ⓒ Ⓓ Ⓔ	22. Ⓐ Ⓑ Ⓒ Ⓓ Ⓔ
3. Ⓐ Ⓑ Ⓒ Ⓓ Ⓔ	8. Ⓐ Ⓑ Ⓒ Ⓓ Ⓔ	13. Ⓐ Ⓑ Ⓒ Ⓓ Ⓔ	18. Ⓐ Ⓑ Ⓒ Ⓓ Ⓔ	23. Ⓐ Ⓑ Ⓒ Ⓓ Ⓔ
4. Ⓐ Ⓑ Ⓒ Ⓓ Ⓔ	9. Ⓐ Ⓑ Ⓒ Ⓓ Ⓔ	14. Ⓐ Ⓑ Ⓒ Ⓓ Ⓔ	19. Ⓐ Ⓑ Ⓒ Ⓓ Ⓔ	24. Ⓐ Ⓑ Ⓒ Ⓓ Ⓔ
5. Ⓐ Ⓑ Ⓒ Ⓓ Ⓔ	10. Ⓐ Ⓑ Ⓒ Ⓓ Ⓔ	15. Ⓐ Ⓑ Ⓒ Ⓓ Ⓔ	20. Ⓐ Ⓑ Ⓒ Ⓓ Ⓔ	25. Ⓐ Ⓑ Ⓒ Ⓓ Ⓔ

VERBAL ANALOGIES TEST

75 Minutes   75 Questions

Directions: *In the following questions, you are to determine the relationship between the first pair of capitalized words and then decide which of the answer choices shares a similar relationship with the third capitalized word. Parts A and B of this test are written in mathematical form (expressed as proportion problems). Part A's questions have four answer choices, Part B's questions have five. Part C is written so that relationships are expressed with "is to" and "as."*

Part A

10 Minutes   25 Questions

1. GUN : SHOTS :: KNIFE :

   (A) run
   (B) cuts
   (C) hat
   (D) bird

2. EAR : HEAR :: EYE :

   (A) table
   (B) hand
   (C) see
   (D) foot

3. FUR : MAMMAL :: FEATHERS :

   (A) bird
   (B) neck
   (C) feet
   (D) bill

4. HANDLE : HAMMER :: KNOB :

   (A) key
   (B) room
   (C) shut
   (D) door

5. SHOE : FOOT :: HAT :

   (A) coat
   (B) nose
   (C) head
   (D) collar

6. WATER : DRINK :: BREAD :

   (A) cake
   (B) coffee
   (C) eat
   (D) pie

7. FOOD : MAN :: GASOLINE :

   (A) gas
   (B) oil
   (C) automobile
   (D) spark

8. EAT : FAT :: STARVE :

   (A) thin
   (B) food
   (C) bread
   (D) thirsty

9. MAN : HOUSE :: BIRD :

   (A) fly
   (B) insect
   (C) worm
   (D) nest

10. GO : COME :: SELL :

    (A) leave
    (B) buy
    (C) money
    (D) papers

11. PENINSULA : LAND :: BAY :

    (A) boats
    (B) pay
    (C) ocean
    (D) colony

12. HOUR : MINUTE :: MINUTE :

    (A) hour
    (B) week
    (C) second
    (D) short

13. ABIDE : DEPART :: STAY :

    (A) over
    (B) home
    (C) play
    (D) leave

14. JANUARY : FEBRUARY :: JUNE :

    (A) July
    (B) May
    (C) month
    (D) year

15. BOLD : TIMID :: ADVANCE :

    (A) proceed
    (B) retreat
    (C) campaign
    (B) soldiers

16. ABOVE : BELOW :: TOP :

    (A) spin
    (B) bottom
    (C) surface
    (D) side

17. LION : ANIMAL :: ROSE :

    (A) smell
    (B) leaf
    (C) plant
    (D) thorn

18. TIGER : CARNIVOROUS :: HORSE :

    (A) cow
    (B) nervous
    (C) omnivorous
    (D) herbivorous

19. SAILOR : NAVY :: SOLDIER :

    (A) gun
    (B) cap
    (C) hill
    (D) army

20. PICTURE : SEE :: SOUND :

    (A) noise
    (B) music
    (C) hear
    (D) bark

21. SUCCESS : JOY :: FAILURE :

    (A) sadness
    (B) success
    (C) fail
    (D) work

22. HOPE : DESPAIR :: HAPPINESS :

    (A) frolic
    (B) fun
    (C) joy
    (D) sadness

23. PRETTY : UGLY :: ATTRACT :

    (A) fine
    (B) repel
    (C) nice
    (D) draw

24. PUPIL : TEACHER :: CHILD :

    (A) parent
    (B) dolly
    (C) youngster
    (D) obey

25. CITY : MAYOR :: ARMY :

    (A) navy
    (B) soldier
    (C) general
    (D) private

Part B

10 Minutes   25 Questions

1. REMUNERATIVE : PROFITABLE :: FRAUDLENT :

    (A) lying
    (B) slander
    (C) fallacious
    (D) plausible
    (E) reward

2. AX : WOODSMAN :: AWL :

    (A) cut
    (B) hew
    (C) plumber
    (D) pierce
    (E) cobbler

3. SURGEON : SCALPEL :: BUTCHER :

    (A) mallet
    (B) cleaver
    (C) chisel
    (D) wrench
    (E) medicine

4. CAT : FELINE :: HORSE :

    (A) equine
    (B) tiger
    (C) quadruped
    (D) carnivore
    (E) vulpine

5. ADVERSITY : HAPPINESS :: VEHEMENCE :

    (A) misfortune
    (B) gaiety
    (C) troublesome
    (D) petulance
    (E) serenity

6. NECKLACE : ADORNMENT :: MEDAL :

    (A) jewel
    (B) metal
    (C) bravery
    (D) bronze
    (E) decoration

7. GUN : HOLSTER :: SWORD :

    (A) pistol
    (B) scabbard
    (C) warrior
    (D) slay
    (E) plunder

8. ARCHEOLOGIST : ANTIQUITY :: ICHTHYOLOGIST :

    (A) theology
    (B) ruins
    (C) horticulture
    (D) marine life
    (E) mystic

9. SHOE : LEATHER :: HIGHWAY :

    (A) passage
    (B) road
    (C) asphalt
    (D) trail
    (E) journey

10. SERFDOM : FEUDALISM :: ENTREPRENEUR :

    (A) laissez faire
    (B) captain
    (C) radical
    (D) agriculture
    (E) capitalism

11. FIN : FISH :: PROPELLER :

    (A) automobile
    (B) airplane
    (C) grain elevator
    (D) water
    (E) canoe

12. PULP : PAPER :: HEMP :

    (A) rope
    (B) baskets
    (C) yarn
    (D) cotton
    (E) wood

13. SKIN : MAN :: HIDE :

    (A) scales
    (B) fur
    (C) animal
    (D) hair
    (E) fish

14. RAIN : DROP :: SNOW :

    (A) ice
    (B) cold
    (C) zero
    (D) flake
    (E) sleet

15. WING : BIRD :: HOOF :

    (A) dog
    (B) foot
    (C) horse
    (D) girl
    (E) horseshoe

16. CONSTELLATION : STAR :: ARCHIPELAGO :

    (A) continent
    (B) peninsula
    (C) country
    (D) island
    (E) river

17. ACCOUNTANCY : BOOKKEEPING :: COURT REPORTING :

    (A) law
    (B) judgment
    (C) stenography
    (D) lawyer
    (E) judge

18. ABSENCE : PRESENCE :: STABLE :

    (A) steady
    (B) secure
    (C) safe
    (D) changeable
    (E) influential

19. RUBBER : FLEXIBILITY :: PIPE :

    (A) iron
    (B) copper
    (C) pliability
    (D) elasticity
    (E) rigidity

20. SAFETY VALVE : BOILER :: FUSE :

    (A) motor
    (B) house
    (C) wire
    (D) city
    (E) factory

21. SCHOLARLY : UNSCHOLARLY :: LEARNED :

    (A) ignorant
    (B) wise
    (C) skilled
    (D) scholarly
    (E) literary

22. IMMIGRANT : ARRIVAL :: EMIGRATION :

    (A) leaving
    (B) alienation
    (C) native
    (D) welcoming
    (E) emigrant

23. GOVERNOR : STATE :: GENERAL :

    (A) lieutenant
    (B) navy
    (C) army
    (D) captain
    (E) admiral

24. LETTER CARRIER : MAIL :: MESSENGER :

    (A) value
    (B) dispatches
    (C) easy
    (D) complicated
    (E) fast

25. CLOTH : COAT :: GINGHAM :

    (A) doll
    (B) cover
    (C) washable
    (D) dress
    (E) dressmaker

Part C

10 Minutes   25 Questions

1. BOAT is to DOCK as AIRPLANE is to

   (A) wing
   (B) strut
   (C) engine
   (D) wind
   (E) hangar

2. OAT is to BUSHEL as DIAMOND is to

   (A) gram
   (B) hardness
   (C) usefulness
   (D) carat
   (E) ornament

3. MEDICINE is to EXAMINATION as LAW is to

   (A) jurist
   (B) court
   (C) interrogation
   (D) contract
   (E) suit

4. PARENT is to COMMAND as CHILD is to

   (A) obey
   (B) will
   (C) women
   (D) love
   (E) achieve

5. CAPTAIN is to VESSEL as DIRECTOR is to

   (A) touring party
   (B) board
   (C) travel
   (D) orchestra
   (E) musician

6. FATHER is to DAUGHTER as UNCLE is to

   (A) son
   (B) daughter
   (C) son-in-law
   (D) niece
   (E) aunt

7. PISTOL is to TRIGGER as MOTOR is to

   (A) wire
   (B) dynamo
   (C) amperes
   (D) barrel
   (E) switch

8. CUBE is to PYRAMID as SQUARE is to

   (A) box
   (B) solid
   (C) pentagon
   (D) triangle
   (E) cylinder

9. PROFIT is to SELLING as FAME is to

   (A) buying
   (B) cheating
   (C) bravery
   (D) praying
   (E) loving

10. BINDING is to BOOK as WELDING is to

    (A) box
    (B) tank
    (C) chair
    (D) wire
    (E) pencil

11. GYMNASIUM is to HEALTH as SCHOOL is to

    (A) sick
    (B) study
    (C) books
    (D) knowledge
    (E) library

12. RIGHT is to WRONG as SUCCEED is to

    (A) aid
    (B) profit
    (C) fail
    (D) error
    (E) gain

13. INDIAN is to AMERICA as ABORIG-
INE is to

    (A) Hindustan
    (B) Mexico
    (C) soil
    (D) magic
    (E) Australia

14. WEALTH is to MERCENARY as GOLD
is to

    (A) lucre
    (B) miner
    (C) fame
    (D) eleemosynary
    (E) South Africa

15. BOTTLE is to BRITTLE as TIRE is to

    (A) elastic
    (B) scarce
    (C) rubber
    (D) spheroid
    (E) automobile

16. SOPRANO is to HIGH as BASS is to

    (A) violin
    (B) good
    (C) low
    (D) fish
    (E) soft

17. OLFACTORY is to NOSE as TACTILE is
to

    (A) tacit
    (B) bloody
    (C) finger
    (D) handkerchief
    (E) stomach

18. STREET is to HORIZONTAL as BUILD-
ING is to

    (A) tall
    (B) brick
    (C) broad
    (D) vertical
    (E) large

19. ALLEGIANCE is to LOYALTY as
TREASON is to

    (A) obedience
    (B) rebellion
    (C) murder
    (D) felony
    (E) homage

20. CANVAS is to PAINT as MOLD is to

    (A) clay
    (B) cloth
    (C) statue
    (D) art
    (E) aesthetic

21. FISH is to FIN as BIRD is to

    (A) wing
    (B) five
    (C) feet
    (D) beak
    (E) feathers

22. CONQUEST is to ASCENDANCY as
DEFEAT is to

    (A) omission
    (B) frustration
    (C) censure
    (D) subjugation
    (E) mastery

23. SOLUTION is to MYSTERY as COM-
PLETION is to

    (A) puzzle
    (B) books
    (C) college
    (D) school
    (E) detective

24. ALUMNUS is to ALUMNA as PRINCE is to

    (A) castle
    (B) king
    (C) knight
    (D) country
    (E) princess

25. OCCULT is to OVERT as SECRET is to

    (A) abstract
    (B) outward
    (C) science
    (D) tarry
    (E) concealed

Answer Key

PART A

1. B	6. C	11. C	16. B	21. A
2. C	7. C	12. C	17. C	22. D
3. A	8. A	13. D	18. D	23. B
4. D	9. D	14. A	19. D	24. A
5. C	10. B	15. B	20. C	25. C

PART B

1. C	6. E	11. B	16. D	21. A
2. E	7. B	12. A	17. C	22. A
3. B	8. D	13. C	18. D	23. C
4. A	9. C	14. D	19. E	24. B
5. E	10. E	15. C	20. A	25. D

PART C

1. E	6. D	11. D	16. C	21. A
2. D	7. E	12. C	17. C	22. D
3. C	8. D	13. E	18. D	23. A
4. A	9. C	14. A	19. B	24. E
5. B	10. B	15. A	20. A	25. B

Let's Put You to the Test

Now that you have thoroughly reviewed the various kinds of verbal-ability items and are familiar with the test-taking strategies associated with them, let's put you to the test.

Pay strict attention to the time allotted for each section of the test and do your best to adhere to the time limits. Read the directions for each part of the test before attempting to answer any of the items.

This test has three parts: A—Synonyms; B—Antonyms; C—Verbal Analogies. The total time allotted for this test is 50 minutes. Have extra pencils available in case of point breakage, so as not to lose testing time.

An answer key is provided at the end of the test so that you can evaluate your performance. Remember, this is a simulation of the "real thing," so be honest with yourself and save the glance at the answer key until after you have completed the test.

Answer Sheet
Final Verbal Ability Examination

PART A
SYNONYMS

1. Ⓐ Ⓑ Ⓒ Ⓓ	8. Ⓐ Ⓑ Ⓒ Ⓓ	15. Ⓐ Ⓑ Ⓒ Ⓓ	22. Ⓐ Ⓑ Ⓒ Ⓓ	29. Ⓐ Ⓑ Ⓒ Ⓓ
2. Ⓐ Ⓑ Ⓒ Ⓓ	9. Ⓐ Ⓑ Ⓒ Ⓓ	16. Ⓐ Ⓑ Ⓒ Ⓓ	23. Ⓐ Ⓑ Ⓒ Ⓓ	30. Ⓐ Ⓑ Ⓒ Ⓓ
3. Ⓐ Ⓑ Ⓒ Ⓓ	10. Ⓐ Ⓑ Ⓒ Ⓓ	17. Ⓐ Ⓑ Ⓒ Ⓓ	24. Ⓐ Ⓑ Ⓒ Ⓓ	31. Ⓐ Ⓑ Ⓒ Ⓓ
4. Ⓐ Ⓑ Ⓒ Ⓓ	11. Ⓐ Ⓑ Ⓒ Ⓓ	18. Ⓐ Ⓑ Ⓒ Ⓓ	25. Ⓐ Ⓑ Ⓒ Ⓓ	32. Ⓐ Ⓑ Ⓒ Ⓓ
5. Ⓐ Ⓑ Ⓒ Ⓓ	12. Ⓐ Ⓑ Ⓒ Ⓓ	19. Ⓐ Ⓑ Ⓒ Ⓓ	26. Ⓐ Ⓑ Ⓒ Ⓓ	33. Ⓐ Ⓑ Ⓒ Ⓓ
6. Ⓐ Ⓑ Ⓒ Ⓓ	13. Ⓐ Ⓑ Ⓒ Ⓓ	20. Ⓐ Ⓑ Ⓒ Ⓓ	27. Ⓐ Ⓑ Ⓒ Ⓓ	34. Ⓐ Ⓑ Ⓒ Ⓓ
7. Ⓐ Ⓑ Ⓒ Ⓓ	14. Ⓐ Ⓑ Ⓒ Ⓓ	21. Ⓐ Ⓑ Ⓒ Ⓓ	28. Ⓐ Ⓑ Ⓒ Ⓓ	35. Ⓐ Ⓑ Ⓒ Ⓓ

PART B
ANTONYMS

1. Ⓐ Ⓑ Ⓒ Ⓓ	9. Ⓐ Ⓑ Ⓒ Ⓓ	17. Ⓐ Ⓑ Ⓒ Ⓓ	25. Ⓐ Ⓑ Ⓒ Ⓓ	33. Ⓐ Ⓑ Ⓒ Ⓓ
2. Ⓐ Ⓑ Ⓒ Ⓓ	10. Ⓐ Ⓑ Ⓒ Ⓓ	18. Ⓐ Ⓑ Ⓒ Ⓓ	26. Ⓐ Ⓑ Ⓒ Ⓓ	34. Ⓐ Ⓑ Ⓒ Ⓓ
3. Ⓐ Ⓑ Ⓒ Ⓓ	11. Ⓐ Ⓑ Ⓒ Ⓓ	19. Ⓐ Ⓑ Ⓒ Ⓓ	27. Ⓐ Ⓑ Ⓒ Ⓓ	35. Ⓐ Ⓑ Ⓒ Ⓓ
4. Ⓐ Ⓑ Ⓒ Ⓓ	12. Ⓐ Ⓑ Ⓒ Ⓓ	20. Ⓐ Ⓑ Ⓒ Ⓓ	28. Ⓐ Ⓑ Ⓒ Ⓓ	36. Ⓐ Ⓑ Ⓒ Ⓓ
5. Ⓐ Ⓑ Ⓒ Ⓓ	13. Ⓐ Ⓑ Ⓒ Ⓓ	21. Ⓐ Ⓑ Ⓒ Ⓓ	29. Ⓐ Ⓑ Ⓒ Ⓓ	37. Ⓐ Ⓑ Ⓒ Ⓓ
6. Ⓐ Ⓑ Ⓒ Ⓓ	14. Ⓐ Ⓑ Ⓒ Ⓓ	22. Ⓐ Ⓑ Ⓒ Ⓓ	30. Ⓐ Ⓑ Ⓒ Ⓓ	38. Ⓐ Ⓑ Ⓒ Ⓓ
7. Ⓐ Ⓑ Ⓒ Ⓓ	15. Ⓐ Ⓑ Ⓒ Ⓓ	23. Ⓐ Ⓑ Ⓒ Ⓓ	31. Ⓐ Ⓑ Ⓒ Ⓓ	39. Ⓐ Ⓑ Ⓒ Ⓓ
8. Ⓐ Ⓑ Ⓒ Ⓓ	16. Ⓐ Ⓑ Ⓒ Ⓓ	24. Ⓐ Ⓑ Ⓒ Ⓓ	32. Ⓐ Ⓑ Ⓒ Ⓓ	40. Ⓐ Ⓑ Ⓒ Ⓓ

PART C
VERBAL ANALOGIES

1. Ⓐ Ⓑ Ⓒ Ⓓ   6. Ⓐ Ⓑ Ⓒ Ⓓ   11. Ⓐ Ⓑ Ⓒ Ⓓ   16. Ⓐ Ⓑ Ⓒ Ⓓ   21. Ⓐ Ⓑ Ⓒ Ⓓ

2. Ⓐ Ⓑ Ⓒ Ⓓ   7. Ⓐ Ⓑ Ⓒ Ⓓ   12. Ⓐ Ⓑ Ⓒ Ⓓ   17. Ⓐ Ⓑ Ⓒ Ⓓ   22. Ⓐ Ⓑ Ⓒ Ⓓ

3. Ⓐ Ⓑ Ⓒ Ⓓ   8. Ⓐ Ⓑ Ⓒ Ⓓ   13. Ⓐ Ⓑ Ⓒ Ⓓ   18. Ⓐ Ⓑ Ⓒ Ⓓ   23. Ⓐ Ⓑ Ⓒ Ⓓ

4. Ⓐ Ⓑ Ⓒ Ⓓ   9. Ⓐ Ⓑ Ⓒ Ⓓ   14. Ⓐ Ⓑ Ⓒ Ⓓ   19. Ⓐ Ⓑ Ⓒ Ⓓ   24. Ⓐ Ⓑ Ⓒ Ⓓ

5. Ⓐ Ⓑ Ⓒ Ⓓ   10. Ⓐ Ⓑ Ⓒ Ⓓ   15. Ⓐ Ⓑ Ⓒ Ⓓ   20. Ⓐ Ⓑ Ⓒ Ⓓ   25. Ⓐ Ⓑ Ⓒ Ⓓ

FINAL VERBAL ABILITY EXAMINATION

50 Minutes   100 Questions

Part A—Synonyms

35 Minutes   35 Questions

Directions: *In each of the sentences below, one word is in italics. Following each sentence are four words or phrases. For each sentence, select the word or phrase that best corresponds in meaning to the italicized word.*

1. It has been recommended that this system be used in place of the *traditional* type.

   (A) unfamiliar
   (B) usual
   (C) flexible
   (D) general

2. On many teams, a player may face a *penalty* for irresponsible or unruly behavior.

   (A) arrangement
   (B) gratification
   (C) punishment
   (D) precaution

3. He used the *allotted* study time to complete his assignments.

   (A) authorized
   (B) designated
   (C) agreed
   (D) alerted

4. The Senate passed the farmland *preservation* bill.

   (A) maintenance
   (B) strategem
   (C) exordium
   (D) incumbency

5. It was apparent that he had attempted to *concoct* an alibi.

   (A) inculcate
   (B) conceal
   (C) reveal
   (D) fabricate

6. The City Council could have avoided this *sanction* by passing the ordinance.

   (A) preliminary plan
   (B) obliteration
   (C) veneration
   (D) penalty

7. The superior court judge *imposed* the sentence.

   (A) indicated
   (B) granted
   (C) perpetuated
   (D) inflicted

8. The soldiers retreated to a position of *comparative* safety.

   (A) objective
   (B) relative
   (C) subjective
   (D) scientific

9. Geologists *assure* us that our earth is a few billion years old.

   (A) guarantee
   (B) instruct
   (C) deny
   (D) assail

10. It has been said that he is a *connoisseur* of fine wines.

   (A) expert on
   (B) taster of
   (C) procurer of
   (D) vendor of

11. He *spurned* the name that had won him this dishonor.

   (A) lauded
   (B) extolled
   (C) acclaimed
   (D) repudiated

12. The well-dressed gentleman bowed *ceremoniously*.

   (A) without ritual
   (B) disrespectfully
   (C) serenely
   (D) formally

13. *Instinctively* cautious

   (A) briskly
   (B) sullenly
   (C) automatically
   (D) swiftly

14. The annual parade *traversed* this magnificent city from the east to the west side.

   (A) was patronized
   (B) extended
   (C) crossed
   (D) augmented

15. *Enraptured* by the beauty of the mountains, they had not spoken for twenty minutes.

   (A) summoned
   (B) impeded
   (C) exonerated
   (D) entranced

16. The results of the experiment upheld the *contention* of those who supported the hypothesis.

   (A) realization
   (B) contiguity
   (C) argument
   (D) exhilaration

17. The *consensus* of the group

   (A) stipulation
   (B) regulation
   (C) conviction
   (D) collective opinion

18. If the members of the council were *directed* to analyze the data further, they were

   (A) requested
   (B) corrected
   (C) encouraged
   (D) instructed

19. Mayan magnificence *abounds* in the small resort village of Kailuum.

   (A) is remote
   (B) is abundant
   (C) is significant
   (D) is inadequate

20. If enthusiasm for the project *waxed* under the direction of a newly appointed administrator, the level of excitement

   (A) stirred
   (B) waned
   (C) vanished
   (D) increased

21. *Void* of intellectual stimuli

   (A) composed
   (B) in excess
   (C) empty
   (D) full

22. An *illusion* of space

   (A) apparition
   (B) vision
   (C) impression
   (D) dream

23. Security was *risked* to attain maximum career satisfaction.

   (A) ventured
   (B) squandered
   (C) exhausted
   (D) wasted

24. The fruit was *pared* and sliced for the salad.

   (A) divided
   (B) rinsed
   (C) peeled
   (D) sectioned

25. An extraordinary floral arrangement *accented* the table setting.

    (A) called attention to
    (B) embellished
    (C) beautified
    (D) made acceptable

26. The introduction *delineates* the book's content and format.

    (A) discredits
    (B) describes
    (C) sanctions
    (D) endorses

27. With the signing of the contract, the *transaction* was completed.

    (A) business proceeding
    (B) tribulation
    (C) redemption
    (D) obligation

28. The receptionist *confirmed* the appointment.

    (A) canceled
    (B) rescheduled
    (C) verified
    (D) recorded

29. *Provisions* were made for the immediate transport of supplies.

    (A) orders
    (B) arrangements
    (C) contracts
    (D) funds

30. If the engine was *malfunctioning* at the time, it was

    (A) operative
    (B) operating incorrectly
    (C) firing
    (D) igniting

31. The clients were shocked at the *fraudulent* practices of the contractors.

    (A) thorough
    (B) extensive
    (C) legal
    (D) deceitful

32. The employer questioned the *competence* of his staff. The employer was not sure about their

    (A) honesty
    (B) punctuality
    (C) credibility
    (D) ability

33. The reading list included an *anthology* by a famous author.

    (A) collection of literary selections
    (B) annotated bibliography
    (C) archaeological study
    (D) autobiography

34. We listened *intently* to the lecture.

    (A) with dismay
    (B) with doubt
    (C) with belief
    (D) with concentration

35. Smiled *wryly*

    (A) deceptively
    (B) nastily
    (C) ironically
    (D) delightedly

Part B—Antonyms

15 Minutes   40 Questions

Directions: *For each of the following test items, select the word that is opposite in meaning to the term printed in capital letters.*

1. IMPERIOUS

   (A) submissive
   (B) valuable
   (C) pointed
   (D) positive

2. CAPRICIOUS

   (A) whimsical
   (B) judicious
   (C) steadfast
   (D) tranquil

3. CANTANKEROUS

   (A) pleasant
   (B) dubious
   (C) effective
   (D) awkward

4. FORBEARANCE

   (A) indulgence
   (B) pliancy
   (C) politeness
   (D) impatience

5. HAPHAZARD

   (A) inefficient
   (B) premeditated
   (C) unsatisfactory
   (D) blundering

6. INEFFABLE

   (A) forgettable
   (B) exquisite
   (C) unorganized
   (D) race

7. CHIMERICAL

   (A) philosophical
   (B) elite
   (C) factual
   (D) unimpressive

8. REPRESS

   (A) reserve
   (B) liberate
   (C) thrust
   (D) precipitate

9. ABOMINABLE

   (A) agreeable
   (B) loathsome
   (C) sufficient
   (D) degrading

10. UNETHICAL

   (A) vulgar
   (B) feasible
   (C) pompous
   (D) scrupulous

11. ANTECEDENT

   (A) previous
   (B) subsequent
   (C) foregoing
   (D) propitious

12. PONDEROUS

   (A) delicate
   (B) potent
   (C) supportive
   (D) massive

13. SUPPLICATION

   (A) worship
   (B) compassion
   (C) entreaty
   (D) disdain

14. POSITIVE

   (A) negative
   (B) sensitive
   (C) diplomatic
   (D) popular

15. RENEGADE

    (A) constant
    (B) extricate
    (C) obedient
    (D) heretical

16. DISREGARD

    (A) disown
    (B) respond
    (C) revoke
    (D) recover

17. WRATH

    (A) delight
    (B) travail
    (C) frivolity
    (D) detriment

18. TEDIOUS

    (A) ungainly
    (B) imperative
    (C) stimulating
    (D) suitable

19. EMBODY

    (A) impel
    (B) fuse
    (C) dissociate
    (D) collect

20. DEFERRABLE

    (A) urgent
    (B) furtive
    (C) inclined
    (D) deniable

21. HOMOGENOUS

    (A) invariable
    (B) homosexual
    (C) importunate
    (D) heterogenous

22. ADHERENT

    (A) disciple
    (B) repudiator
    (C) soothsayer
    (D) hypocrite

23. CRUDE

    (A) barbarous
    (B) refined
    (C) obscure
    (D) covetous

24. DAFT

    (A) cynical
    (B) sharp
    (C) prevalent
    (D) sensible

25. GRAPHIC

    (A) vague
    (B) illustrative
    (C) forcible
    (D) glacial

26. DEVASTATE

    (A) tolerate
    (B) obstruct
    (C) renovate
    (D) promote

27. STRINGENT

    (A) exacting
    (B) tough
    (C) influential
    (D) flexible

28. ACQUIESCE

    (A) contest
    (B) invest
    (C) dismiss
    (D) supply

29. BREVITY

    (A) abbreviation
    (B) length
    (C) ramification
    (D) delusion

30. FLAUNT

    (A) disavow
    (B) conserve
    (C) blight
    (D) astonish

31. CULTIVATE

    (A) restore
    (B) stifle
    (C) reinstate
    (D) nurture

32. DILATE

    (A) negate
    (B) abet
    (C) constrict
    (D) suspend

33. BEFITTING

    (A) enhancing
    (B) conciliatory
    (C) inappropriate
    (D) elegant

34. COHERENT

    (A) illogical
    (B) consecutive
    (C) cognizant
    (D) courtly

35. PALTRY

    (A) political
    (B) complaisant
    (C) clever
    (D) impressive

36. BUCOLIC

    (A) urbane
    (B) gallant
    (C) valiant
    (D) functional

37. EXTRAVAGANT

    (A) coarse
    (B) superior
    (C) frugal
    (D) typical

38. LENIENCY

    (A) indulgence
    (B) severity
    (C) embroilment
    (D) inequality

39. MANIFEST

    (A) latent
    (B) oblivious
    (C) terminal
    (D) languid

40. PLEBEIAN

    (A) congenial
    (B) ignoble
    (C) scientific
    (D) patrician

Part C—Verbal Analogies

10 Minutes   25 Questions

Directions: *In the following questions you are to determine the relationship between the first pair of capitalized words and then decide which of the answer choices shares a similar relationship with the third capitalized word.*

1. CAT is to DOG as TIGER is to

    (A) wild
    (B) fur
    (C) wolf
    (D) bovine

2. SALINE is to SALT as SWEET is to

    (A) sugar
    (B) stale
    (C) bread
    (D) insipid

3. FLANNEL is to WOOL as LINEN is to

(A) cotton
(B) flax
(C) silk
(D) rayon

4. CONTEMPORARY is to PRESENT as POSTERITY is to

(A) past
(B) present
(C) future
(D) ancient

5. MOON is to EARTH as EARTH is to

(A) space
(B) moon
(C) sky
(D) sun

6. ACUTE is to CHRONIC as INTENSE is to

(A) sardonic
(B) tonic
(C) persistent
(D) pretty

7. VALLEY is to GORGE as MOUNTAIN is to

(A) freshet
(B) cliff
(C) steep
(D) high

8. EAST is to WEST as NORTHWEST is to

(A) southeast
(B) southwest
(C) north
(D) northeast

9. GASOLINE is to PETROLEUM as SUGAR is to

(A) oil
(B) cane
(C) plant
(D) sweet

10. AGGRAVATE is to TEASE as FONDLE is to

(A) vex
(B) wound
(C) embrace
(D) pursuit

11. LATITUDE is to LONGITUDE as WARP is to

(A) weave
(B) woof
(C) thread
(D) line

12. EDGE is to CENTER as EFFUSIVE is to

(A) unemotional
(B) exuberant
(C) eclectic
(D) eccentricity

13. DISCIPLE is to MENTOR as PROSELYTE is to

(A) opinion
(B) expedition
(C) leader
(D) football

14. SOPHISTICATION is to FINESSE as INEPTITUDE is to

(A) inefficiency
(B) artistry
(C) trickiness
(D) insatiability

15. CAPTAIN is to STEAMSHIP as PRINCIPAL is to

(A) interest
(B) school
(C) agent
(D) concern

16. DIME is to SILVER as PENNY is to

(A) mint
(B) copper
(C) currency
(D) value

17. REVERT is to REVERSION as SYMPA-THIZE is to

    (A) sympathetic
    (B) symposium
    (C) sympathy
    (D) sympathizer

18. REGRESSIVE is to REGRESS as STER-ILE is to

    (A) sterilization
    (B) sterilize
    (C) sterility
    (D) sterilizer

19. DOWN is to UP as AGE is to

    (A) year
    (B) youth
    (C) snow
    (D) date

20. I is to MINE as MAN is to

    (A) men
    (B) his
    (C) man's
    (D) mine

21. DISLOYAL is to FAITHLESS as IMPERFECTION is to

    (A) faithful
    (B) depression
    (C) foible
    (D) decrepitude

22. NECKLACE is to PEARLS as CHAIN is to

    (A) locket
    (B) prisoner
    (C) links
    (D) clasp

23. DRIFT is to SNOW as DUNE is to

    (A) hill
    (B) rain
    (C) sand
    (D) hail

24. DILIGENT is to UNREMITTING as COMPLETE is to

    (A) pretentious
    (B) diametric
    (C) adamant
    (D) dietetic

25. SCHOONER is to VESSEL as PERSIM-MON is to

    (A) machine
    (B) fruit
    (C) engine
    (D) vehicle

Answer Key

PART A

1. **B**	8. **B**	15. **D**	22. **C**	29. **B**
2. **C**	9. **A**	16. **C**	23. **A**	30. **B**
3. **B**	10. **A**	17. **D**	24. **C**	31. **D**
4. **A**	11. **D**	18. **D**	25. **A**	32. **D**
5. **D**	12. **D**	19. **B**	26. **B**	33. **A**
6. **D**	13. **C**	20. **D**	27. **A**	34. **D**
7. **D**	14. **C**	21. **C**	28. **C**	35. **C**

PART B

1. **A**	9. **A**	17. **A**	25. **A**	33. **C**
2. **C**	10. **D**	18. **C**	26. **C**	34. **A**
3. **A**	11. **B**	19. **C**	27. **D**	35. **D**
4. **D**	12. **A**	20. **A**	28. **A**	36. **A**
5. **B**	13. **D**	21. **D**	29. **B**	37. **C**
6. **A**	14. **A**	22. **B**	30. **A**	38. **B**
7. **C**	15. **C**	23. **B**	31. **B**	39. **A**
8. **B**	16. **B**	24. **D**	32. **C**	40. **D**

PART C

1. **C**	6. **C**	11. **B**	16. **B**	21. **C**
2. **A**	7. **B**	12. **A**	17. **C**	22. **C**
3. **B**	8. **A**	13. **C**	18. **B**	23. **C**
4. **C**	9. **B**	14. **A**	19. **B**	24. **B**
5. **D**	10. **C**	15. **B**	20. **C**	25. **B**

UNIT II   MATHEMATICS

MATHEMATICS REVIEW

The review of mathematics in this section and the numerical ability tests include the following: basic quantitative problems involving addition, subtraction, multiplication, and division; calculations including decimals, fractions, percentages, and measurements; basic operations in algebra and geometry; and quantitative comparison question-types. Throughout the exercises, emphasis is placed on verbal problems in order to prepare you for the interpretations and methods required for problem-solving. The explanatory answers and problem solutions provide a variety of opportunities to review or to learn the numerical processes included on the prenursing examinations.

    Study the guidelines listed below, which provide the major mathematics concepts needed for successful performance on your examination.

Guidelines for Mathematical Calculations

1. **Whole numbers** have place-value based on units of ten (decimal system). Therefore, it is extremely important that all whole numbers, including zeros, are lined up correctly in columns when adding and subtracting.

2. The **average** of a set of given numbers is the sum of the given numbers divided by the number of given numbers.

   Example:

   The average of the numbers 10, 14, 17, and 23 is

   $$\frac{10 + 14 + 17 + 23}{4} = 16$$

3. Use division to determine the value of one quantity when the value of several quantities is given. (All quantities have the same value).

   Example:

   Three loaves of bread cost $2.40. How much will one loaf cost?

   Divide 3 into $2.40; the answer is 80 cents.

4. Use multiplication to determine the value of several quantities with the same value if the value of one quantity is given.

Example:

If one loaf of bread costs 80 cents, how much will three loaves cost? Multiply 3 times 80 cents; the answer is $2.40.

5. The **square** of a number is the product obtained when a number is multiplied by itself.

Example:

$4^2 = 4 \times 4 = 16$

6. The **square root** $(\sqrt{})$ of a given number is the number that yields the given number when multiplied by itself.

Example:

$\sqrt{16} = 4$, since $4 \times 4 = 16$

7. The square of any whole number is called a **perfect square**. Conversely, the square root of a perfect square is a whole number.

Example:

$4^2 = 16$ (a perfect square); thus $\sqrt{16} = 4$.

8. If a number is not a perfect square, you can approximate the square root of the number when a calculator is not available. One method of approximating the square root of a number is given below.

Example:

Approximate the square root of 90 $(\sqrt{90})$.

1. Estimate the square root of the given number. Since 90 is between 81 and 100, the square root of 90 will be between 9 and 10. A possible estimate is 9.30.

2. Divide the given number by the estimated square root.

$90 \div 9.30 = 9.68$

3. Find the average of the resulting quotient and the estimated square root.

$\dfrac{9.68 + 9.30}{2} = 9.49$ (9.49 is the first approximation for $\sqrt{90}$.)

4. Divide the given number by the average (first approximation) found above.

$90 \div 9.49 = 9.48$

5. Find the average of the divisor (first approximation) and the quotient found in step 4.

$\dfrac{9.49 + 9.48}{2} = 9.485$

The approximate square root of 90 is 9.485.

6. This process may be repeated to get a more accurate estimate of the square root of a number.

9. To add or subtract **radicals** (numbers expressed as square roots), the **radicands** (numbers under the radical) must be the same.

Example:

$$4\sqrt{12} + 3\sqrt{12} = 7\sqrt{12}$$

If the radicands are *not* the same, simplify the radicals and then see if they can be combined.

Example:

$$
\begin{aligned}
&3\sqrt{12} - 8\sqrt{3} \\
&= 3\sqrt{4 \times 3} - 8\sqrt{3} &&(\text{12 can be factored as } 4 \times 3.) \\
&= 3 \times 2\sqrt{3} - 8\sqrt{3} &&(\text{Take } \sqrt{4}, \text{ which equals 2.}) \\
&= 6\sqrt{3} - 8\sqrt{3} \\
&= -2\sqrt{3}
\end{aligned}
$$

10. To reduce fractions to lowest terms, factor the numerator and denominator and cancel the common factors.

Example:

$$\frac{35}{55} = \frac{7 \times 5}{11 \times 5} = \frac{7}{11}$$

11. When subtracting decimals, make sure both numbers have the same number of decimal places. If they don't, add zeros to the number with fewer decimal places until it has the same number of decimal places as the other number.

Example:

Subtract 2.715 from 4.

Note: When adding and subtracting decimals, the numbers should be lined up so decimals are under each other.

$$
\begin{array}{r}
4.000 \\
-2.715 \\
\hline
1.285
\end{array}
$$

12. When multiplying, be certain to include all zeros and keep the columns in line.

Example:

$$
\begin{array}{r}
3600 \\
\times \quad 507 \\
\hline
25200 \\
0000 \\
18000 \\
\hline
1,825,200
\end{array}
$$

13. When a decimal is changed to a fraction, the digits after the decimal point become the numerator. The denominator is 1 and as many zeros as there are decimal places. (The denominator can also be determined by raising 10 to a power. The power is the number of decimal places in the number.)

Example:

$$0.540 = \frac{540}{1000}$$ (Note that $1,000 = 10^3$. There are 3 decimal places in the number so the power is 3.)

14. A **polygon** is a simple closed plane figure made up of line segments.

a. Polygons with three sides are called **triangles**.

If the lengths of two sides of a triangle are equal, the triangle is called an **isosceles** triangle.

When all three sides of a triangle have the same length, the triangle is called an **equilateral** triangle.

b. Polygons with four sides are called **quadrilaterals**.

A **square** is a quadrilateral with all four sides equal.

A **rectangle** is a quadrilateral with opposite sides equal.

c. To find the **perimeter** (*P*) of a figure, add the lengths of all its sides.

Triangle P = sum of the three sides $\boldsymbol{P = a + b + c}$
Rectangle $P = 2 \times$ Length $+ 2 \times$ Width $\boldsymbol{P = 2L + 2W}$
Square $\boldsymbol{P = 4 \times S}$, where S = length of each side.
Circle   The circumference (*C*) is the distance around a circle.

The circumference of a circle is equal to $\pi \times$ the diameter: $\boldsymbol{C = \pi \times d}$.

Point O is the center of the given circle. Points P, R, and S are points on the circle.

A **chord** of a circle is any segment with its two end points on the circle. $\overline{MN}$ is a chord of the given circle.

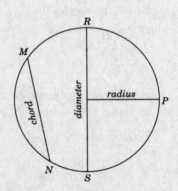

A **radius** of a circle is a segment from the center of the circle to any point on the circle. $\overline{OP}$ is a radius of the circle.

A **diameter** of a circle is a chord that passes through the center of a circle. $\overline{RS}$ is a diameter of the given circle.

All radii of a circle have the same length. A diameter of a given circle is always twice the radius of the circle.

Example: If the length of radius $\overline{OP}$ = 7 cm, the diameter $\overline{RS}$ = 14 cm.

15. a. To find the **area** (A) of plane figures:

Square $\qquad A = (\text{side})^2 \qquad \boldsymbol{A = S^2}$

Rectangle $\qquad A = \text{Base} \times \text{Height, or} \qquad \boldsymbol{A = L \times W}$

Triangle $\qquad A = \frac{1}{2}\,\text{Base} \times \text{Height, or} \quad \boldsymbol{A = \frac{1}{2}\,bh}$

Circle $\qquad A = \pi \times (\text{radius})^2, \text{ or} \qquad \boldsymbol{A = \pi\,r^2}$

b. The **areas of other polygons** may be found by dividing the polygon into nonoverlapping triangles and/or quadrilaterals (squares, rectangles) and then adding the areas of the triangles and quadrilaterals.

Nonoverlapping triangles and quadrilaterals may be obtained by drawing diagonals of the polygon. A **diagonal** of a polygon is a line segment joining two nonconsecutive vertices of a polygon. $\overline{BE}$ is a diagonal of polygon ABCDE.

Example: Given polygon ABCDE with the measurements indicated, draw diagonal $\overline{BE}$ to divide the polygon into a triangle, △BAE, and a rectangle, BEDC.

Area of △BAE = 1/2 × 10 × 4 = 20 sq in.

Area of ☐BEDC = 2 × 10 = 20 sq in.

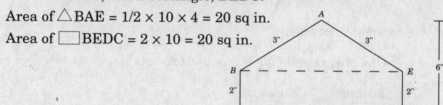

Since 20 + 20 = 40, the area of polygon ABCDE = 40 sq in.

16. **Similar triangles** have the same shape. The angles of one similar triangle are equal to the angles of the other. The ratios of corresponding sides of similar triangles are equal.

Example: The two given triangles are similar (measures of corresponding angles are equal).

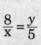
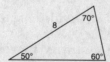
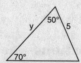

$\dfrac{8}{x} = \dfrac{y}{5}$

17. A right triangle is a triangle with a right angle. The side of the triangle that is opposite the right angle is called the **hypotenuse**.

Pythagorean Theorem: The square of the hypotenuse of a triangle is equal to the sum of the squares of the other two sides.

$$c^2 = a^2 + b^2$$

Example: Find the hypotenuse of the right triangle given below:

The two sides of the triange are 5 and 12. The hypotenuse (c) can be found with the use of the Pythagorean theorem.

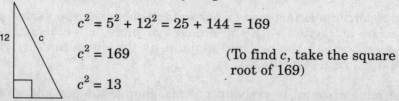

$c^2 = 5^2 + 12^2 = 25 + 144 = 169$

$c^2 = 169 \qquad\qquad$ (To find c, take the square root of 169)

$c^2 = 13$

18. **Parallel** lines are two lines that do not intersect (have no points in common). The slopes of two parallel lines are equal.

    Perpendicular lines are two lines that intersect at right angles. The slopes of two perpendicular lines have a product of –1.

19. A **ratio** is the comparison of two numerical quantities by division.

    Example   A box contains 3 red balls and 2 blue balls. The ratio of blue to red balls in the box is 2 to 3 or 2/3.

20. A **proportion** is a statement that two ratios are equivalent.

    Example   The ratio of 4 to x is equivalent to the ratio of 5 to 10.
    $$\frac{4}{x} = \frac{5}{10}$$

    a. **Direct proportions**—One quantity increases ($\uparrow$) or decreases ($\downarrow$) as the other increases or decreases. In other words, the direction of the changes is the same for both factors. (x increases as y increases or x decreases as y decreases.)

    Example: (Increase:)

    One orange sells for 15 cents. How much will six oranges cost?

    $$\frac{1 \text{ orange}}{15\cent} = \frac{6 \text{ oranges}}{y\cent}$$

    Cross multiply: $1y = 6 \times 15$ $y = 90\cent$

    Example: (Decrease:)

    Six oranges cost 90 cents. How much would one orange cost?

    $$\frac{6 \text{ oranges}}{90\cent} = \frac{1 \text{ orange}}{y\cent}$$

    Cross multiply: $6y = 90\cent$ $y = 15\cent$ (Divide both sides by 6.)

    b. **Inverse proportions**—As one quantity increases ($\uparrow$), another quantity decreases ($\downarrow$), and vice versa. In other words, the direction of the changes is opposite. As x increases y decreases; or as x decreases, y increases.

    Example: A 5-pound bag of dog food lasts one week when the dog is given 2 servings per day. How long would this bag last if the dog were to receive 3 servings per day?
    $$\frac{3}{2} = \frac{7}{y} \quad 3y = 14 \quad y = 4.6$$

    (As the number of meals increases, the number of days the dog food lasts decreases).

21. To find a percentage increase or percentage decrease in a verbal problem, write a fraction with the amount of increase or decrease as the numerator and the original amount as the denominator. Then change fraction to percentage.

22. To determine discount in verbal problems, change the percentage to a fraction or decimal, multiply by the original cost, and deduct this amount from the original cost.

23. For verbal problems dealing with commission and taxes, multiply the total value of the goods or services by the percentage of tax or commission.

24. For **operations with signed numbers** (+ or –):

    Addition

    • For numbers with the same sign, add and keep the same sign in the answer.

    • For numbers with different signs, subtract and give the answer the sign of the higher number.

    Subtraction

    • Combine the two signs of the bottom number (taking the subtraction sign as a negative sign, [– and – = +] [– and + = –]. Then use the rules for addition.

    Examples:
    $$-4 - (-2) = -4 + 2 = -2$$
    $$-4 - (+2) = -4 - 2 = -6$$

    Multiplication

    • The product of an odd number of negative numbers is negative.

    • The product of an even number of negative numbers is positive.

    Examples:
    $$(-3)(-2)(-5) = -30$$
    $$(-4)(-2)(-3)(-5) = 90$$

    Division

    • If the two numbers have the same sign, the answer is positive; if otherwise, it is negative.

25. For **literal expressions** (problems with letters instead of numbers) use the same processes as you would for numbers.

    Example: How many inches are in x yards and x feet?

    $$y \text{ yd.} \times \frac{36 \text{ in.}}{\text{yd.}} = 36y \text{ in.} \quad x \text{ ft.} \times \frac{12 \text{ in.}}{\text{ft.}} = 12x \text{ in.}$$

26. Problems involving **metric** measurements (other than conversions within the metric system) are solved using the same techniques as problems with English measurement units.

    The basic metric units of measure are:

    Length–Meter   Weight–Gram
    Volume–Liter   Temperature–Celsius

27. A **prime number** is any whole number other than 0 or 1 that is only divisible by itself and 1.

    Example: 17 is a prime number since it is only divisible by 1 and 17.

28. The symbols < and > are used to represent the inequalities "less than" and "greater than." Various statements of inequality are expressed by the following:

    a. $a < b$ means a is less than b.
        $7 < 12$ 7 is less than 12.

    b. $a \leq b$ means a is either less than or equal to b.
        $5 \leq 9$ 5 is less than or equal to 9.

    c. $a > b$ means a is greater than b.
          18 > 14   18 is greater than 14.

    d. $a \geq b$ means a is either greater than or equal to b.
          $3 \geq 3$ 3 is greater than or equal to 3.

    e. $a < b \leq c$ means a is less than b and b is less than or equal to c.
          $-1 < 3 \leq 5$ -1 is less than 3 and 3 is less than or equal to 5.
          $2 \leq x < 5$ x is a number that is greater than or equal to 2 and is less than 5.

29. Units of measurement for angles are called **degrees**.
An **acute angle** has a measure that is less than 90°.
A **right angle** has a measure of exactly 90°.
    (Perpendicular lines form right angles.)
An **obtuse angle** has a measure that is greater than 90°.
Two angles are **complementary** if the sum of their measures is 90°.
Two angles are **supplementary** if the sum of their measure is 180°.
If the exterior sides of a pair of adjacent angles form a straight line, the two adjacent angles are supplementary.

Examples: If $\overrightarrow{AB} \perp \overleftrightarrow{DC}$ ($\overrightarrow{AB}$ is perpendicular to $\overleftrightarrow{DC}$), then

∠ABF and ∠FBC are complementary angles.
(∠ABF and ∠FBC = 90°)

∠EBD and ∠EBC are supplementary angles.
(∠EBD and ∠EBC = 180°)

∠FBC is an acute angle.

30. The sum of the measures of the three angles of a triangle is 180°. If the measures of two angles of a triangle are given, the measure of the third angle can be found by subtracting the sum of the measures of the two known angles from 180°.

Example: If ∠A = 40° and ∠B = 60°, then ∠C

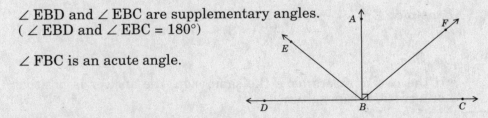

= 180° − (∠A + ∠B)
= 180° − (40° + 60°)
= 180° − 100°
= 80°

31. The total degree measure of a circle is 360°.

    a. A **central angle** of a circle is an angle whose vertex is the center of the circle. If a central angle represents $1/n$ of a circle, the measure of the central angle is $1/n \times 360°$.

        Angle ∠AOB is a central angle in the circle below.

    b. A **minor arc** of a circle consists of two points A and B where the sides of a central angle intersect the circle plus all points of the circle that lie in the interior of the central angle.

        The minor arc $\overarc{AB}$ is indicated in the given circle.

    c. A **major arc** of a circle consists of points A and B and all points on the circle that lie in the exterior of the central angle.

        The major arc $\overarc{AB}$ is indicated in the circle below.

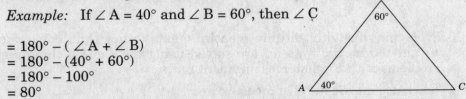

d. An **inscribed angle** of a circle is an angle whose vertex is on the circle and whose rays intersect the circle in two points different from the vertex. The measure of an inscribed angle equals one-half the measure of its intercepted arc.

∠ ACB is an inscribed angle of the given circle. The measure of ∠ ACB is one-half the measure of the central angle, ∠ AOB.

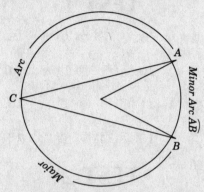

32. **Defined functions**. Certain questions may include a special sign such as "*" or "#" that is defined for you. The sign tells you to perform a specific function or operation. This kind of problem tests your ability to learn and apply a new concept.

Example: For all numbers, $a * b = \dfrac{a}{b} + 2$. What is $6 * 3$?

$$6 * 3 = \frac{6}{3} + 2$$
$$= 2 + 2$$
$$= 4$$

Answer Sheet
Mathematics

TEST 1

1. Ⓐ Ⓑ Ⓒ Ⓓ   5. Ⓐ Ⓑ Ⓒ Ⓓ   9. Ⓐ Ⓑ Ⓒ Ⓓ   13. Ⓐ Ⓑ Ⓒ Ⓓ   17. Ⓐ Ⓑ Ⓒ Ⓓ

2. Ⓐ Ⓑ Ⓒ Ⓓ   6. Ⓐ Ⓑ Ⓒ Ⓓ   10. Ⓐ Ⓑ Ⓒ Ⓓ   14. Ⓐ Ⓑ Ⓒ Ⓓ   18. Ⓐ Ⓑ Ⓒ Ⓓ

3. Ⓐ Ⓑ Ⓒ Ⓓ   7. Ⓐ Ⓑ Ⓒ Ⓓ   11. Ⓐ Ⓑ Ⓒ Ⓓ   15. Ⓐ Ⓑ Ⓒ Ⓓ   19. Ⓐ Ⓑ Ⓒ Ⓓ

4. Ⓐ Ⓑ Ⓒ Ⓓ   8. Ⓐ Ⓑ Ⓒ Ⓓ   12. Ⓐ Ⓑ Ⓒ Ⓓ   16. Ⓐ Ⓑ Ⓒ Ⓓ   20. Ⓐ Ⓑ Ⓒ Ⓓ

TEST 2

1. Ⓐ Ⓑ Ⓒ Ⓓ   5. Ⓐ Ⓑ Ⓒ Ⓓ   9. Ⓐ Ⓑ Ⓒ Ⓓ   13. Ⓐ Ⓑ Ⓒ Ⓓ   17. Ⓐ Ⓑ Ⓒ Ⓓ

2. Ⓐ Ⓑ Ⓒ Ⓓ   6. Ⓐ Ⓑ Ⓒ Ⓓ   10. Ⓐ Ⓑ Ⓒ Ⓓ   14. Ⓐ Ⓑ Ⓒ Ⓓ   18. Ⓐ Ⓑ Ⓒ Ⓓ

3. Ⓐ Ⓑ Ⓒ Ⓓ   7. Ⓐ Ⓑ Ⓒ Ⓓ   11. Ⓐ Ⓑ Ⓒ Ⓓ   15. Ⓐ Ⓑ Ⓒ Ⓓ   19. Ⓐ Ⓑ Ⓒ Ⓓ

4. Ⓐ Ⓑ Ⓒ Ⓓ   8. Ⓐ Ⓑ Ⓒ Ⓓ   12. Ⓐ Ⓑ Ⓒ Ⓓ   16. Ⓐ Ⓑ Ⓒ Ⓓ   20. Ⓐ Ⓑ Ⓒ Ⓓ

TEST 3

1. Ⓐ Ⓑ Ⓒ Ⓓ   5. Ⓐ Ⓑ Ⓒ Ⓓ   9. Ⓐ Ⓑ Ⓒ Ⓓ   13. Ⓐ Ⓑ Ⓒ Ⓓ   17. Ⓐ Ⓑ Ⓒ Ⓓ

2. Ⓐ Ⓑ Ⓒ Ⓓ   6. Ⓐ Ⓑ Ⓒ Ⓓ   10. Ⓐ Ⓑ Ⓒ Ⓓ   14. Ⓐ Ⓑ Ⓒ Ⓓ   18. Ⓐ Ⓑ Ⓒ Ⓓ

3. Ⓐ Ⓑ Ⓒ Ⓓ   7. Ⓐ Ⓑ Ⓒ Ⓓ   11. Ⓐ Ⓑ Ⓒ Ⓓ   15. Ⓐ Ⓑ Ⓒ Ⓓ   19. Ⓐ Ⓑ Ⓒ Ⓓ

4. Ⓐ Ⓑ Ⓒ Ⓓ   8. Ⓐ Ⓑ Ⓒ Ⓓ   12. Ⓐ Ⓑ Ⓒ Ⓓ   16. Ⓐ Ⓑ Ⓒ Ⓓ   20. Ⓐ Ⓑ Ⓒ Ⓓ

TEST 4

1. Ⓐ Ⓑ Ⓒ Ⓓ   8. Ⓐ Ⓑ Ⓒ Ⓓ   14. Ⓐ Ⓑ Ⓒ Ⓓ   20. Ⓐ Ⓑ Ⓒ Ⓓ   26. Ⓐ Ⓑ Ⓒ Ⓓ

2. Ⓐ Ⓑ Ⓒ Ⓓ   9. Ⓐ Ⓑ Ⓒ Ⓓ   15. Ⓐ Ⓑ Ⓒ Ⓓ   21. Ⓐ Ⓑ Ⓒ Ⓓ   27. Ⓐ Ⓑ Ⓒ Ⓓ

3. Ⓐ Ⓑ Ⓒ Ⓓ   10. Ⓐ Ⓑ Ⓒ Ⓓ   16. Ⓐ Ⓑ Ⓒ Ⓓ   22. Ⓐ Ⓑ Ⓒ Ⓓ   28. Ⓐ Ⓑ Ⓒ Ⓓ

4. Ⓐ Ⓑ Ⓒ Ⓓ   11. Ⓐ Ⓑ Ⓒ Ⓓ   17. Ⓐ Ⓑ Ⓒ Ⓓ   23. Ⓐ Ⓑ Ⓒ Ⓓ   29. Ⓐ Ⓑ Ⓒ Ⓓ

5. Ⓐ Ⓑ Ⓒ Ⓓ   12. Ⓐ Ⓑ Ⓒ Ⓓ   18. Ⓐ Ⓑ Ⓒ Ⓓ   24. Ⓐ Ⓑ Ⓒ Ⓓ   30. Ⓐ Ⓑ Ⓒ Ⓓ

6. Ⓐ Ⓑ Ⓒ Ⓓ   13. Ⓐ Ⓑ Ⓒ Ⓓ   19. Ⓐ Ⓑ Ⓒ Ⓓ   25. Ⓐ Ⓑ Ⓒ Ⓓ   31. Ⓐ Ⓑ Ⓒ Ⓓ

7. Ⓐ Ⓑ Ⓒ Ⓓ

MATHEMATICS TEST 1

15 Minutes   20 Questions

Directions: *Each problem in this test involves a certain amount of logical reasoning and thinking on your part, besides simple computations, to help you find the solution. Read each problem carefully and choose the correct answer from the four choices that follow. Blacken the corresponding space on your answer sheet.*

1. Find the interest on $25,800 for 144 days at six percent per annum. Base your calculations on a 360-day year.

   (A) $619.20
   (B) $619.02
   (C) $691.02
   (D) $691.20

2. Arthur can shovel snow from a sidewalk in 60 minutes and Jack can do it in 30 minutes. How many minutes will it take them to do the job together?

   (A) 90
   (B) 15
   (C) 30
   (D) 20

3. The visitors' section of a courtroom seats 105 people. The court is in session six hours per day. On one particular day, 485 people visited the court and were given seats. What is the average length of time spent by each visitor in the court? Assume that as soon as a person leaves his seat it is immediately filled and that at no time during the day is one of the 105 seats vacant. Express your answer in hours and minutes.

   (A) 1 hour 20 minutes
   (B) 1 hour 18 minutes
   (C) 1 hour 30 minutes
   (D) 2 hours

4. If copy paper costs $14.50 per ream and a five percent discount is allowed for cash, how many reams can be purchased for $690 cash? Do not round off cents in your calculations.

   (A) 49 reams
   (B) 60 reams
   (C) 50 reams
   (D) 53 reams

5. How many hours are there between 8:30 A.M. today and 3:15 A.M. tomorrow?

   (A) $17\frac{3}{4}$ hours
   (B) $18\frac{3}{4}$ hours
   (C) $18\frac{2}{3}$ hours
   (D) $18\frac{1}{2}$ hours

6. How many days are there from September 19 to December 25 (*inclusive*)?

   (A) 98 days
   (B) 96 days
   (C) 89 days
   (D) 90 days

7. A clerk is requested to file 800 cards. If he can file cards at the rate of 80 cards an hour, the number of cards remaining to be filed after seven hours of work is

   (A) 40
   (B) 240
   (C) 140
   (D) 260

8. If your monthly electricity bill increases from $80 to $90, the percentage of increase is, most nearly,

   (A) 10 percent
   (B) $11\frac{1}{9}$ percent
   (C) $12\frac{1}{2}$ percent
   (D) $14\frac{1}{7}$ percent

9. If there are 245 sections in a city containing five boroughs, the average number of sections for each of the five boroughs is

(A) 50 sections
(B) 49 sections
(C) 47 sections
(D) 59 sections

10. If, in that same city, a section has 45 miles of street to plow after a snowstorm and nine plows are used, each plow will cover an average of how many miles?

(A) 7 miles
(B) 6 miles
(C) 8 miles
(D) 5 miles

11. If a crosswalk plow engine is run five minutes a day for ten days in a given month, how long will it run in the course of this month?

(A) 50 minutes
(B) $1\frac{1}{2}$ hours
(C) 1 hour
(D) 30 minutes

12. If the department uses 1500 men in manual street cleaning and half as many more to load and drive trucks, the total number of men used is

(A) 2200
(B) 2520
(C) 2050
(D) 2250

13. If an inspector issued 182 summonses in the course of seven hours, his hourly average of summonses issued was

(A) 23 summonses
(B) 26 summonses
(C) 25 summonses
(D) 28 summonses

14. If, of 186 summonses issued, 100 were issued to first offenders, then there were how many summonses issued to other than first offenders?

(A) 68
(B) 90
(C) 86
(D) 108

15. A truck going at a rate of 40 miles an hour will reach a town 80 miles away in how many hours?

(A) 1 hour
(B) 3 hours
(C) 2 hours
(D) 4 hours

16. If a barrel has a capacity of 100 gallons, how many gallons will it contain when it is two-fifths full?

(A) 20 gallons
(B) 60 gallons
(C) 40 gallons
(D) 80 gallons

17. If a monthly salary of $3000 is subject to a 20 percent tax, the net salary is

(A) $2000
(B) $2400
(C) $2500
(D) $2600

18. If $1000 is the cost of repairing 100 square yards of pavement, the cost of repairing one square yard is

(A) $10
(B) $150
(C) $100
(D) $300

19. If a woman's base pay is $3000 per month, and it is increased by a monthly bonus of $350 and a seniority increment of $250 this month, her total salary for the month is

(A) $3600
(B) $3500
(C) $3000
(D) $3700

20. If an annual salary of $21,600 is increased by a bonus of $7200 and by a service increment of $1200, the total pay rate is

(A) $29,600
(B) $39,600
(C) $26,900
(D) $30,000

Answer Key

1.	A	11.	A
2.	D	12.	D
3.	B	13.	B
4.	C	14.	C
5.	B	15.	C
6.	A	16.	C
7.	B	17.	B
8.	C	18.	A
9.	B	19.	A
10.	D	20.	D

Explanatory Answers

1. **(A)** *Interest = Principal × Rate × Time*

   Note: 6% = 0.06

   144 days = $\dfrac{144}{360}$ year

   $$I = P \times R \times T$$
   $$= \$25{,}800 \times 0.06 \times \frac{144}{360}$$
   $$= \frac{\$222{,}912}{360}$$
   $$= \$619.20$$

2. **(D)** Let n = number of minutes in which they can do the job together. Arthur can do $\frac{1}{60}$ of the job in one minute, so in n minutes he can do $\frac{n}{60}$ of the job. Jack can do $\frac{1}{30}$ of the job in one minute and $\frac{n}{30}$ of the job in n minutes. Together, in n minutes they can do the complete job.

   $\dfrac{n}{60} + \dfrac{n}{30} = 1$

   $n + 2n = 60$ multiplying both sides by 60 (the lowest common denominator)

   $3n = 60$ combine like terms

   $n = 20$ divide by 3

   They can do the job together in 20 minutes.

3. **(B)** Total seats = 105
   Total time = 6 hours
   Total people involved = 486.

   105 seats × 6 hours = 630 seating hours

   To find the average seating time, divide

   630 ÷ 485 = 1.3 hours

   Now change the 0.3 hours to minutes (1 hour = 60 minutes).

   $0.3 \cancel{\text{hour}} \times \dfrac{60 \text{ minutes}}{1 \cancel{\text{hour}}}$

   = 18 minutes

   The amount is 1 hour 18 minutes.

4. **(C)** Paper per ream = $14.50
   Discount = 5% or 0.05
   Total cash = $690.00

   First, find the discount on the paper per ream when paying cash.

   $14.50 × 0.05 = 0.725 cents

   Our price per ream is $14.50 − 0.725 = $13.775. Given $690 to spend, divide to find how much paper can be purchased.

   $690.00 ÷ $13.775/ream = 50

   50 reams for $688.75

5. **(B)** Use simple logic on this problem.

From	To	
8:30 A.M. →	8:30 P.M. =	12 hours
8:30 P.M. →	3:30 A.M. =	7 hours
	Total =	19 hours

   But this is 15 minutes too much.

   Note: Change one of the hours to minutes—1 hour = 60 minutes.

   45 minutes = $\frac{45}{60}$ hours or $\frac{3}{4}$ hours.

   18 hours 60 minutes
   −   15 minutes
   ―――――――――――――
   18 hours 45 minutes

   $18\frac{3}{4}$ is the total number of hours.

6. **(A)** Again, use logic.

Month	Number of days/month	
September	from 19 to 30	12 days
October	31 days	31 days
November	30 days	30 days
December	from 1 to 25	25 days
		98 days

   Note: Remember that 19 September and 25 December are included.

   Total = 98 days inclusive

7. **(B)** Total to be filed = 800 cards
   Rate cards can be filed = 80 cards per hour

   How many cards were filed in the first seven hours?

$7 \times 80 = 560$ cards were filed.

Subtract to find the remaining cards to be filed.

$800 - 560 = 240$

240 cards remain unfiled.

8. **(C)** From \$80 to \$90 there is a \$10 increase; the percentage of increase is found by dividing the amount of increase by the original amount:

$10 \div 80 = 0.125$ or $12\frac{1}{2}\%$

Note: $0.125 = 12.5\%$ or $12\frac{1}{2}\%$

Percentage of increase $= 12\frac{1}{2}\%$

9. **(B)** To find the *average* number of sections per borough, divide:

245 sections $\div$ 5 boroughs $= 49$

49 sections/borough

10. **(D)** Total miles $\quad = 45$
Number of plows $= 9$

To find the *average* number of miles, divide:

45 miles $\div$ 9 plows $= 5$ miles/plow.

Average $= 5$ miles

11. **(A)** Total time per day $\quad = 5$ minutes
Total days per month $= 10$ days
Total time per month $=$

$5 \dfrac{\text{minutes}}{\cancel{\text{day}}} \times 10 \dfrac{\cancel{\text{days}}}{\text{month}} = 50$

50 minutes/month

12. **(D)** Total number
for street cleaning $\qquad = \quad 1500$
Half that number
load and drive $\qquad = \quad +\ \underline{750}$
$\qquad\qquad\qquad\qquad\qquad\qquad 2250$

2250 men used

13. **(B)** Total summonses in seven hours $=$ 182

To find the *average* number of summonses per hour, divide:

182 summonses $\div$ 7 hours $= 26$

Average $= 26$ summonses/hour

14. **(C)** Total issued $\qquad\qquad = \qquad 186$
Subtract:
First offenders $\qquad\quad = \quad -\underline{100}$
Other-than-first offenders $= \qquad 86$

15. **(C)** If it takes one truck one hour to go 40 miles, it will take two hours to go 80 miles.

$2 \ \cancel{\text{hours}} \times 40 \ \dfrac{\text{miles}}{\cancel{\text{hour}}} = 80$ miles

16. **(C)** If the total capacity is 100 gallons, then

$\dfrac{2}{5}$ of $100 = \dfrac{2}{5} \times 100$

$\qquad\qquad = \dfrac{200}{5}$

$\qquad\qquad = 40$ gallons

17. **(B)** Total salary $= \$3000$
Tax $\qquad\quad = 20\%$ or $.20$

First, find the amount of the 20% tax by multiplying:

$\$3000 - .20 = \$600$

Now subtract the tax from the salary to find the net:

$\$3000 - \$600 = \$2400$

$\$2400 =$ net pay

18. **(A)** Total cost $= \$1000$
Total square yards $= 100$

Find the cost per square yard by dividing:

$\$1000 \div 100$ square yards $= \$10$

$\$10$/square yard

19. **(A)** Base pay $\qquad = \quad \$3000$
Bonus $\qquad\quad = \ +\ 350$
Sr. Increment $\quad +\ \underline{250}$
Total pay $\qquad = \quad \$3600$

20. **(D)** Annual salary $= \$21,600$
Bonus $\qquad\quad = \quad 7200$
Increment $\quad = \quad \underline{1200}$
Total pay $\qquad = \$30,000$

MATHEMATICS TEST 2

15 Minutes   20 Questions

Directions: *Each problem in this test involves a certain amount of logical reasoning and thinking on your part, besides simple computations, to help you find the solution. Read each problem carefully and choose the correct answer from the four choices that follow. Blacken the corresponding space on your answer sheet.*

1. A sanitation man is 40 feet behind a sanitation truck. There is a second sanitation truck 90 feet behind the first truck. How much closer is the man to the first truck than to the second?

   (A) 30 feet
   (B) 50 feet
   (C) 10 feet
   (D) 70 feet

2. If a flushing machine has a capacity of 1260 gallons, how many gallons will it contain when it is two-thirds full?

   (A) 809 gallons
   (B) 750 gallons
   (C) 630 gallons
   (D) 840 gallons

3. If a man's salary is $2500 a month and there are 23 working days in the month, he earns approximately how much for each day he works that month?

   (A) $108.70
   (B) $150.00
   (C) $112.50
   (D) $186.70

4. If an employee earns $160.00 a week and has deductions of $8.00 for the pension fund, $12.00 for medical insurance, and $29.60 withholding tax, his take-home pay will be

   (A) $110.40
   (B) $108.60
   (C) $102.00
   (D) $98.40

5. A city department uses 25 twenty-cent, 35 thirty-cent, and 350 forty-cent metered postage units each day. The total cost of stamps used by the department in a five-day period is

   (A) $29.50
   (B) $155.00
   (C) $290.50
   (D) $777.50

6. A city department issued 12,000 applications in 1979. The number of applications that the department issued in 1977 was 25 percent greater than the number it issued in 1979. If the department issued 10 percent fewer applications in 1975 than it did in 1977, the number it issued in 1975 was

   (A) 16,500
   (B) 13,500
   (C) 9900
   (D) 8100

7. A clerk can add 40 columns of figures in an hour by using an adding machine and 20 columns of figures an hour without using an adding machine. The total number of hours it would take him to add 200 columns if he does three-fifths of the work by machine and the rest without the machine is

   (A) 6
   (B) 7
   (C) 8
   (D) 9

8. In 1975, a city department bought 500 dozen pencils at 40 cents per dozen. In 1978, only 75 percent as many pencils were bought as were bought in 1975, but the price was 20 percent higher than the 1975

price. The total cost of the pencils bought in 1978 was

(A) $180
(B) $187.50
(C) $240
(D) $250.00

9. A clerk is assigned to check the accuracy of the entries on 490 forms. He checks 40 forms an hour. After working one hour on this task, he is joined by another clerk, who checks these forms at the rate of 35 an hour. The total number of hours required to do the entire assignment is

(A) 5
(B) 6
(C) 7
(D) 8

10. Assume that there are a total of 420 employees in a city agency. 30 percent of the employees are clerks and one-seventh are typists. The difference between the number of clerks and the number of typists is

(A) 60
(B) 66
(C) 186
(D) 360

11. Assume that a duplicating machine produces copies of a bulletin at a cost of 12 cents per copy. The machine produces 120 copies of the bulletin per minute. If the cost of producing a certain number of copies was $36, how many minutes did it take the machine to produce this number of copies?

(A) 10 minutes
(B) 6 minutes
(C) 2.5 minutes
(D) 1.2 minutes

12. The average number of reports filed per day by a clerk during a five-day week was 720. She filed 610 reports the first day, 720 reports the second day, 740 reports the third day, and 755 reports the fourth day. The number of reports she filed the fifth day was

(A) 748
(B) 165
(C) 775
(D) 565

13. A city department employs 1400 people, of whom 35 percent are clerks and one-eighth are stenographers. The number of employees in the department who are neither clerks nor stenographers is

(A) 640
(B) 665
(C) 735
(D) 750

14. Assume that there are 190 papers to be filed and that Clerk A and Clerk B are assigned to file these papers. If Clerk A files 40 papers more than Clerk B, then the number of papers that Clerk A files is

(A) 75
(B) 110
(C) 115
(D) 150

15. A stock clerk had on hand the following items:

500 pads, worth $0.04 each
130 pencils, worth $0.03 each
50 dozen rubber bands, worth $0.02 a dozen

If, from this stock, he issued 125 pads, 45 pencils, and 48 rubber bands, the value of the remaining stock would be

(A) $6.43
(B) $8.95
(C) $17.63
(D) $18.47

16. Joe can paint a fence in three hours and his friend can paint the fence in four hours. How long will it take them to do the job if they work together?

(A) 7 hours
(B) $\frac{15}{7}$ hours
(C) $1\frac{5}{7}$ hours
(D) 2 hours

17. A department head hired a total of 60 temporary employees to handle a seasonal increase in the department's workload.

The following lists the number of temporary employees hired, their rates of pay, and the duration of their employment:

One-third of the total were hired as clerks, each at the rate of $9750 a year, for two months.

30 percent of the total were hired as office-machine operators, each at the rate of $11,500 a year, for four months.

22 stenographers were hired, each at the rate of $10,200 a year, for three months.

The total amount paid to these temporary employees was approximately

(A) $178,000
(B) $157,600
(C) $52,200
(D) $48,500

18. Assume that there are 2300 employees in a city agency. Also assume that five percent of these employees are accountants; that 80 percent of the accountants have college degrees; and that one-half of the accountants who have college degrees have five years of experience. Then the number of employees in the agency who are accountants with college degrees and five years of experience is

(A) 46
(B) 51
(C) 460
(D) 920

19. If a monthly salary of $3000 is subject to a $425 tax deduction, the net salary is

(A) $2557.00
(B) $2755.00
(C) $2575.00
(D) $2555.00

20. A sanitation worker who reports 45 minutes early for 8:00 A.M. duty will report at

(A) 7:00 A.M.
(B) 7:30 A.M.
(C) 6:15 A.M.
(D) 7:15 A.M.

Answer Key

1.	**C**	11.	**C**
2.	**D**	12.	**C**
3.	**A**	13.	**C**
4.	**A**	14.	**C**
5.	**D**	15.	**D**
6.	**B**	16.	**C**
7.	**B**	17.	**B**
8.	**A**	18.	**A**
9.	**C**	19.	**C**
10.	**B**	20.	**D**

Explanatory Answers

1. **(C)**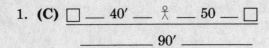

   The second truck is 90 feet − 40 feet = 50 feet from the man. The first truck is 40 feet from the man. The first truck is 50 feet − 40 feet = 10 feet closer than the second truck.

2. **(D)** Total capacity = 1260 gallons

   $\frac{2}{3}$ of 1260 is $\frac{2}{3} \times 1260$

   $$= \frac{2520}{3}$$

   $$= 840 \text{ gallons}$$

3. **(A)** Salary per month = $2500
   Days worked = 23

   To find the earnings per day, divide:

   $2500/month ÷ 23 days/month = $108.70/day

   or

   $$\frac{\$2500}{month} \div \frac{23 \text{ days}}{month}$$

   $$= \frac{\$2500}{\cancel{month}} \times \frac{\cancel{month}}{23 \text{ days}}$$

   $$\frac{\$2500}{23 \text{ days}} = \$108.70/day$$

4. **(A)**

Total earnings	=	$160.00
Deductions	=	8.00 pension
	=	12.00 medical insurance
	=	29.60 withholding tax
	=	$49.60 total deductions

   The take-home pay can be found by subtracting the total deduction from the salary.

   $160.00 − $49.60 = $110.40

   Take-home pay = $110.40

5. **(D)**

Stamps per day	Cost per day
25/day × $0.20 =	5.00
35/day × $0.30 =	10.50
350 × $0.40 =	140.00
Total cost/day	$155.50

   For five days, 5 × $155.50 = $777.50

   Total cost = $777.50

6. **(B)** Number of applications issued in 1979 = 12,000

   In 1977, 25 percent more were issued, or:

   0.25 × 12,000 = 3000 more in 1977

   So there were 3000 + 12,000 = 15,000 issued in 1977.

   In 1975, ten percent fewer were issued than in 1977, or:

   0.10 × 15,000 = 1500 fewer were issued in 1975.

   The number issued in 1975 is

   15,000 − 1500 = 13,500

   13,500 issued.

7. **(B)** If three-fifths of the 200 are done by machine, then:

   $$\frac{3}{5} \times 200 = \frac{600}{5} = 120$$

   columns will be done by the machine. To find the number done by hand, subtract:

   200 − 120 = 80 will be done by hand.

   To find the time it takes to do the 120 columns by machine and the 80 columns by hand, divide:

   120 columns ÷ 40 columns per hour = 3 hours
   80 columns ÷ 20 columns per hour = 4 hours
   Total time = 7 hours

8. **(A)** Total number of pencils bought in 1975 was 500 dozen at 40 cents a dozen; in 1978, 75 percent of the 500 dozen were bought at a 20 percent increase in price.

First, find how many pencils were bought in 1978. Do this by multiplying:

$500 \times 0.75 = 375$ dozen were bought in 1978

Now find the price per dozen. You know that it was 20 percent more than 40 cents:

$\$0.40 \times 0.20$ increase $= \$0.08$ or 8¢ increase in price.

So the price per dozen is:

40¢ + 8¢ = 48¢ or $0.48

To find the cost, multiply the number of dozens of pencils by the cost per dozen.

375 dozen $\times \$0.48$/dozen $= \$180$

Total cost for 1978 = $180.

9. **(C)** During the first hour, 40 forms were checked, leaving 450 to be checked:

$490 - 40 = 450$

The two clerks working together can check 75 forms.

Now find the time it takes to do the 450 forms. Do this by dividing:

450 forms $\div$ 75 forms/hour = 6 hours

It takes six hours to do the 450 and one hour for the first 40 forms:

6 hours + 1 hour = 7 hours to do the job.

A total of 7 hours is needed.

10. **(B)** Total employed = 420
If 30 percent are clerks,

$420 \times 0.30 = 126$ clerks

$\frac{1}{7}$ are typists:

$420 \times \frac{1}{7} = 60$ typists

The difference is $126 - 60 = 66$.

11. **(C)** Cost = 12¢ per copy
Time = 120 copies per minute

To find the number of copies produced, divide:

$36 \div 0.12 = 300$ copies

To find the number of minutes, divide:

300 copies $\div$ 120 copies/minute = 2.5 minutes

12. **(C)** If the average number of reports filed for five days was 720, then

5 days $\times$ 720 reports/day = 3600 reports for the five-day period.

For four days:

$610 + 720 + 740 + 755 = 2825$ reports were filed.

Subtract:

$3600 - 2825 = 775$ need to be filed the fifth day to get an average of 720 for the five-day period.

13. **(C)** Total employees = 1400

35% clerks = $1400 \times .35 = 490$ clerks

$\frac{1}{8}$ stenos = $1400 \times \frac{1}{8} = 175$ stenos

Together ($490 + 175 = 665$), there are 665 clerks and stenographers. To find how many employees are neither, subtract:

$1400 - 665 = 735$

Answer = 735 other employees

14. **(C)** If clerk A files 40 more than clerk B, then take 40 papers aside:

$190 - 40 = 150$

There are now 150 papers to be filed; each will file half of the 150 papers:

$150 \div 2 = 75$ papers

Clerk A files 75 + 40 = 115.
Clerk B files 75.

15. **(D)** Stock on hand and cost per item:

		cost
500 pads × 0.04/pad		= $20.00
130 pencils × 0.03/pencil		= $3.90
50 dozen rubber bands × 0.02/ dozen		= $1.00
		$24.90

value of stock on hand

If we issue the items below,

125 pads × $0.04	=	5.00
45 pencils × .03	=	1.35
48 rubber bands or 4 dozen × .02	=	.08
		$6.43

To find the value of the remaining stock, subtract:

$24.90 − $6.43 = $18.47

Value = $18.47

16. **(C)** Let t be the amount of time for both to do the job. If Joe does $\frac{t}{3}$ part of the job, and his friend does $\frac{t}{4}$ part of the job, then

$$\frac{t}{3} + \frac{t}{4} = 1 \text{ (the whole job)}$$

$4t + 3t = 12$ multiply lowest common denominator by 12

$7t = 12$ combine like terms

$t = \frac{12}{7}$ divide by 7.

$t = 1\frac{5}{7}$ hours

17. **(B)** Total employees = 60

$\frac{1}{3} \times 60$ = 20 clerks

30% × 60,

or $0.30 \times 60 = \begin{matrix} 18 \text{ office machine} \\ 38 \text{ operators} \end{matrix}$

$60 - 38$ = 22 stenos

To find their *rate per month*, divide their monthly salaries by 12, because there are 12 months in a year:

clerks	$\frac{\$9750}{12} = \$812.50$
OMOs	$\frac{\$11,500}{12} = \$958.33$
stenos	$\frac{\$10,200}{12} = \$850.00$

Now find the salary for all employees for the time they worked:

If 20 clerks worked two months, total pay equals:

20 × 2 × $812.50 = $32,500.00

If 18 OMOs worked four months, total pay equals:

18 × 4 × $958.33 = $68,999.76

If 22 stenos worked three months, total pay equals:

22 × 3 × $850.00 = $56,100.00

Total salaries = $157,599.76. This amount can be rounded off to $157,600.00

18. **(A)** 5 percent of 2300 are accountants:

0.05 × 2300 = 115

80 percent of the 115 accountants have college degrees:

0.80 × 115 = 92

One-half of the 92 have five years experience:

$\frac{1}{2} \times 92 = 46$

46 employees have all three qualifications.

19. **(C)** $3000 is subject to $425 tax. The net can be found by subtracting:

$3000 − $425 = $2575

20. **(D)** A sanitation worker who reports 45 minutes early for 8:00 A.M. duty reports

      7 hours 60 minutes
      −   45 minutes
      _____
      7 hours 15 minutes

Note: 1 hour = 60 minutes
        8 hours = 7 hours 60 minutes

This worker reports at 7:15 A.M.

MATHEMATICS TEST 3

15 Minutes   20 Questions

Directions: *Each problem in this test involves a certain amount of logical reasoning and thinking on your part, besides simple computations, to help you find the solution. Read each problem carefully and choose the correct answer from the four choices that follow. Blacken the corresponding space on your answer sheet.*

1. If the average cost of sweeping a square foot of a small town's street is $0.75, the cost of sweeping 100 square feet is

   (A) $7.50
   (B) $750
   (C) $75
   (D) $70

2. If a sanitation department scow is towed at the rate of three miles an hour, how many hours will it need to go 28 miles?

   (A) 10 hours 30 minutes
   (B) 12 hours
   (C) 9 hours 20 minutes
   (D) 9 hours 15 minutes

3. If a man is 60 feet away from a sanitation truck, how many feet nearer is he to the truck than a second truck that is 100 feet away?

   (A) 60 feet
   (B) 40 feet
   (C) 50 feet
   (D) 20 feet

4. A clerk divided his 35-hour work-week as follows:

   One-fifth of his time in sorting mail; one-half of his time in filing letters; and one-seventh of his time in reception work.

   The rest of his time was devoted to messenger work. The percentage of time spent on messenger work by the clerk during the week was most nearly

   (A) 6 percent
   (B) 10 percent
   (C) 14 percent
   (D) 16 percent

5. A city department has set up a computing unit and has rented five computing machines at a yearly rental of $1400 per machine. In addition, the cost to the department for the maintenance and repair of each of these machines is $100 per year. Five computing machine operators, each receiving an annual salary of $30,000 and a supervisor, who receives $38,000 a year, have been assigned to the unit. This unit will perform the work previously performed by ten employees whose combined salary was $324,000 a year. On the basis of these facts, the savings that will result from the operation of this computing unit for five years will be most nearly

   (A) $500,000
   (B) $947,500
   (C) $640,000
   (D) $950,000

6. Joe can do a certain job in eight days. After working alone for four days, he is joined by Mary, and together they finish the work in two more days. How long would it take Mary alone?

   (A) 5 days
   (B) 6 days
   (C) 7 days
   (D) 8 days

7. Six gross of special drawing pencils were purchased for use in a city department. If the pencils were used at the rate of 24 a week, the maximum number of weeks that the six gross of pencils would last is

   (A) 6 weeks
   (B) 12 weeks
   (C) 24 weeks
   (D) 36 weeks

8. A stock clerk had 600 pads on hand. He then issued three-eighths of his supply of pads to Division X, one-fourth to Division Y, and one-sixth to Division Z. The number of pads remaining in stock is

   (A) 48
   (B) 125
   (C) 240
   (D) 475

9. Typist A can do a job in three hours. Typist B can do the same job in five hours. How long would it take both, working together, to do the job?

   (A) 5 hours
   (B) $3\frac{1}{2}$ hours
   (C) $1\frac{7}{8}$ hours
   (D) $1\frac{5}{8}$ hours

10. After gaining 50 percent of his original capital, a man had capital of $18,000. Find the original capital.

   (A) $12,200.00
   (B) $13,100.00
   (C) $12,000.00
   (D) $12,025.00

11. A cogwheel having eight cogs plays into another cogwheel having 24 cogs. When the small wheel has made 42 revolutions, how many has the larger wheel made?

   (A) 14
   (B) 20
   (C) 16
   (D) 10

12. A student worked 30 days at a part-time job. He paid two-fifths of his earnings for room and board and had $81 left. What was his daily wage?

   (A) $4.50
   (B) $5.00
   (C) $5.50
   (D) $6.25

13. A dealer bought motorcycles for $4000. He sold them for $6200, making $50 on each motorcycle. How many motorcycles were there?

   (A) 40
   (B) 38
   (C) 43
   (D) 44

14. An organization had one-fourth of its capital invested in goods, two-thirds of the remainder in land, and the remainder, $1224, in cash. What was the capital of the firm?

   (A) $4986.00
   (B) $4698.00
   (C) $4896.00
   (D) $4869.00

15. A and B together earn $2100. If B is paid one-fourth more than A, how many dollars should B receive?

   (A) $1166.66
   (B) $1162.66
   (C) $1617.66
   (D) $1167.66

16. If a boat is bought for $21,500 and sold again for $23,650, what is the percentage of gain?

   (A) 8 percent
   (B) 15 percent
   (C) 20 percent
   (D) 10 percent

17. A person owned five-sixths of a piece of property and sold three-fourths of her share for $1800. What was the value of the property?

   (A) $2808.00
   (B) $2880.00
   (C) $2088.00
   (D) $2880.80

18. A lot costing $21,250 leases for $1900 a year. The taxes and other expenses are $300 per year. Find the percentage of net income on the investment.

   (A) $7\frac{1}{2}$ percent
   (B) 6 percent
   (C) 4 percent
   (D) 10 percent

19. B owned 75 shares of stock in a building association worth $50 each. The association declared a dividend of eight percent, payable in stock. How many shares did he then own?

    (A) 81 shares
    (B) 80 shares
    (C) 90 shares
    (D) 85 shares

20. It requires four men three days to take an inventory; the weekly salary of each is as follows:

    A—$250, B—$130, C—$120, D—$90.

    Calculate the cost of taking the inventory, assuming that there are five full working days in a week.

    (A) $119.00
    (B) $196.00
    (C) $354.00
    (D) $588.00

ANSWER KEY

1.	C	11.	A
2.	C	12.	A
3.	B	13.	D
4.	D	14.	C
5.	C	15.	A
6.	D	16.	D
7.	D	17.	B
8.	B	18.	A
9.	C	19.	A
10.	C	20.	C

Explanatory Answers

1. **(C)** If it cost $0.75 to sweep one square foot, to find the cost for 100 square feet, multiply:

   100 square feet × 0.75 square foot
   = $75

   Total cost = $75

2. **(C)** It takes one hour to tow a scow three miles. Find the time to tow the scow 28 miles by dividing:

   28 miles ÷ 3 miles/hour

   $= 9\dfrac{1}{3}$ hours

   $\dfrac{1}{3}$ hour × 60 minutes/hour

   = 20 minutes

   Note: 1 hour = 60 minutes. To change hours to minutes, multiply by 60 minutes/hour.

   It takes nine hours, 20 minutes to tow the scow 28 miles.

3. **(B)** ☐---60 ft.-------- 👤   ☐
   --------------------100 ft.--

Truck to the other truck	100 feet
Truck to the man	−60 feet
	40 feet

   The difference is 40 feet.

4. **(D)** A clerk works 35 hours per week. $\frac{1}{5}$ of his time is used to sort mail:

   $\dfrac{1}{5}$ × 35 = 7 hours

   $\frac{1}{2}$ of his time is used to file letters:

   $\dfrac{1}{2}$ × 35 = $17\dfrac{1}{2}$ hours

   $\frac{1}{7}$ of his time is used for reception work.

   $\dfrac{1}{7}$ × 35 = 5 hours

   Total = $29\frac{1}{2}$ hours

   $29\frac{1}{2}$ hours was used for the above. To find the time left for messenger work, subtract $35 - 29\frac{1}{2} = 5\frac{1}{2}$ hours.

Now to find what percentage of 35 is $5\frac{1}{2}$, divide:

   $5.5 \div 35 = 0.16$ or 16%

Note: $5\frac{1}{2} = 5.5$

16% remains for messenger work.

5. **(C)** *Item*

5 machines— $1400/year	5 × 1400	$7000
Maintenance, repairs—$100/ machine	5 × 100	$500
5 operators' annual salary —$30,000	5 × 30,000	$150,000
Supervisor's annual salary —$38,000	1 × 38,000	$38,000
	total cost	$195,500

   If ten employees were paid a total of $324,000, find the savings by subtracting:

   $324,000 − $195,500 = $128,500 one year's savings

   To find the savings for five years, multiply:

   $128,500 × 5 = $642,500

   This amount *rounds off to* (is nearest) $640,000

6. **(D)** If Joe can do the job alone in eight days, then he can do $\frac{1}{8}$ in one day and $\frac{6}{8}$ or $\frac{3}{4}$ in six days.

   Let n be the number of days it would take Mary to do the job alone. Then:

   $\dfrac{1}{n}$ is the part of the job she can do in one day and $\dfrac{2}{n}$ is the part of the job she can do

   in the two days she works with Joe.

Now, the sum of parts done by Joe and Mary equal one whole job:

$$\frac{3}{4} + \frac{2}{n} = 1$$

$3n + 8 = 4n$ multiply by the lowest common denominator (LCD), $4n$

$8 = 4n - 3n$ subtract $3n$ from both sides of the equation

$8 = n$ subtract like terms

$n = 8$

Mary alone could do the job in 8 days.

7. **(D)** One gross = 144 pencils
6 gross = 144/gross × 6 gross = 864 pencils (on hand)
If 24 pencils are used each week, divide to find the number of weeks they will last:

$$864 \div 24/\text{week} = 36 \text{ weeks}$$

Supplies would last 36 weeks.

8. **(B)** From a total of 600 pads on hand:

$$\frac{3}{8} \times 600 = 225 \text{ for Div. X}$$

$$\frac{1}{4} \times 600 = 150 \text{ for Div. Y}$$

$$\frac{1}{6} \times 600 = \underline{100} \text{ for Div. Z}$$

Total to be issued 475
The number left $600 - 475 = 125$

125 remain.

9. **(C)** A can do one-third of the job in one hour. B can do one-fifth of the job in one hour. Together they can do $\frac{1}{3} + \frac{1}{5}$ of the job in one hour. Let t be the time it takes for both to do the job. Together, they can do $\frac{1}{t}$ of the job in one hour. Thus:

$$\frac{1}{3} + \frac{1}{5} = \frac{1}{t}$$

$5t + 3t = 15$ multiply lowest common denominator by the $15t$ or $3 \times 5 \times t$.

$8t = 15$ add like terms

$t = \frac{15}{8}$ divide both sides by 8

$t = 1\frac{7}{8}$ hour

10. **(C)** Let x be the unknown original capital and $0.50x$ be 50 percent of the unknown capital.
Therefore:

$x + .50x = \$18,000$
$1.50x = \$18,000$ add like terms

$$\frac{1.50x}{1.50} = \frac{\$18,000}{1.50}$$ divide both sides by 1.50

$x = \$12,000$

$12,000 is the original amount of the capital.

11. **(A)** If the cogs on two wheels are sized and spaced the same, the smaller of the two wheels will turn faster than the larger one—the fewer cogs a wheel has, the more revolutions it makes. The number of cogs is, therefore, inversely proportional to the number of revolutions:

cogs $\dfrac{8}{24}$ = $\dfrac{x}{42}$ revolutions

$$\frac{8}{24} \times \frac{x}{42}$$

$24x = 8(42)$ cross-multiply

$24x = 336$ multiply like terms (8×42)

$$\frac{24x}{24} = \frac{336}{24}$$ divide both sides by 24

$x = 14$ revolutions

12. **(A)** If two-fifths of his salary was used, then three-fifths was left; three-fifths of his salary is $81. Now, since his salary is unknown, let x represent it:

$$\frac{3}{5} \times x = \$81$$

$$x = \$81 \div \frac{3}{5} \quad \text{divide both sides by } \tfrac{3}{5}$$

$$x = \$81 \times \frac{5}{3} \quad \text{invert and multiply}$$

$$x = \$135$$

His salary is \$135 for 30 days of work. To find the *daily wage*, divide the salary by 30:

$$\$135 \div 30 \text{ days} = \$4.50/\text{day}$$

Daily wage = \$4.50

13. **(D)** To find the number of motorcycles purchased, first subtract his original purchase price from the selling price:

$$\$6200 - \$4000 = \$2200 \text{ profit}$$

Since the profit was \$2200, and the profit on each motorcycle was \$50, the number of motorcycles sold is:

$$\$2200 \text{ profit} \div 50 \text{ profit/motorcycle} = 44 \text{ motorcycles sold}$$

14. **(C)** $\frac{1}{4}$ in *goods* (given)

$$\frac{2}{3} \times \frac{3}{4} = \frac{1}{2} \quad \text{in } land \text{ (because } \tfrac{3}{4} \text{ is the remainder after the goods are invested).}$$

$\frac{1}{4}$ is left in *cash*, because if,

$\frac{1}{4}$ is in goods $+ \frac{1}{2}$ is in land, $\frac{3}{4}$ is invested, leaving $\frac{1}{4}$ for cash.

If $\frac{1}{4}$, which is the cash, is valued at \$1224,

$$\frac{1}{4} \text{ in goods} = \$1224$$

$\frac{1}{2}$ is twice as much as $\frac{1}{4}$:

$$\frac{1}{2} \text{ in land} = \$2448$$

$$\frac{1}{4} \text{ in cash} = \underline{\$1224}$$
$$\$4896$$

Total capital = \$4896

15. **(A)** Let A equal the amount A earned, and B equal the amount B earned.

Together, they earned $A + B = \$2100$.

If B is paid $\frac{1}{4}$ more than A, then A's salary plus $\frac{1}{4}$ of A's salary is equal to B's salary. Express this as follows:

$$B = A + \tfrac{1}{4}A$$

$$4B = 4A + A \quad \text{multiply by 4}$$

$$-5A + 4B = 0 \quad \text{transpose the } A \text{ terms}$$

Now you have two equations with two unknowns. Use the elimination method to find B's salary:

$$
\begin{aligned}
A + B &= \quad \$2100 \quad &\text{multipy} \\
-5A + 4B &= \qquad\quad 0 \quad &\text{the first} \\
5A + 5B &= \$10{,}500 \quad &\text{equation} \\
-5A + 4B &= \qquad\quad 0 \quad &\text{by 5.} \\
\hline
9B &= \$10{,}500 \quad &\text{add the two equations} \\
B &= \$1166.67 \\
&\text{or } \$1166\tfrac{2}{3} \quad &\text{now divide by 9}
\end{aligned}
$$

Note: $0.67 = \frac{2}{3}$

16. **(D)** The boat costs \$21,500 and was sold for \$23,650. Subtract:

$$\$23{,}650 - \$21{,}500 = \$2150$$

\$2150 was gained. To find the percentage gained, divide the amount gained by the original amount:

$$\$2150 \div \$21{,}500 = 0.10 \text{ or } 10\%$$

Percentage gained = 10%

17. **(B)** $\frac{5}{6} \times \frac{3}{4} = \frac{5}{8}$ of the property costs \$1800

Then, letting y represent the value of the property,

$$\frac{5}{8} \times y = \$1800$$

$$y = \$1800 \div \frac{5}{8} \quad \text{divide both sides by } \tfrac{5}{8}$$

$$y = \$1800 \times \frac{8}{5} \quad \text{invert and multiply}$$

Therefore, $2880 is the price of the property.

18. **(A)** A lot costs $21,250.

$1900 is received for lease
-300 is deducted for expenses
$1600 is net income

To find what percentage $1600 is of the cost of the lot, divide:

$1600 \div 21,250 = 0.075$ or $7\frac{1}{2}\%$

$7\frac{1}{2}\%$ = percentage of cost

19. **(A)** Total shares currently owned = 75. Values per share = $50.

To find the value of the stock, multiply 75 $\times$ $50 = $3750

To find 8%, multiply the stock value by 0.08.

$3750 \times 0.08 = $300 (dividend)

Given $300, divide by $50 to see how many additional shares of stock can be purchased:

$300 \div 50 = 6$ shares

Therefore, he now owns $75 + 6 = 81$ shares.

20. **(C)** First, find the salary each man is paid for one day. To do so, divide their salaries by 5 days:

	salary/ day		salary/ 3 days
A $\frac{\$250}{5}$ =	$50.00	$\times 3$ =	$150
B $\frac{\$130}{5}$ =	$26.00	$\times 3$ =	$78
C $\frac{\$120}{5}$ =	$24.00	$\times 3$ =	$72
D $\frac{\$90}{5}$ =	$18.00	$\times 3$ =	$54 / $354

Total salaries for 3 days = $354

MATHEMATICS TEST 4

22 Minutes   31 Questions

Directions: *Each problem in this test involves a certain amount of logical reasoning and thinking on your part, besides simple computations, to help you find the solution. Read each problem carefully and choose the correct answer from the choices that follow. Blacken the corresponding space on your answer sheet.*

1. In simplest form, $-11 - (-2)$ is

   (A) 7
   (B) 9
   (C) -11
   (D) -9

2. Find the average of 6.47, 5.89, 3.42, 0.65, 7.09.

   (A) 5.812
   (B) 4.704
   (C) 3.920
   (D) 4.705

3. $\dfrac{456.3}{0.89}$ equals

   (A) $513\frac{13}{89}$

   (B) 512.70

   (C) 513.89

   (D) $512\frac{59}{89}$

4. Add 5 hours 13 minutes; 3 hours 49 minutes; and 24 minutes. The sum is

   (A) 9 hours 26 minutes
   (B) 8 hours 16 minutes
   (C) 9 hours 76 minutes
   (D) 8 hours 6 minutes

5. Two numbers are in the ratio of 18:47. If the smaller number is 126, the larger number is

   (A) 376
   (B) 144
   (C) 235
   (D) 329

6. Change 0.3125 to a fraction.

   (A) $\frac{3}{64}$

   (B) $\frac{1}{16}$

   (C) $\frac{1}{64}$

   (D) $\frac{5}{16}$

7. Divide $\frac{7}{8}$ by $\frac{7}{8}$.

   (A) 1

   (B) 0

   (C) $\frac{7}{8}$

   (D) $\frac{49}{64}$

8. In the series 5, 8, 13, 20, the next number should be

   (A) 23
   (B) 26
   (C) 29
   (D) 32

9. What is interest on $300 at 6 percent for ten days? (Assume year = 360 days)

   (A) $0.50
   (B) $1.50
   (C) $2.50
   (D) $5.50

10. If the scale on a map indicates that one and one-half inches equals 500 miles, then five inches on the map will represent approximately

    (A) 1800 miles
    (B) 1700 miles
    (C) 1300 miles
    (D) 700 miles

11. $\frac{1}{2}$ percent equals

(A) 0.002
(B) 0.020
(C) 0.005
(D) 0.050

12. If an employee drew $260, which was 20 percent of her bonus, her entire bonus was

(A) $2300
(B) $2600
(C) $1600
(D) $1300

13. If a kilogram equals about 35 ounces, the number of grams in one ounce is approximately

(A) 29
(B) 30
(C) 31
(D) 32

14. The price per gross of items that sell at the rate of 20 for 30 cents is

(A) $2.16
(B) $1.80
(C) $3.60
(D) $2.40

15. If sound travels at the rate of 1100 feet per second, in one-half minute it will travel about

(A) 6 miles
(B) 8 miles
(C) 10 miles
(D) 3 miles

16. If a kilometer is about five-eighths of a mile, two miles are about

(A) 1.6 kilometers
(B) 3.2 kilometers
(C) 2.4 kilometers
(D) 3.75 kilometers

17. A lecture hall which is 25 feet wide and 75 feet long has a perimeter equal to

(A) 1750 feet
(B) 200 yards
(C) 66 $\frac{2}{3}$ yards
(D) 1875 feet

18. After deducting a discount of $16\frac{2}{3}$ percent, the price of a blouse was $35. The list price was

(A) $37.50
(B) $38
(C) $41.75
(D) $42

19. The number of decimal places in the product of 0.4266 and 0.3333 is

(A) 8
(B) 4
(C) 14
(D) none of these

20. What is the cost of 5500 powder puffs at $50 per thousand?

(A) $385
(B) $550
(C) $275
(D) $285

21. 572 divided by 0.52 is

(A) 1100
(B) 110
(C) 11.10
(D) 11,000

22. 200 percent of 800 equals

(A) 2500
(B) 16
(C) 1600
(D) 4

23. The average of a seventh-grade baseball team that won ten games and lost five games is

(A) 0.667
(B) 0.500
(C) 0.333
(D) 0.200

24. The number of cubic feet of soil needed for a flower box three feet long, eight inches wide, and one foot deep is

(A) 24
(B) 12
(C) $4\frac{2}{3}$
(D) 2

25. At $1250 per hundred, 228 watches will cost

    (A) $2850

    (B) $36,000

    (C) $2880

    (D) $360

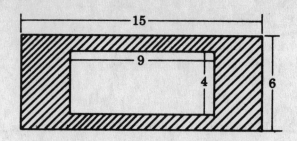

26. The area of the shaded portion of the rectangle above right is

    (A) 54 square inches

    (B) 90 square inches

    (C) 45 square inches

    (D) 36 square inches

27. On February 12, 1989, the age of a boy who was born on March 15, 1979, will be

    (A) 10 years 10 months 3 days

    (B) 9 years 9 months 27 days

    (C) 10 years 1 month 3 days

    (D) 9 years 10 months 27 days

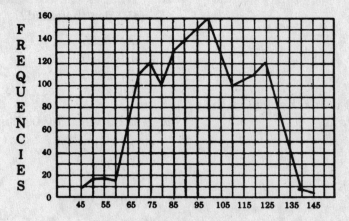

INTELLIGENCE QUOTIENTS (IQs)

Questions 28 to 31 are based on the above graph.

28. The number of pupils having the highest IQ is about

    (A) 5

    (B) 160

    (C) 145

    (D) 20

29. The number of pupils having an IQ of 75 is about

    (A) 130

    (B) 100

    (C) 120

    (D) 110

30. The number of pupils having an IQ of 80 is identical with the number of pupils having an IQ of

    (A) 100

    (B) 68

    (C) 110

    (D) 128

31. The IQ that has the greatest frequency is

    (A) 100

    (B) 95

    (C) 105

    (D) 160

Answer Key

1.	**D**	12.	**D**	22.	**C**
2.	**B**	13.	**A**	23.	**A**
3.	**B**	14.	**A**	24.	**D**
4.	**A**	15.	**A**	25.	**A**
5.	**D**	16.	**B**	26.	**A**
6.	**D**	17.	**C**	27.	**D**
7.	**A**	18.	**D**	28.	**A**
8.	**C**	19.	**A**	29.	**C**
9.	**A**	20.	**C**	30.	**C**
10.	**B**	21.	**A**	31.	**A**
11.	**C**				

Explanatory Answers

1. **(D)** $-11 - (-2)$
   $= -11 + 2$
   $= -9$

2. **(B)** $6.47 + 5.89 + 3.42 + .65 + 7.09$
   $= 23.52$

   To find the average, divide the sum by five (the number of terms involved).

   $23.52 \div 5 = 4.704$

   Average $= 4.704$

3. **(B)**
$$
\begin{array}{r}
512.69\frac{59}{89} \\
.89\overline{)456.30.00} \\
445 \\
\hline
113 \\
89 \\
\hline
240 \\
178 \\
\hline
620 \\
534 \\
\hline
860 \\
801 \\
\hline
59 \text{ remainder}
\end{array}
$$

   $512.69 \frac{59}{89}$ rounds off to 512.70.

4. **(A)**
$$
\begin{array}{r}
5 \text{ hours } 13 \text{ minutes} \\
3 \text{ hours } 49 \text{ minutes} \\
+ \phantom{3 \text{ hours }} 24 \text{ minutes} \\
\hline
8 \text{ hours } 86 \text{ minutes}
\end{array}
$$

   Since there are 60 minutes in one hour, then 86 minutes = 60 minutes + 26 minutes or 1 hour and 26 minutes.

   So,
   8 hours and 86 minutes = 9 hours and 26 minutes.

5. **(D)**
$$\frac{18}{47} \diagdown \diagup \frac{126}{x}$$
   $18x = 47(126)$ cross-multiply
   $18x = 5922$
   $x = 329$ divide by 18

6. **(D)** $0.3125 = \dfrac{3125}{1,000} = \dfrac{5}{16}$

7. **(A)** $\dfrac{7}{8} \div \dfrac{7}{8}$

   $= \dfrac{7}{8} \times \dfrac{8}{7}$ invert the second term and multiply

   $= 1$

8. **(C)** 5, 8, 13, 20. To each number, add the next odd number to determine the next number in the series.

Series		Odd Number		
5	+	3	=	8
8	+	5	=	13
13	+	7	=	20
20	+	9	=	29

   29 will be the next number.

9. **(A)** $Interest = \dfrac{Principal \times Rate}{\times Time}$

   $= \$300 \times 0.06 \times \dfrac{10}{360}$

   $= \dfrac{\$180}{360} = \dfrac{\$1}{2}$

   $= \$.50$

10. **(B)** First, find the number of $1\frac{1}{2}$ inch units there are in five inches. Do this by dividing:

    $5 \div 1\frac{1}{2}$
    $= 5 \div \frac{3}{2}$ change $1\frac{1}{2}$ to $\frac{3}{2}$
    $= 5 \times \frac{2}{3}$ invert and multiply
    $= \frac{10}{3}$

    Now find the total miles by multiplying:

    $500 \times \dfrac{10}{3} = 1666.67$

    Five inches represents approximately 1700 miles.

11. **(C)** $\dfrac{1}{2\%} = 0.5\%$ or $\dfrac{0.5}{100} = 0.005$

12. **(D)** $260 is 20% of the bonus.
    Write this in equation form. Let the bonus be x.

    $\$260 = .20x$

    $\dfrac{260}{.20} = \dfrac{.20x}{.20}$ divide by 0.20

    $\$1300 = x$

    Her entire bonus was $1300.

13. **(A)** 1 kilogram = 35 ounces

Find how many grams there are in 1 ounce.

Note: 1 kilogram = 1000 grams
           1000 grams = 35 ounces

$$1 \text{ ounce} \times \frac{1000 \text{ grams}}{35 \text{ ounces}}$$
$$= \frac{1000 \text{ grams}}{35}$$
$$= 28.6 \text{ or } 29 \text{ grams in one ounce}$$

14. **(A)** 1 gross = 144

If 20 items sell for $0.30, find how many groups of 20 there are in 144:

144 ÷ 20 = 7.2 groups of 20

To find the cost, multiply by $0.30

7.2 × $0.30 = $2.16

The price multiplied per gross = $2.16

15. **(A)** First, find the number of seconds there are in one-half minute:

$\frac{1}{2} \times$ 60 sec/min = 30 seconds.

Since sound travels 1100 feet per second, it will travel:

30 sec. × 1100 ft. = 33,000 ft.

Change the 33,000 feet to miles (1 mile = 5280 feet).

$$33,000 \text{ feet} \times \frac{1 \text{ mile}}{5280 \text{ feet}}$$
$$= 6.25$$

Round off: 6.25 miles = about 6 miles

16. **(B)** 1 kilometer = $\frac{5}{8}$ mile

$$2 \text{ miles} \times \frac{1 \text{ kilometer}}{5/8 \text{ mile}}$$
$$= 2 \text{ miles} \times \frac{1 \text{ kilometer}}{\frac{5}{8} \text{ mile}}$$
$$= 2 \text{ miles} \times \frac{8 \text{ kilometers}}{5 \text{ meters}}$$
$$= 3.2 \text{ kilometers}$$

Two miles = about 3.2 kilometers

17. **(C)** Perimeter of a rectangle (the hall is shaped like a rectangle) is:

$$Perimeter = 2 \ length \ + \ 2 \ width$$
$$= 2(75) + 2(25)$$
$$= 150 + 50$$
$$= 200 \text{ feet}$$

The perimeter is 200 feet.

Now change 200 feet to yards (3 feet = 1 yard).

$$200 \text{ feet} \times \frac{1 \text{ yard}}{3 \text{ feet}} = 66\tfrac{2}{3} \text{ yards}$$

18. **(D)** Let the price of a blouse be x. Then:

$$x - 16\tfrac{2}{3}\%x = 35$$

$\frac{2}{3} = 0.67$, so 16.6770% = 0.1667.

$x - 0.1667x = \$35$	Change the percent to a decimal
$0.8333x = \$35$	combine like terms
$x = \$42$	divide by 0.8333

List price was $42.

19. **(A)** To find the number of decimal places in the product of two numbers, find the sum of the number of digits to the right of the decimal of each number.

0.4266   has 4 digits to the right.
0.3333   has 4 digits to the right.

There should be 8 digits in the product.

20. **(C)** 5.5 thousand × $50 thousand = $275

21. **(A)**
```
          1100.
  .52,)572,00,
      52
      52
      52
      00
      00
```

Answer: 1100

22. **(C)** 200 percent of 800

2.00 × 800 = 1600

23. **(A)** The total games played was 15. To find their average, divide games won by total played:

    $$10 \div 15 = 0.667$$

    Their average is 0.667

24. **(D)** To find the soil needed, first change the 8 inches to feet, so all units will be the same.

    $$8 \text{ inches} \times \frac{1 \text{ foot}}{12 \text{ inches}} = 0.67 \text{ feet}$$

    Now multiply all units.

    $$3 \text{ feet} \times 0.67 \text{ feet} \times 1 \text{ foot} = 2 \text{ cubic feet}$$

    2 cubic feet of soil will be needed to fill the box.

25. **(A)** Find the price for one watch by dividing:

    1250 (per hundred) $\div 100$
    $= \$12.50$ (price of one watch)

    To find the cost of 228, multiply the number of watches by the price per watch.

    228 watches $\times \$12.50$ per watch
    $= \$2850$

    The cost of the watches will be $2850.

26. **(A)** Find the area of the small rectangle and subtract its area from the large rectangle to determine the shaded area.

    Large rectangle

    A = *length* $\times$ *width*
    $= 6 \times 15$
    $= 90$ square inches

    Small rectangle

    A = *length* $\times$ *width*
    $= 4 \times 9$
    $= 36$ square inches

    $90 - 36 = 54$ square inches

    The area of the shaded area is 54 square inches.

27. **(D)**

From	To
March 15, 1979 ...	March 15, 1988
March 15, 1988 ...	Jan. 15, 1989
Jan. 15, 1989	Feb. 12, 1989

    Time

    9 years
    10 months
    27 days

    His age will be 9 years 10 months 27 days.

28. **(A)** On the chart, each line represents ten units. The highest IQ is about halfway on the first line, which is half of ten.

    So the answer is five.

29. **(C)** Locate IQ on base and trace to horizontal intersection.

30. **(C)** There are 100 students with an IQ of 80. Looking across the chart we see that there are also 100 students with an IQ of 110.

31. **(A)** Highest point on the graph, an IQ of 100.

Answer Sheet
Mathematics—Quantitative Comparisons

TEST 5

1. Ⓐ Ⓑ Ⓒ Ⓓ   8. Ⓐ Ⓑ Ⓒ Ⓓ   15. Ⓐ Ⓑ Ⓒ Ⓓ   22. Ⓐ Ⓑ Ⓒ Ⓓ

2. Ⓐ Ⓑ Ⓒ Ⓓ   9. Ⓐ Ⓑ Ⓒ Ⓓ   16. Ⓐ Ⓑ Ⓒ Ⓓ   23. Ⓐ Ⓑ Ⓒ Ⓓ

3. Ⓐ Ⓑ Ⓒ Ⓓ   10. Ⓐ Ⓑ Ⓒ Ⓓ   17. Ⓐ Ⓑ Ⓒ Ⓓ   24. Ⓐ Ⓑ Ⓒ Ⓓ

4. Ⓐ Ⓑ Ⓒ Ⓓ   11. Ⓐ Ⓑ Ⓒ Ⓓ   18. Ⓐ Ⓑ Ⓒ Ⓓ   25. Ⓐ Ⓑ Ⓒ Ⓓ

5. Ⓐ Ⓑ Ⓒ Ⓓ   12. Ⓐ Ⓑ Ⓒ Ⓓ   19. Ⓐ Ⓑ Ⓒ Ⓓ   26. Ⓐ Ⓑ Ⓒ Ⓓ

6. Ⓐ Ⓑ Ⓒ Ⓓ   13. Ⓐ Ⓑ Ⓒ Ⓓ   20. Ⓐ Ⓑ Ⓒ Ⓓ   27. Ⓐ Ⓑ Ⓒ Ⓓ

7. Ⓐ Ⓑ Ⓒ Ⓓ   14. Ⓐ Ⓑ Ⓒ Ⓓ   21. Ⓐ Ⓑ Ⓒ Ⓓ   28. Ⓐ Ⓑ Ⓒ Ⓓ

TEST 6

1. Ⓐ Ⓑ Ⓒ Ⓓ   4. Ⓐ Ⓑ Ⓒ Ⓓ   7. Ⓐ Ⓑ Ⓒ Ⓓ   10. Ⓐ Ⓑ Ⓒ Ⓓ

2. Ⓐ Ⓑ Ⓒ Ⓓ   5. Ⓐ Ⓑ Ⓒ Ⓓ   8. Ⓐ Ⓑ Ⓒ Ⓓ   11. Ⓐ Ⓑ Ⓒ Ⓓ

3. Ⓐ Ⓑ Ⓒ Ⓓ   6. Ⓐ Ⓑ Ⓒ Ⓓ   9. Ⓐ Ⓑ Ⓒ Ⓓ   12. Ⓐ Ⓑ Ⓒ Ⓓ

TEST 7

1. Ⓐ Ⓑ Ⓒ Ⓓ   6. Ⓐ Ⓑ Ⓒ Ⓓ   11. Ⓐ Ⓑ Ⓒ Ⓓ   16. Ⓐ Ⓑ Ⓒ Ⓓ

2. Ⓐ Ⓑ Ⓒ Ⓓ   7. Ⓐ Ⓑ Ⓒ Ⓓ   12. Ⓐ Ⓑ Ⓒ Ⓓ   17. Ⓐ Ⓑ Ⓒ Ⓓ

3. Ⓐ Ⓑ Ⓒ Ⓓ   8. Ⓐ Ⓑ Ⓒ Ⓓ   13. Ⓐ Ⓑ Ⓒ Ⓓ   18. Ⓐ Ⓑ Ⓒ Ⓓ

4. Ⓐ Ⓑ Ⓒ Ⓓ   9. Ⓐ Ⓑ Ⓒ Ⓓ   14. Ⓐ Ⓑ Ⓒ Ⓓ   19. Ⓐ Ⓑ Ⓒ Ⓓ

5. Ⓐ Ⓑ Ⓒ Ⓓ   10. Ⓐ Ⓑ Ⓒ Ⓓ   15. Ⓐ Ⓑ Ⓒ Ⓓ   20. Ⓐ Ⓑ Ⓒ Ⓓ

MATHEMATICS TEST 5

Quantitative Comparisons

35 Minutes   28 Questions

Common Information: *In each question, information concerning one or both of the quantities to be compared is given in the ITEM column. A symbol that appears in any column represents the same thing in Column A as it does in Column B.*

FIGURES: Assume that the position of points, angles, regions, and so forth, are in the order shown; that the lines shown as straight are indeed straight; that figures lie in a plane unless otherwise indicated. Figures accompanying questions are intended to provide information you can use in answering the questions. However, unless a note states that a figure is drawn to scale, you should solve the problems by using your knowledge of mathematics, NOT by estimating sizes by sight or by measurement.

Directions: *For each of the following questions, two quantities are given: one in Column A and one in Column B. Compare the two quantities and mark your answer sheet with the correct, lettered conclusion. These are your options:*

A: *if the quantity in Column A is the greater;*

B: *if the quantity in Column B is the greater;*

C: *if the two quantities are equal;*

D: *if the relationship cannot be determined from the information given.*

ITEM	Column A	Column B
1.	$\angle x$	$\angle y$

Isosceles $\triangle ABC$
$\angle CAB = \angle ACB$

	ITEM	Column A	Column B

2.   Area of △DEC   Area of △AED + Area △EBC

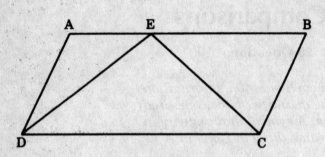

Parallelogram ABCD
E a point on AB

3. $x = -1$ $x^3 + x^2 - x + 1$ $x^3 - x^2 + x - 1$

4.   The edge of a cube whose volume is 27.   The edge of a cube whose total surface area is 54.

5. $\dfrac{\frac{1}{2} + \frac{1}{3}}{\frac{2}{3}}$ $\dfrac{\frac{2}{3}}{\frac{1}{2} + \frac{1}{3}}$

6. x is a given number.   Area of a circle radius = x^3 Area of a circle radius = $3x$

7. $\frac{1}{4}^{-2}$ 4^2

8. 0.02 $\sqrt{0.02}$

9. $(AB)^2$ $(AC)^2 + 5(CB)$

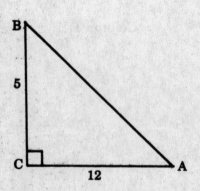

Right △ABC

10.   Area of circle with radius 7.   Area of equilateral triangle with side 14.

ITEM	Column A	Column B

11.
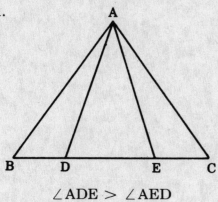

∠ADE > ∠AED

Column A: B

Column B: ∠C

12.
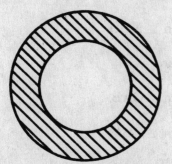

Radius of large circle = 10

Radius of small circle = 7

Column A: Area of shaded portion.

Column B: Area of small circle.

13.
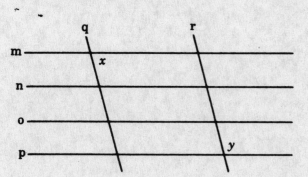

m ∥ n ∥ o ∥ p
and q ∥ r

Column A: ∠x

Column B: ∠y

14.　$a < 0 < b$　　a^2　　$b/2$

15.　$t < 0 < r$　　t^2　　r

ITEM	Column A	Column B

Diagram for problems 16-20

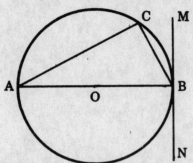

MN tangent to circle O

at point B and $\angle A = 30°$

16.	m $\angle ACB$	m $\angle NBO$
17.	arc CB	arc AC
18.	m $\angle CBM$	m $\angle CAB$
19.	m $\angle CBA$	m $\angle CBM$
20.	$\overline{AO} + \overline{AC}$	$\overline{BO} + \overline{BC}$

Diagram for problems 21-25

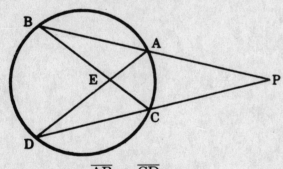

$\overline{AB} = \overline{CD}$

arc BD = 160°

arc AC = 40°

21.	m $\angle APC$	m $\angle ABC$
22.	m $\angle BED$	m $\angle BEA$
23.	m $\angle BAD$	m $\angle DCB$
24.	m $\angle BCP$	m $\angle AEC$ + m $\angle ADC$
25.	arc DC + AC	arc BD

ITEM	Column A	Column B
26.	75% of $\frac{3}{4}$	0.09×6
27.	4% of 0.003	3% of 0.004
28.	$\angle$ BCA	$\angle$ FEG

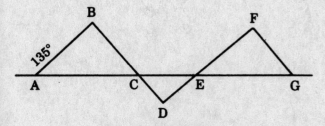

Intersecting straight lines

$AB \perp CB$, $CD = ED$

Answer Key

1.	D	8.	C	15.	D	22.	A
2.	C	9.	C	16.	C	23.	C
3.	A	10.	A	17.	B	24.	B
4.	C	11.	D	18.	C	25.	B
5.	A	12.	A	19.	A	26.	A
6.	D	13.	D	20.	A	27.	C
7.	C	14.	D	21.	A	28.	C

Explanatory Answers

1. **(D)** The value of $\angle x$ or $\angle y$ cannot be determined unless the measure of at least one angle is known.

2. **(C)** Area of $\triangle DEC = \frac{1}{2}\ base \times height$.
Area of parallelogram $= base \times height$.
Area of $\triangle ADE + \triangle EBC =$ area of the whole parallelogram $- \triangle DEC = base \times height - \frac{1}{2}\ base \times height = \frac{1}{2}\ base \times height$.

3. **(A)**
$$x^3 + x^2 - x + 1 = (-1)^3 + (-1)^2 - (-1) + 1$$
$$= -1 + 1 + 1 + 1$$
$$= 2$$
$$x^3 - x^2 + x - 1 = (-1)^3 - (-1)^2 + (-1) - 1$$
$$= -1 - 1 - 1 - 1$$
$$= -4$$

4. **(C)** A cube has six surfaces, each one's area e^2
$$e^3 = 27 \qquad 6e^2 = 54$$
$$e = 3 \qquad e^2 = 9$$
$$e = 3$$

5. **(A)** $\dfrac{1/2 + 1/3}{2/3} = \dfrac{\dfrac{3 + 2}{6}}{2/3}$

$$= \dfrac{\dfrac{5}{6}}{2/3}$$

$$= \dfrac{\dfrac{15}{12}}{1}$$

$$= \dfrac{15}{12}$$

$\dfrac{2/3}{1/2 + 1/3} = \dfrac{2/3}{\dfrac{3 + 2}{6}}$

$$= \dfrac{2/3}{\dfrac{5}{6}}$$

$$= \dfrac{\dfrac{12}{15}}{1}$$ multiply numerator and denominator by $\frac{6}{5}$

$$= \dfrac{12}{15}$$

$$\dfrac{15}{12} > \dfrac{12}{15}$$

6. **(D)** Area of circle $x^3 = \pi(x^3)^2$
$$= \pi x^6$$
Area of circle radius $3x = \pi(3x)^2$
$$= 9\pi x^2$$
We cannot know whether πx^6 or $9\pi x^2$ is larger unless we know the value of x.

7. **(C)** $\quad (1/4)^{-2} = \dfrac{1}{(1/4)^2} \qquad 4^2 = 16$
$$= \dfrac{1}{\dfrac{1}{16}}$$
$$= 16$$

8. **(B)** $\quad 0.02 = \sqrt{0.0004}$
$$\sqrt{0.02} > \sqrt{0.0004}$$

9. **(C)** By the Pythagorean theorem,
$$(AB)^2 = (AC)^2 + (BC)^2$$
However,
$$(BC)^2 = 5^2 = 25 \text{ and } 5CB = 5 \cdot 5 = 25$$
Therefore, $(BC)^2 = 5CB$
$$(AB)^2 = (AC)^2 + 5CB$$
(Substituting $5CB$ for $(BC)^2$ in the Pythagorean theorem)

10. **(A)** Area of circle radius $7 = \pi r^2 = \pi(7)^2 = 49\pi$

Area of equilateral $\triangle$ with side of 14:

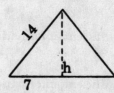

A line from one vertex to the midpoint of the opposite side is perpendicular to the opposite side. It is, therefore, the height of the triangle. Let the length of this line be h. Then, by the Pythagorean theorem, $7^2 + h^2 = 14^2$.
$$h^2 = 14^2 - 7^2 = 14$$
$$h^2 = 3 \times 7 \times 7$$
$$h = 7\sqrt{3}$$

Area of $\triangle = \frac{1}{2}\ base \times height$
$$= \frac{1}{2}(14)\,(7\sqrt{3})$$
Area of $\triangle = (7)\,7\sqrt{3}$
$$= 49\sqrt{3}$$

Is 49π bigger than $49\sqrt{3}$?
$\pi = 3.14$
Therefore, $\pi > \sqrt{3}$

Therefore, $49\pi > 49\sqrt{3}$ and $A > B$

11. **(D)** Not enough information is given to determine the values of the angles.

12. **(A)** $\begin{pmatrix} \text{Area of} \\ \text{shaded} \\ \text{portion} \end{pmatrix} = \begin{pmatrix} \text{Area of} \\ \text{larger} \\ \text{circle} \end{pmatrix} - \begin{pmatrix} \text{Area of} \\ \text{smaller} \\ \text{circle} \end{pmatrix}$

$$= (10^2) - (7^2)$$
$$= 100 - 49$$
$$= 51$$

$\begin{pmatrix} \text{Area of} \\ \text{smaller} \\ \text{circle} \end{pmatrix} = r^2$

$$= (7^2)$$
$$= 49$$

$51 > 49$

13. **(D)**

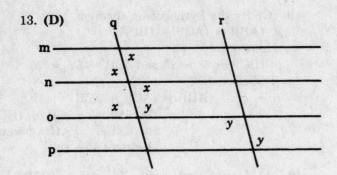

All that can be determined is that x and y are supplementary.

14. **(D)** There is insufficient information to determine an answer.

15. **(D)** There is insufficient information to determine an answer.

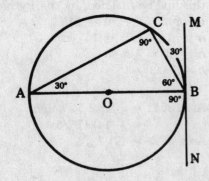

16. **(C)** m $\angle$ACB = 90°   m $\angle$NBO = 90°

A tangent to a circle is perpendicular to the radius of the circle at their point of contact. An inscribed angle is equal to one-half its intercepted arc. Therefore m $\angle$ACB = 90°.

17. **(B)** arc AC = 120°   arc CB = 60°

An inscribed angle is equal to one-half its intercepted arc.

18. **(C)** m $\angle$CBM = 30°   m $\angle$CAB = 30°

19. **(A)** m $\angle$CBA = 60°   m $\angle$CBM = 30°

20. **(A)** $\overline{AO} = \overline{BO}$ all radii in the same circle are equal.

$\overline{AC} > \overline{BC}$ in a triangle the greater side lies opposite the greater angle.

$\overline{AO} + \overline{AC} > \overline{BO} + \overline{BC}$

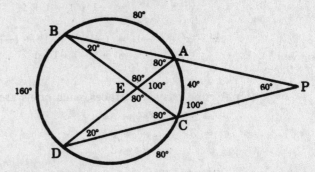

21. **(A)** m $\angle$APC = 60°   m $\angle$ABC = 20°

22. **(A)** m $\angle$BED = 100°   m $\angle$BEA = 80°

23. **(C)** m $\angle$BAD = 80°   m $\angle$DCB = 80°

24. **(B)** m $\angle$BCP = 100°
     m $\angle$AEC + m $\angle$ADC = 100° + 20°
                            = 120°

25. **(B)** arc DC + arc AC = 80° + 40° = 120°
                 arc BD = 160°

26. **(A)** 75% of $\frac{3}{4}$ = .75 × .75   .09 × 6 = .54
                     = .5625

27. **(C)** 4% of 0.003 = 0.04 × .003
                         = 0.00012

3% of 0.004 = 0.03 × 0.004
                         = 0.00012

28. **(C)**

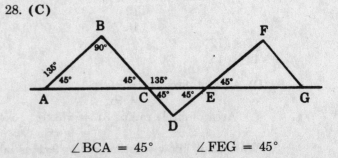

$\angle$BCA = 45° $\angle$FEG = 45°

MATHEMATICS TEST 6

Quantitative Comparisons

15 Minutes   12 Questions

Common Information: *In each question, information concerning one or both of the quantities to be compared is given in the ITEM column. A symbol that appears in any column represents the same thing in Column A as it does in Column B.*

FIGURES: Assume that the position of points, angles, regions, and so forth, are in the order shown; that the lines shown as straight are indeed straight; that figures lie in a plane unless otherwise indicated. Figures accompanying questions are intended to provide information you can use in answering the questions. However, unless a note states that a figure is drawn to scale, you should solve the problems by using your knowledge of mathematics, and NOT by estimating sizes by sight or by measurement.

DIRECTIONS: *For each of the following questions, two quantities are given: one in Column A and one in Column B. Compare the two quantities and mark your answer sheet with the correct lettered conclusion. These are your options:*

A: *if the quantity in Column A is the greater;*
B: *if the quantity in Column B is the greater;*
C: *if the two quantities are equal;*
D: *if the relationship cannot be determined from the information given.*

ITEM	Column A	Column B
1. $a > 0$ $x > 0$	$a + x$	$a - x$
2.	The average of 17, 19, 21, 23, 25	The average of 16, 18, 20, 22, 24

125

ITEM	Column A	Column B

3.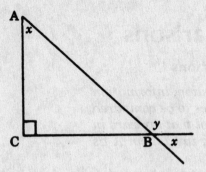

Column A: $2x$

Column B: y

4. $0 < a < 12$
   $0 < b < 12$

Column A: a

Column B: b

5. $4a - 4b = 20$

Column A: a

Column B: b

6.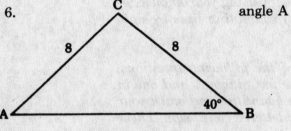

Column A: angle A

Column B: angle B

7. $a/9 = b^2$

Column A: a

Column B: b

8.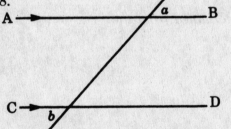

AB ∥ CD

Column A: a

Column B: b

9.

Column A: $3 + 24(3 - 2)$

Column B: $27 + 5(0)(5)$

10.

Column A: AM

Column B: BM

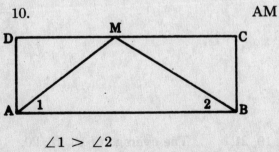

$\angle 1 > \angle 2$

	ITEM	Column A	Column B

11.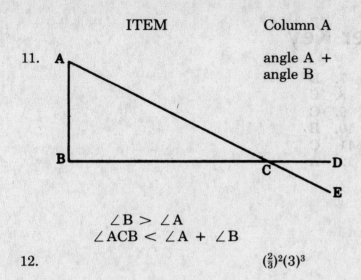

angle A + angle B

angle ACD

$$\angle B > \angle A$$
$$\angle ACB < \angle A + \angle B$$

12.

$(\frac{2}{3})^2(3)^3$

$(3)^2(\frac{2}{3})^3$

Answer Key

1.	A	7.	D
2.	A	8.	C
3.	B	9.	C
4.	D	10.	B
5.	A	11.	C
6.	C	12.	A

Explanatory Answers

1. **(A)** The statement $a > 0$ and $x > 0$ implies both a and x are positive. The sum of two positive numbers is always greater than their difference.

2. **(A)** The averages of Column A and Column B are 21 and 20 respectively.

3. **(B)** Angle ABC = x (vertical angles are equal). Since $\angle C = 90°$, $\angle A + \angle ABC = 90°$ (180° in a $\triangle$). Therefore, $2x = 90°$, and $x = 45°$. Angle ABC and $\angle y$ are supplementary; hence $y = 135°$. Therefore, $y > 2x$.

4. **(D)** Impossible to determine because a could be any number between 0 and 12 and b any number between 0 and 10.

5. **(A)** $4a - 4b = 20$
$$a - b = 5$$
$$a - 5 = b$$
For all values of a and b, $a > b$.

6. **(C)** Angles opposite equal sides of a triangle are equal.

7. **(D)** Impossible to determine because b could be positive or negative.

8. **(C)** If two parallel lines are cut by a transversal, the alternate exterior angles are equal.

9. **(C)** Column A and Column B both equal 27.

10. **(B)** The greater side lies opposite the greater angle.

11. **(C)** The exterior angle of a triangle is equal to the two interior nonadjacent angles.

12. **(A)** The value of Column A is 12 and the value of Column B is $2\frac{2}{3}$. Therefore, A > B.

MATHEMATICS TEST 7

Quantitative Comparisons

30 Minutes   20 Questions

Common Information: *In each question, information concerning one or both of the quantities to be compared is given in the ITEM column. A symbol that appears in any column represents the same thing in Column A as it does in Column B.*

FIGURES: Assume that the position of points, angles, regions, and so forth, are in the order shown; that the lines shown as straight are indeed straight; that figures lie in a plane unless otherwise indicated. Figures accompanying questions are intended to provide information you can use in answering the questions. However, unless a note states that a figure is drawn to scale, you should solve the problems by using your knowledge of mathematics, NOT by estimating sizes by sight or by measurement.

Directions: *For each of the following questions, two quantities are given: one in Column A and one in Column B. Compare the two quantities and mark your answer sheet with the correct, lettered conclusion. These are your options:*

A: *if the quantity in Column A is the greater;*
B: *if the quantity in Column B is the greater;*
C: *if the two quantities are equal;*
D: *if the relationship cannot be determined from the information given.*

ITEM	Column A	Column B
1.	5% of 34	The number that 34 is 5% of

2.

$1 < 2$

	Column A	Column B
2.	IR	IT

		Column A	Column B
3.	$4 > x > -3$	$x/3$	$3/x$

ITEM	Column A	Column B
4.	$\frac{2}{3} + \frac{3}{7}$	$\frac{16}{21} - \frac{3}{7}$
5.	$\angle A + \angle B$	$\angle 2$

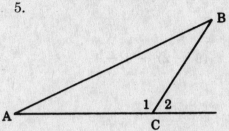

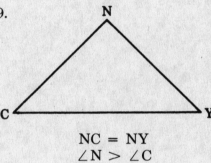

$$\angle A > \angle B$$
$$\angle 1 < \angle A + \angle B$$

6.	y = an odd integer	The numerical value of y^2	The numerical value of y^3
7.		$8 + (6 \div 3) - 7(2)$	$6 + (8 \div 2) - 7(3)$
8.		$\frac{3}{4}$ of $\frac{9}{9}$	$\frac{9}{9} \times \frac{3}{4}$
9.		NC	CY

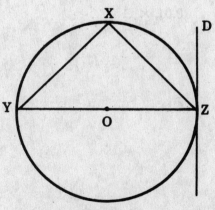

$$NC = NY$$
$$\angle N > \angle C$$

10.	$\angle YXZ$	$\angle DZY$

△XYZ is inscribed in circle 0
and DZ is tangent to circle 0.

11.	A given chord in a given circle.	The radius of the same circle.

	Column A	Column B

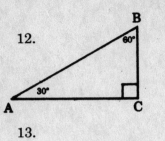 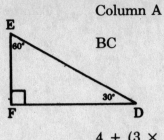

12. BC   FD

13. $4 + (3 \times 2) - 7$ $(8 \div 2) + 3 - 1$

14. 50% of $\frac{4}{5}$ $\frac{4}{5}$ of $\frac{1}{2}$

15. AB   CD

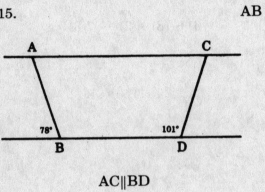

AC‖BD

16. $0.01 \div .1$ $0.01 \times .1$

17. AB   CD

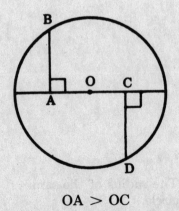

OA > OC

ITEM	Column A	Column B
18.	The number that 6 is 20% of	10% of 300
19. $3x + 2y = -1$ $2x + 3y = 1$	The numerical value of x	The numerical value of y
20.	AC	CB

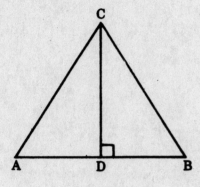

CD ⊥ AB
∠A > ∠B

Answer Key

1.	**B**	11.	**D**
2.	**A**	12.	**D**
3.	**D**	13.	**B**
4.	**A**	14.	**C**
5.	**C**	15.	**A**
6.	**D**	16.	**A**
7.	**A**	17.	**B**
8.	**C**	18.	**C**
9.	**B**	19.	**B**
10.	**C**	20.	**B**

Explanatory Answers

1. **(B)** 5% of 34 = 34 × 0.05 = 1.7
   The number that 34 is 5% of =
   5% of n = 34
   0.05 n = 34
   $$n = \frac{34}{0.05}$$

   $$n = 0.05\overline{\smash{)}34.00.}$$
   $$\begin{array}{r} 680. \\ \hline 34.00. \\ 30 \\ \hline 40 \\ 40 \\ \hline 00 \\ 00 \end{array}$$

   $n = 680$
   $680 > 1.7$

2. **(A)** In a triangle the greater side lies opposite the greater angle. $\angle 2 > \angle 1$ (given)
   IR > IT

3. **(D)** Since x could be any number from -3 to 4, the values of the fractions are impossible to determine.

4. **(A)** $\frac{2}{3} + \frac{3}{7} = \frac{14}{21} + \frac{9}{21}$

   $$= \frac{23}{21}$$

   $$\frac{16}{21} - \frac{3}{7} = \frac{16}{21} - \frac{9}{21}$$

   $$= \frac{7}{21}$$

5. **(C)**

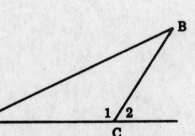

   $\angle 2 = \angle A + \angle B$ (an exterior angle of a triangle is equal to the sum of the two interior remote angles)

6. **(D)** There is not enough information given; y could equal 1, which would make both quantities equal; or y could be greater than 1, which would make y^3 greater than y^2. If y were a negative integer, then y^2 would be greater than y^3.

7. **(A)** $8 + (6 \div 3) - 7(2) = 8 + 2 - 14$
   $$= 10 - 14$$
   $$= -4$$

   $6 + (8 \div 2) - 7(3) = 6 + 4 - 21$
   $$= 10 - 21$$
   $$= -11$$

8. **(C)** $\frac{3}{4} \cdot \frac{9}{9} = \frac{3}{4}$

   $$\frac{9}{9} \cdot \frac{3}{4} = \frac{3}{4}$$

9. **(B)**

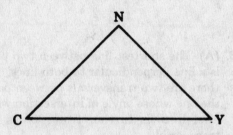

   NC = NY given
   $\angle C = \angle Y$ angles opposite equal sides are equal
   $\angle N > \angle C$ given
   $\angle N > \angle Y$ substitution
   CY > NC the greater side lies opposite the greater angle

10. **(C)**

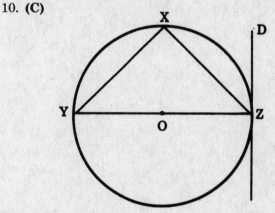

   $\angle YXZ = 90°$ an angle inscribed in a semicircle equals 90°
   $\angle DZY = 90°$ a radius is perpendicular to a tangent at their point of contact

11. **(D)** Impossible to determine from the information given. The radius could be less than, equal to, or greater than the chord.

12. **(D)** Since there are three unknown sides on both triangles, the length of BC or FD is impossible to determine.

13. **(B)** $4 + 3 \times 2 - 7 = 4 + 6 - 7$
$$= 10 - 7$$
$$= 3$$
$$8 \div 2 + 3 - 1 = 4 + 3 - 1$$
$$= 7 - 1$$
$$= 6$$

14. **(C)** 50% of $\dfrac{4}{5} = \dfrac{1}{2} \times \dfrac{4}{5}$
$$= \dfrac{2}{5}$$
$$\dfrac{4}{5} \text{ of } \dfrac{1}{2} = \dfrac{4}{5} \times \dfrac{1}{2}$$
$$= \dfrac{2}{5}$$

15. **(A)** The shortest line between two parallel lines is a line perpendicular to both lines. Therefore if there are two transversals between parallel lines, the one whose angle of intersection with the parallel lines is further from 90° is the longer transversal.
$$\angle B = 90° - 78° = 12°$$
$$\angle D = 101° - 90° = 11°$$
$$\therefore AB > CD$$

16. **(A)** $0.01 \div 0.1 = 0.1$
$$0.01 \times 0.1 = 0.001$$

17. **(B)** If two perpendiculars are drawn from the circumference of a circle to a diameter of the same circle the one that is closer to the center of the circle will be longer.

18. **(C)** The number that 6 is 20% of:
$$20\% \text{ of } n = 6$$
$$0.20n = 6$$
$$n = 6 \div 0.2$$
$$n = 30$$
$$10\% \times 300:$$
$$0.10 \times 300$$
$$= 30$$

19. **(B)** $3(3x + 2y = -1)$
$\underline{2(2x + 3y = 1)}$
$9x + 6y = -3)$
$4x + 6y = 2)$
$5x = -5)$
$x = -1)$

$$3x + 2y = -1$$
$$3(-1) + 2y = -1$$
$$-3 + 2y = -1$$
$$2y = 2$$
$$y = 1$$

20. **(B)** $\angle A > \angle B$ given

CB > AC In a triangle the greater side lies opposite the greater angle

Answer Sheet
Final Mathematics Examination
PART ONE
GENERAL MATHEMATICS

1. Ⓐ Ⓑ Ⓒ Ⓓ   11. Ⓐ Ⓑ Ⓒ Ⓓ   21. Ⓐ Ⓑ Ⓒ Ⓓ   31. Ⓐ Ⓑ Ⓒ Ⓓ

2. Ⓐ Ⓑ Ⓒ Ⓓ   12. Ⓐ Ⓑ Ⓒ Ⓓ   22. Ⓐ Ⓑ Ⓒ Ⓓ   32. Ⓐ Ⓑ Ⓒ Ⓓ

3. Ⓐ Ⓑ Ⓒ Ⓓ   13. Ⓐ Ⓑ Ⓒ Ⓓ   23. Ⓐ Ⓑ Ⓒ Ⓓ   33. Ⓐ Ⓑ Ⓒ Ⓓ

4. Ⓐ Ⓑ Ⓒ Ⓓ   14. Ⓐ Ⓑ Ⓒ Ⓓ   24. Ⓐ Ⓑ Ⓒ Ⓓ   34. Ⓐ Ⓑ Ⓒ Ⓓ

5. Ⓐ Ⓑ Ⓒ Ⓓ   15. Ⓐ Ⓑ Ⓒ Ⓓ   25. Ⓐ Ⓑ Ⓒ Ⓓ   35. Ⓐ Ⓑ Ⓒ Ⓓ

6. Ⓐ Ⓑ Ⓒ Ⓓ   16. Ⓐ Ⓑ Ⓒ Ⓓ   26. Ⓐ Ⓑ Ⓒ Ⓓ   36. Ⓐ Ⓑ Ⓒ Ⓓ

7. Ⓐ Ⓑ Ⓒ Ⓓ   17. Ⓐ Ⓑ Ⓒ Ⓓ   27. Ⓐ Ⓑ Ⓒ Ⓓ   37. Ⓐ Ⓑ Ⓒ Ⓓ

8. Ⓐ Ⓑ Ⓒ Ⓓ   18. Ⓐ Ⓑ Ⓒ Ⓓ   28. Ⓐ Ⓑ Ⓒ Ⓓ   38. Ⓐ Ⓑ Ⓒ Ⓓ

9. Ⓐ Ⓑ Ⓒ Ⓓ   19. Ⓐ Ⓑ Ⓒ Ⓓ   29. Ⓐ Ⓑ Ⓒ Ⓓ   39. Ⓐ Ⓑ Ⓒ Ⓓ

10. Ⓐ Ⓑ Ⓒ Ⓓ   20. Ⓐ Ⓑ Ⓒ Ⓓ   30. Ⓐ Ⓑ Ⓒ Ⓓ   40. Ⓐ Ⓑ Ⓒ Ⓓ

PART TWO
QUANTITATIVE COMPARISONS

1. Ⓐ Ⓑ Ⓒ Ⓓ   7. Ⓐ Ⓑ Ⓒ Ⓓ

2. Ⓐ Ⓑ Ⓒ Ⓓ   8. Ⓐ Ⓑ Ⓒ Ⓓ

3. Ⓐ Ⓑ Ⓒ Ⓓ   9. Ⓐ Ⓑ Ⓒ Ⓓ

4. Ⓐ Ⓑ Ⓒ Ⓓ   10. Ⓐ Ⓑ Ⓒ Ⓓ

5. Ⓐ Ⓑ Ⓒ Ⓓ   11. Ⓐ Ⓑ Ⓒ Ⓓ

6. Ⓐ Ⓑ Ⓒ Ⓓ   12. Ⓐ Ⓑ Ⓒ Ⓓ

FINAL MATHEMATICS EXAMINATION

60 Minutes   54 Questions

Part I–General Mathematics

40 Minutes   42 Questions

1. Jane Doe borrowed $225,000 for five years at $13\frac{1}{2}$ percent. The annual interest charge was

   (A) $1667
   (B) $6000
   (C) $30,375
   (D) $39,375

2. A junior salesman gets a commission of 14 percent on his sales. If he wants his commission to amount to $140, he will have to sell merchandise totaling

   (A) $1960
   (B) $10
   (C) $1000
   (D) $100

3. On a list price of $200, the difference between a single discount of 25 percent and successive discounts of 20 percent and 5 percent is

   (A) $0
   (B) $48
   (C) $8
   (D) $2

4. A worked five days on overhauling an old car. B worked four days more to finish the job. After the sale of the car, the net profit was $243. They wanted to divide the profit on the basis of the time spent by each. A's share of the profit was

   (A) $108
   (B) $135
   (C) $127
   (D) $143

5. If cloth costs $42\frac{1}{2}$ cents per yard, how many yards can be purchased for $76.50?

   (A) 220
   (B) 180
   (C) 190
   (D) 230

6. A fashionable dress shop offers a 20 percent discount on selected items. For a dress marked at $280, what is the discount price?

   (A) $224.00
   (B) $232.00
   (C) $248.00
   (D) $261.00

7. If A takes six days to do a task and B takes three days to do the same task, working together they should do the same task in

   (A) $2\frac{2}{3}$ days
   (B) 2 days
   (C) $2\frac{1}{3}$ days
   (D) $2\frac{1}{2}$ days

8. The area of a mirror 40 inches long and 20 inches wide is approximately

   (A) 8.5 square feet
   (B) 5.5 square feet
   (C) 8.0 square feet
   (D) 2.5 square feet

9. $\frac{2}{3}$ plus $\frac{1}{8}$ equals

   (A) $\frac{37}{72}$
   (B) $\frac{82}{72}$
   (C) $\frac{3}{11}$
   (D) $\frac{19}{24}$

10. A student has received two grades of 90 and two grades of 80 in an English course. Assuming the grades are weighed equally, what is the student's average for the course?

    (A) 90
    (B) 87
    (C) 85
    (D) 84

11. If a man has only quarters and dimes totaling $2.00, the number of quarters *cannot* be

    (A) 2
    (B) 4
    (C) 6
    (D) 3

12. The number that increased by one-sixth of itself yields 182 is

    (A) 156
    (B) 176
    (C) 148
    (D) 160

13. $0.16\frac{3}{4}$ written as a percent is

    (A) $16\frac{3}{4}$ percent
    (B) $16.\frac{3}{4}$ percent
    (C) $0.016\frac{3}{4}$ percent
    (D) $0.0016\frac{3}{4}$ percent

14. $40 reduced by three-eighths of itself is

    (A) $25
    (B) $65
    (C) $15
    (D) $55

15. $1296.53 minus $264.87 is

    (A) $1232.76
    (B) $1032.76
    (C) $1031.66
    (D) $1132.53

16. $12\frac{1}{2}$ minus $6\frac{1}{4}$ is

    (A) $5\frac{3}{4}$
    (B) $6\frac{1}{4}$
    (C) $6\frac{1}{2}$
    (D) $5\frac{1}{2}$

17. Men's handkerchiefs cost $1.29 for three. The cost per dozen handkerchiefs is

    (A) $7.74
    (B) $3.87
    (C) $14.48
    (D) $5.16

18. Add: $\frac{1}{4}, \frac{7}{12}, \frac{3}{8}, \frac{1}{2}, \frac{5}{6}$.

    (A) $2\frac{1}{2}$
    (B) $2\frac{13}{24}$
    (C) $2\frac{3}{4}$
    (D) $2\frac{15}{24}$

19. A floor is 25 feet wide by 36 feet long. To cover this floor with carpet will require

    (A) 100 square yards
    (B) 300 square yards
    (C) 900 square yards
    (D) 25 square yards

20. 72 divided by 0.0009 is

    (A) 0.125
    (B) 800
    (C) 80,000
    (D) 80

21. 345 safety pins at $4.15 per hundred will cost

    (A) $0.1432
    (B) $1.4320
    (C) $14.32
    (D) $143.20

22. The number that decreased by one-fifth of itself yields 132 is

    (A) 165
    (B) 198
    (C) 98
    (D) 88

23. 285 is 5 percent of

    (A) 1700
    (B) 7350
    (C) 1750
    (D) 5700

24. A store sold jackets for $65 each. The jackets cost the store $50 each. The percentage of increase of selling price over cost is

    (A) 40 percent
    (B) $33\frac{1}{2}$ percent
    (C) $33\frac{1}{3}$ percent
    (D) 30 percent

25. The denominator of a fraction is 20 more than the numerator. What is the numerator if the fraction is equivalent to $\frac{3}{5}$.

    (A) 12
    (B) 30
    (C) -50
    (D) 10

26. Which statement below is true about the inequality of $2 < \times \leq 7$.

    (A) $X < 2$
    (B) $X = 2$
    (C) X is greater than 7
    (D) $X > 2$

27. $\frac{x}{5} - 4 = 11$. Find the value of x.

    (A) 75
    (B) 3
    (C) 35
    (D) 59

28. A punch recipe for a half gallon (64 ounces) of punch requires one pint (16 ounces) of grape juice. How many quarts (1 quart = 32 ounces) of grape juice are required for $2\frac{1}{2}$ gallons of the punch.

    (A) 5 quarts
    (B) 10 quarts
    (C) $1\frac{1}{4}$ quarts
    (D) $2\frac{1}{2}$ quarts

29. Mrs. Bowler got up at 7:00 A.M. last Wednesday morning and went to bed at 11:00 P.M. Wednesday night. During the time that she was up, she spent $\frac{1}{2}$ her time at work, $\frac{1}{8}$ her time bowling with friends, and $\frac{1}{4}$ her time with her family. How much time did she have left for other activities?

    (A) 2 hours
    (B) 4 hours
    (C) 1 hour
    (D) 8 hours

30. If 24 percent of the students who enrolled in an algebra class of 50 students dropped the course before the semester ended, how many students remained in the class?

    (A) 27
    (B) 76
    (C) 12
    (D) 38

31. How many $\frac{3}{4}$-gram tablets are needed for a dosage of $4\frac{1}{2}$ grams?

    (A) 3.75
    (B) 1.5
    (C) 6
    (D) 3

32. $3.6 - 1.2(.8 - .3) + 8 \div .4 =$

    (A) 23
    (B) 20.5
    (C) 50
    (D) 3.2

33. Find .2 percent of 400.

    (A) 80
    (B) 800
    (C) .8
    (D) 2000

34. What percent of a circle is a central angle of 72°?

    (A) 5 percent
    (B) 20 percent
    (C) 72 percent
    (D) 1/5 percent

35. Find the length of the hypotenuse in the triangle below.

    (A) 7
    (B) 5
    (C) 25
    (D) 6

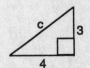

36. What is the width of a rectangle with an area of 63 square feet and a length of 9 feet?

    (A) 22.5 feet
    (B) 7 feet
    (C) 567 feet
    (D) 144 feet

37. If the triangles below are similar, find the length of side x

    (A) 21 inches
    (B) 11 inches
    (C) 13 inches
    (D) $3\frac{6}{7}$ inches

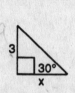 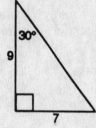

38. If two lines are parallel, the following statements are true:

    (A) The two lines have equal slopes.
    (B) The two lines have one point in common.
    (C) The product of the slopes of the lines is −1.
    (D) The two lines form right angles.

39. If the area of a square is 144 m^2, what is the length of a side of the square?

    (A) 12 m
    (B) 12 m^2
    (C) 72 m
    (D) 72 m^2

40. Find the area of the figure below.

    (A) 40 m
    (B) 46 m
    (C) 80 m^2
    (D) 96 m^2

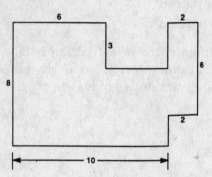

Consider the circle with central angles shown below:

41. What percent of the circle does the central angle of 60° represent? (give answer to the nearest degree)

    (A) 6%
    (B) 60%
    (C) 17%
    (D) 25%

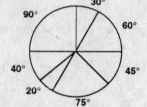

42. If $\frac{1}{12}$ of a family's weekly budget is spent on entertainment and $\frac{1}{8}$ of the budget is spent on gasoline, which central angle represents the total spent on entertainment and gasoline?

    (A) 20
    (B) 45
    (C) 90
    (D) 75

Part II—Quantitative Comparisons

15 Minutes   12 Questions

Common Information: *In each question, information concerning one or both of the quantities to be compared is given in the ITEM column. A symbol that appears in any column represents the same thing in column A as it does in column B.*

FIGURES: Assume that the position of points, angles, regions, and so forth, are in the order shown; that the lines shown as straight are indeed straight; that figures lie in a plane unless otherwise indicated. Figures accompanying questions are intended to provide information you can use in answering the questions. However, unless a note states that a figure is drawn to scale, you should solve the problems by using your knowledge of mathematics, and NOT by estimating sizes by sight or by measurement.

Directions: *For each of the following questions two quantities are given: one in Column A and one in Column B. Compare the two quantities and mark your answer sheet with the correct, lettered conclusion. These are your options:*

A: *if the quantity in Column A is the greater;*
B: *if the quantity in Column B is the greater;*
C: *if the two quantities are equal;*
D: *if the relationship cannot be determined from the information given.*

ITEM	Column A	Column B
1. $n < 0$ $a < 0$	$n + a$	$n - a$
2.	The average of: 22, 24, 26, 28, 30	The average of: 17, 19, 21, 23, 25, 27, 29, 31, 33
3.	$N - C$	$90°$

4. $0 < y < 5$ $0 < n < 7$	y	n
5. $5n - 5a = 25$	n	a

6. In isosceles △NCY:

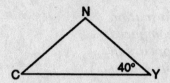

C   Y

7. $\dfrac{m}{2} = c^2$ m c

ITEM	Column A	Column B
8.	c	a

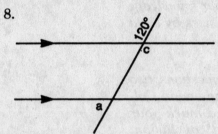

9. 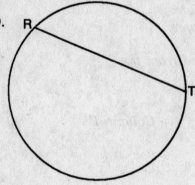   arc RT   chord RT

10. $5 + 16(3 - 2)$ $21 + 5 - 3(4 - 3)(0)$

11. $8[2x - 3(4x - 6) - 9]$ $6[3x - 2(6x - 3) + 2]$

12. h y

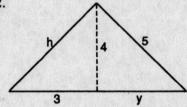

Answer Key

Part I

1. C	9. D	17. D	25. B	33. C	41. C
2. C	10. C	18. B	26. D	34. B	42. D
3. D	11. D	19. A	27. A	35. B	
4. B	12. A	20. C	28. D	36. B	
5. B	13. A	21. C	29. A	37. D	
6. A	14. A	22. A	30. D	38. A	
7. B	15. C	23. D	31. C	39. A	
8. B	16. B	24. D	32. A	40. C	

Part II

1. B	5. A	9. A
2. A	6. D	10. B
3. C	7. D	11. D
4. D	8. A	12. A

Explanatory Answers

Part I

1. **(C)** $I = P \times R \times T$
   $= \$225,000 \times 0.135 \times 1$ (year)
   $= \$30,375$

2. **(C)** 14% of $x = \$140$ Let x be
   $0.04 \times x = \$140$ the total sales
   $x = 1000$ divide by 0.04

3. **(D)** 25% of $\$200 = .25 \times \$200 = \$50$

   Next, first find 20% discount on $200:

   $0.20 \times \$200 = \$40$

   The list price is $\$200 - \$40 = \$160$
   Now take 5% of $160:

   $0.05 \times \$160 = \$8$

   The discount is $48 when taken at 20%
   and 5% successively.
   $\$50 - \$48 = \$2.$

4. **(B)** The job took 9 days to complete.

   A worked 5 days: he completed $\frac{5}{9}$ of the work.
   B worked 4 days: he completed $\frac{4}{9}$ of the work.

   If the net profit was $243, then

   A received $\frac{5}{9} \times \$243 = \$135$

5. **(B)** $\$76.50 \div 42\frac{1}{2}\text{¢/yard}$
   $(42\frac{1}{2}\text{¢} = \$0.425)$
   $= \$76.50 \div \$0.425/\text{yard}$
   $= 180$ yards

6. **(A)** Discount = 20%
   Sale price = 80%

   0.80 of $\$280.00 = \$224.00$

7. **(B)** $\frac{n}{6} + \frac{n}{3} = 1$

   $n + 2n = 6$ multiply by 6
   $3n = 6$ combine like terms
   $n = 2$ divide by 3

8. **(B)** Area of a rectangle is
   $A = length \times width$
   $= 40$ inches $\times$ 20 inches
   $= 800$ square inches

Note: 1 square foot = 144 square inches
   800 square inches
   $\dfrac{800 \text{ square inches}}{144 \text{ square inches}} = 5.5$ square feet

9. **(D)** $\dfrac{2}{3} \times \dfrac{8}{8} = \dfrac{16}{24}$ lowest common denominator is 24

   $+ \quad \dfrac{1}{8} \times \dfrac{3}{3} = \dfrac{3}{24}$

   $\rule{3cm}{0.4pt}$

   $= \dfrac{19}{24}$

10. **(C)** To arrive at the average, add all numbers and divide by total number of grades.

    $\begin{array}{r} 80 \\ 80 \\ 90 \\ \underline{90} \\ 340 \div 4 = 85 \end{array}$

11. **(D)** The number of quarters must be even; otherwise, adding dimes will not give $2.00 *exactly*.
    So the answer cannot be 3, choice (D).

    $3 \times 25\text{¢} = 75\text{¢}$ or 0.75
    $\$2.00 - 0.75 = \$1.25$
    $1.25 cannot be changed to all dimes.

12. **(A)** Let the *number* be x. A *number* increased by $\frac{1}{6}$ of itself is 182. To put this in equation form:

    $x + \dfrac{1}{6x} = 182$
    $6x + x = 1092$ Multiply each term by 6
    $7x = 1092$ Combine like terms
    $x = 156$ Divide by 7

13. **(A)** $.16\frac{3}{4} = 16\frac{3}{4}\%$

    When changing decimals to percents, move the decimal to the right two places.

14. **(A)** $\$40 \times \frac{3}{8} = \$15.$
    $\$40 - \$15 = \$25$

15. **(C)** $\begin{array}{r} \$1296.53 \\ -264.87 \\ \hline \$1031.66 \end{array}$

146

16. **(B)**

$$12\tfrac{1}{2} = 12\tfrac{2}{4}$$
$$-6\tfrac{1}{4} = -6\tfrac{1}{4}$$
$$\overline{\phantom{-6\tfrac{1}{4} =\ } 6\tfrac{1}{4}}$$

Note: $\tfrac{1}{2} \times \tfrac{2}{2} = \tfrac{2}{4}$

17. **(D)** Price per dozen can be found by multiplying the $1.29 by 4. (There are 4 groups of 3 in a dozen.)

$1.25 \times 4 = $5.16

18. **(B)** $\tfrac{1}{4} + \tfrac{7}{12} + \tfrac{3}{8} + \tfrac{1}{2} + \tfrac{5}{6}$

Note: The lowest common denominator is 24. Each fraction needs to be rewritten to an equivalent fraction, so the denominator will be 24.

$$= \frac{6 + 14 + 9 + 12 + 20}{24} = \frac{61}{24}$$

Divide:

$$= 24\overline{)61}\text{ or } 2\tfrac{13}{24}$$
$$\underline{48}$$
$$13$$

19. **(A)** 25 feet $\times$ 36 feet $=$ 900 square feet
Now change 900 square feet to square yards.
Note: 9 square feet $=$ 1 square yard

$$900 \text{ square feet} \times \frac{1 \text{ square yard}}{9 \text{ square feet}}$$

$= 100$ square yards

20. **(C)**

$$.0009\overline{)72.0000} \text{ or } 80{,}000$$
$$80000.$$

21. **(C)** One safety pin cost:
$4.15 $\div$ 100 = $.0415
So 345 costs:
$345 \times 0.0415 = $14.32

22. **(A)** A number, x, that decreased by $\tfrac{1}{5}$ of itself equals 132, can be expressed as:

$$x - \frac{1x}{5} = 132$$

$5x - x = 660$ multiply each term by 5
$4x = 660$ combine like terms
$x = 165$ divide by 4

23. **(D)** $285 = 0.05y$ y is the unknown value
$5700 = y$ divide by 0.05

24. **(D)** $65 - $50 = $15 is the increase, but to find the percentage of increase, we divide the increase by the original amount:
$15 $\div$ $50 = 0.30 or 30%

25. **(B)** Let x represent the numerator of the fraction, then the denominator will be $x + 20$. Since the fraction is equivalent to $\tfrac{3}{5}$, we get

$$\frac{x}{x + 20} = \frac{3}{5}$$

$5x = 3(x + 20)$
$5x = 3x + 60$
$2x = 60$
$x = 30$

26. **(D)** $2 < x \le 7$ means that x is greater than 2 and it is less than or equal to 7.

27. **(A)**

$$\frac{x}{5} - 4 = 11$$

$$\frac{x}{5} - 4 + 4 = 11 + 4$$

$$\frac{x}{5} = 15$$

$$5 \cdot \frac{x}{5} = 5 \cdot 15$$

$$x = 75$$

28. **(D)** Note that one gallon of punch contains 128 ounces (one-half gallon contains 64 ounces). Hence $2\tfrac{1}{2}$ gallons equals 320 ounces. A direct proportion can be used to solve the problem.

Let $x =$ the number of ounces of grape juice needed.

$$\frac{16 \text{ ounces grape}}{64 \text{ ounces punch}} = \frac{x}{320 \text{ ounces punch}}$$
$$\frac{1}{4} = \frac{x}{320}$$

$4x = 320$
$x = 80$ ounces grape juice

Since the answer is to be given in quarts, change 80 ounces to quarts by dividing 80 by 32. (There are 32 ounces in a quart.)
$80 $\div$ 32 = 2.5$, thus 2.5 quarts of grape juice are needed to make $2\tfrac{1}{2}$ gallons of punch.

29. **(A)** There are 16 hours from 7:00 A.M. until 11:00 P.M. Hence Mrs. Bowler was up 16 hours.

Let x = the time Mrs. Bowler had left for other activities, then

$\frac{1}{2}(16) + \frac{1}{8}(16) + \frac{1}{4}(16) + x = 16$

$8 + 2 + 4 + x = 16$

$14 + x = 16$

$x = 2$

30. **(D)** 24 percent of the 50 students dropped the class.
24 percent of 50 = .24 × 50 = 12.

Since 12 students dropped, 50 − 12 or 38 students remained in the class.

31. **(C)** Divide $4\frac{1}{2}$ by $\frac{3}{4}$. (First change $4\frac{1}{2}$ to $\frac{9}{2}$)

$4\frac{1}{2} \div \frac{3}{4} = \frac{9}{2} \times \frac{4}{3} = \frac{36}{6} = 6$

32. **(A)** $3.6 - 1.2(.8 - .3) + 8 \div .4$

$= 3.6 - 1.2(.5) + 8 \div .4$

$= 3.6 - .6 + 8 \div .4$

$= 3.6 - .6 + 20$

$= 3 + 20$

$= 23$

Note that operations must be performed in the correct order. (Parentheses first, then multiplication and division before addition and subtraction.)

33. **(C)** Change .2 percent to a decimal and multiply .2 percent by 400.
.002 × 400 = .800 or .8

34. **(B)** A complete circle has 360°. 72° is $\frac{1}{5}$ of a circle.

$\frac{72}{360} = \frac{1}{5}$

Change $\frac{1}{5}$ to a percent.

$\frac{1}{5}$ = 20 percent. Thus, 72° is 20 percent of a circle.

35. **(B)** Use the Pythagorean theorem
$c^2 = a^2 + b^2$

$c^2 = 3^2 + 4^2$

$c^2 = 9 + 16$

$c^2 = 25$

$c = \sqrt{25}$

$c = 5$

36. **(B)** The formula for the area of a rectangle is $A = LW$. We know the area of the rectangle is 63 and the length is 9 feet. Thus,

$63 \text{ square feet}^2 = 9W \text{ feet}$

$\frac{63 \text{ square feet}}{9 \text{ feet}} = \frac{9W \text{ feet}}{9 \text{ feet}}$

$7 \text{ ft} = W$

37. **(D)** The corresponding sides of similar triangles are proportional. Therefore,

$\frac{3}{7} = \frac{x}{9}$

$7x = 27$

$x = 3\frac{6}{7}$

38. **(A)** Parallel lines have equal slopes, they do not intersect.

39. **(A)** The area of a square is found by squaring a side of the square.

If $A = 144 \; m^2$

$144 \; m^2 = s^2$ where s is a side of the square

$\sqrt{144 \; m^2} = s$

$12 \; m = s$

40. **(C)** Divide the figure into nonoverlapping rectangles. Find the area of each rectangle. Add the areas of the rectangles to get the total area of the figure.

$A = 48m^2 + 20m^2 + 12m^2 = 80m^2$

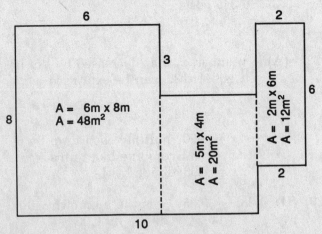

41. **(C)** The entire circle contains 360°. The central angle of 60° represents $\frac{60}{360} = \frac{1}{6}$. Change $\frac{1}{6}$ to a percent by dividing the denominator into the numerator. Thus $\frac{1}{6} = 16\frac{2}{3}\%$. We get 17 when we express $16\frac{2}{3}$ to the nearest whole percent.

42. **(D)** The weekly budget is represented by the entire circle. $\frac{1}{12}$ of the circle represents $\frac{1}{12} \times 360 = 30°$, which is the measure of the central angle for the amount spent on entertainment. $\frac{1}{8}$ of the circle represents $\frac{1}{8} \times 360 = 45°$, which is the measure of the central angle for the amount spent on gasoline. A central angle which represents the total spent on entertainment and gasoline is $30° + 45° = 75°$. (Alternately, $\frac{1}{8} + \frac{1}{12} = \frac{5}{24}$ and $\frac{5}{24} \times 360° = 75°$.)

PART II

1. **(B)** Both n and a are negative because they are both less than 0. Hence $(n - a)$ must be greater than $(n + a)$ because a negative minus a negative is greater than a negative plus a negative.

   $-a > +a$ ($-a$ = positive, $+a$ = negative)

   $n - a > n + a$ (adding n to both sides)

2. **(A)** The average of Column A is 26, while the average of Column B is 25.

3. **(C)**

   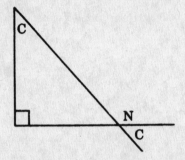

   $\angle N = \angle C = 90°$ an exterior angle is equal to the sum of the interior remote angles

   $\angle N - \angle C = 90°$ when equals are subtracted from equals, the differences are equal

4. **(D)** It is impossible to determine because y could be any number from 0 to 5 and n any number from 0 to 7.

5. **(A)** $5n - 5a = 25$

   $n - a = 5$ equals divided by equals are equals

   $n = a + 5$ equals plus equals are equal

   n is five greater than a.

6. **(D)** An isosceles triangle has two equal angles, but from the information given it is impossible to determine which two angles are actually equal.

7. **(D)** There is insufficient information to determine whether m or c is the greater. By substituting numbers for m and c, we see that either quantity could be greater—for example (1) $m = 2, c = 1$; (2) $m = \frac{1}{8}, c = \frac{1}{4}$.

8. **(A)**

   $\angle c = 120°$ and $\angle a = \angle a_1$ all vertical angles are equal

   $\angle c + \angle a_1 = 180°$ the two interior angles on the same side of a tranversal are supplementary

   $\angle a_1 = 60°$

   $\angle a = 60° < \angle c = 120°$

9. **(A)** The shortest distance between two points is a straight line. Therefore the chord, a straight line, must be shorter than the arc.

10. **(B)** $5 + 16(3 - 2) = 5 + 16(1)$
    $= 5 + 16$
    $= 21$

    $21 + 5 - 3(4 - 3)(0) = 21 + 5 - 0$
    $= 26$

11. **(D)** Since the value of x cannot be determined, the value of Columns A and B remain unknown.

12. **(A)** It can be readily seen that the figure consists of two 3, 4, 5 right triangles. Therefore, $h = 5$ and $y = 3$.

UNIT III   SCIENCE

INTRODUCTION

Living organisms used to be placed into either a plant kingdom or animal kingdom. However, modern classification systems are more sophisticated, and more than two kingdoms are recognized in them. The most widely accepted classification system includes five kingdoms of organisms, as presented below:

Monera   Prokaryotic (cells without a nucleus bounded by a membrane or true, membrane-bound organelles in the cytoplasm), unicellular or colonial, autotrophic or saprotrophic.

                  Includes bacteria and cyanobacteria (formerly called "blue-green algae").

Protista   Eukaryotic (cells with a nucleus bounded by a membrane and with membrane-bound organelles, such as mitochondria or chloroplasts, in the cytoplasm), unicellular or with a simple multicellular body lacking distinct tissues, autotrophic or saprotrophic or phagotrophic.

                  Includes amoebae, flagellates, ciliates, algae (except cyanobacteria), and slime molds.

Fungi   Eukaryotic, usually with a simple multicellular body in the form of a mass of slender filaments (mycelium), sometimes unicellular (e.g., yeasts), lacking chlorophyll, saprophytic, often parasitic.

                  Includes mushrooms and many types of molds.

Animalia   Eukaryotic, multicellular, body usually complex and with many types of true tissues, phagotrophic, sometimes parasitic, usually motile, cells lacking a cell wall.

                  Includes all types of animals such as sponges, worms, arthropods, and vertebrates.

Plantae   Eukaryotic, multicellular, body usually complex and usually with many types of true tissues, possessing chlorophyll, autotrophic, rarely parasitic, never motile, cells always surrounded by a cell wall made of cellulose.

                  Includes flowering plants, conifers, ferns, and mosses.

Regardless of the kingdom in which organisms are classified, all living things have certain characteristics in common. These characteristics sometimes are used to describe life: we can say that any object which exhibits all of these characteristics is alive. Organisms are always made of cells; they respond to stimuli; they produce; they exhibit growth and development; they obtain food and metabolize it for the generation of energy and the synthesis of materials for growth and life; they possess nucleic acid(s); they exhibit some adaptation to environmental conditions.

Organisms are interdependent. This can be exhibited by an indirect relationship, in which two species are adapted to occupying the same habitat, or a direct relationship, such as predation or symbiosis. In addition, organisms may have an effect on the environment, and the environment, in turn, can affect the organisms and the species which are able to live within it.

Organisms are composed of matter; all matter, whether organic or inorganic, obeys certain physical and chemical laws. Thus, the life sciences and the physical sciences are interrelated. The sciences may be described as follows:

Life sciences   The study of living things, including cellular activities; structure and function of tissues; structure and function of organs and of organ systems; psychological behavior and factors affecting all of these, such as heredity, nutrition, and environmental interaction.

Physical sciences   The study of matter and all of the interacting physical and chemical forces that affect matter, life, and the use of the earth's resources for living.

The outline below indicates some of the basic principles of the sciences with special emphasis on the descriptions of the "activities or characteristics of life" as related to humans.

I.   The cell is the basic structural and functional unit of an organism.
    A. All cells have cytoplasm and a cell membrane.
        1. *Prokaryotic cells* lack a nuclear membrane surrounding the DNA.
        2. *Eukaryotic cells* possess a nuclear membrane that surrounds the DNA and separates it from the cytoplasm, creating a well-defined nucleus.
        3. Some types of eukaryotic cells, such as red blood cells of man, lack a nucleus at maturity for functional reasons, but these cells always possess a nucleus during their development.
    B. Typical plant cells lack a centriole, but have plastids and a cell wall, while typical animal cells lack a cell wall and plastids, but possess a centriole.
    C. Reproduction of cells normally involves mitosis, a nuclear process during which nuclear materials, including DNA, are distributed equally to daughter nuclei.
        1. Mitosis may occur without division of the cell, leading to a multinucleate cell.
        2. DNA replicates itself during interphase, before the nucleus enters the mitotic process.
    D. The sum total of cellular functions comprises the functions of the tissues or organ.
        1. The cellular functions are accomplished by one or more parts, or *organelles,* of the cell.
            a. The cell membrane is differentially permeable and functions in regulating the passage of materials into and out of the cell.

(1) Materials may pass through the membrane by osmosis, by diffusion, by active transport, or by some other mechanism.

b. *Mitochondria* are cellular organelles in which food is oxidized for the release of energy.

c. *Plastids* (in plants) are of different types and vary in function.

    (1) *Chloroplasts* are green plastids in which photosynthesis occurs.

    (2) *Chromoplasts* and *leucoplasts* function in storage and other processes.

d. The *endoplasmic reticulum* is a network of branching tubules composed of membrane that functions as an intracellular transport system for many types of materials. It extends throughout the cytoplasm of the cell.

e. *Ribosomes* are organelles in which protein synthesis occurs. They are typically associated with the rough endoplasmic reticulum of the cell; RNA passes over the ribosomes to "line up" the amino acids to form the protein.

f. The *Golgi apparatus* functions in collecting and preparing secretions of the cell for export outside the cell.

g. *Contractile vacuoles* are membranous sacs that maintain a proper concentration of water inside the cell by draining excess water from the cytoplasm and expelling it. They are found in many protists and some animal cells.

h. *Cilia* and *flagella* are slender projections of the cell used for movement. Flagella are longer than cilia, but both have the same internal arrangement of microtubules, the 9 + 2 pattern, and are formed by the same kind of organelle, a *kinetosome.*

i. *Centrioles* are tiny, barrel-shaped organelles similar to kinetosomes that form the *spindle apparatus* that pulls chromosomes to opposite poles of the cell during mitosis or meiosis.

j. *Phagocytic vacuoles,* also called *food vacuoles,* are membranous sacs used by some types of cells to engulf and digest food material. Cells form similar organelles called *autophagic vacuoles* to engulf, digest, and recycle worn-out cytoplasmic organelles.

k. The *nucleus* is the control center of the cell; the nuclear membrane is porous, and materials pass into and out of the nucleus through the nuclear membrane.

    (1) In eukaryotes, DNA is stored in the nucleus.

    (2) *Transcription,* or the biosynthesis of RNA from the DNA, occurs within the nucleus; the RNA travels to the ribosomes where *translation,* or the synthesis of a polypeptide, occurs.

    (3) The *nucleolus,* located within the nucleus, is the site where RNA is manufactured.

II. Animals and plants exhibit organizational levels.

  A. Unicellular organisms are composed of one cell, which accomplishes all of the functions necessary for life.

    1. Unicellular organisms may be prokaryotic, as with bacteria, or eukaryotic, as with protistans.

    a. The first indication of "division of labor" is seen in some colonial unicellular forms, in which specific cells are concerned with the specific functions.

  B. Organisms at the tissue level of organization have well-developed tissues, some of which may be specialized for certain functions, but do not have well-developed organs.

C. The organ level of organization indicates the presence of well-developed organs.

D. Most animals, from round and segmented worms to vertebrates, are characterized by the system level of organization in which organs are arranged to accomplish a multiphase process.

III. All organisms exhibit response to stimuli.

A. Response involves reception of a stimulus, transmission of the impulse, and reaction to the stimulus.

1. In higher animals, such as humans, well-developed sense organs may be involved in the reception of stimuli; these include the skin, eye, ear.

a. Primitive sense organs may be seen in lower animals; in some lower animals, the sense organs may be well developed.

b. Sensory organelles may be seen in some unicellular forms, such as the eyespot of *Euglena*.

2. The transmission of impulses involves nerves or nerve fibers; in humans and other animals, a nervous system is involved in the transmission of impulses.

a. Transmission of nerve impulses is electrical, and involves a difference in the concentration of certain ions, especially potassium and sodium, along the nerve fibers.

3. Reaction to stimuli may involve a change in position, in movement, and in secretory activities. Thus, the skeletal system, muscle system, endocrine glands, and digestive glands may be involved in reactions, as exhibited by humans and other higher animals.

a. Other systems which may be indirectly involved in reactions are the circulatory system, the respiratory system, and the excretory system.

IV. All organisms exhibit reproduction; this keeps the species or population extant. Reproduction may be sexual or asexual.

A. Asexual reproduction occurs by means of mitosis and does not involve a union of reproductive cells (gametes) or gametic nuclei.

1. The following are types of asexual reproduction:

a. *Sporulation* involves the production of asexual reproductive cells (or multicellular units) called spores; these spores develop directly into new individuals.

b. *Binary fission* involves the division of the organism (usually unicellular) into two organisms. In the case of unicellular eukaryotes, binary fission usually involves mitosis.

c. *Multiple fission,* or *fragmentation,* as seen in lower organisms such as filamentous algae, involves the breaking of the organism into smaller units, each of which can develop into a new organism.

d. *Budding* involves the production of an outgrowth or miniature organism which breaks away from the parent and develops into a new adult.

B. Sexual reproduction involves meiosis followed by fertilization, meaning the union of entire reproductive cells (gametes) or gametic nuclei.

1. Several types of sexual reproduction may be described, depending on the morphology of the gametes.

    a. *Isogamy* is reproduction involving fusion of morphologically identical gametes; this is more common among lower plants.

    b. *Heterogamy* is sexual reproduction involving fusion of gametes which differ in size and/or structure.

       (1) One type of heterogamy involves motile gametes differing only in size; this is *anisogamy*.

       (2) The other type of heterogamy involves gametes differing in size and in structure; this is *oogamy*.

          (a) Oogamy is exhibited by man; the gamete produced by the male is the spermatozoon; the gamete produced by the female is the ovum or egg.

          (b) In animals such as man, gametes are produced in gonads: the male gonads are the testes; the female gonads are the ovaries.

             i. Gonads in higher animals, such as man, also have an endocrine function, producing hormones involved with the appearance of secondary sex characteristics and with reproductive cycles.

    c. *Conjugation* is sexual reproduction involving a temporary union of cells for exchange or transmission of nuclei or DNA.

  2. Meiosis is involved in the production of gametes or of spores in the case of most plants.

    a. Gametes are haploid, having one-half the chromosome number characteristic of the zygote of the species.

    b. The diploid number is restored to the zygote (the cells resulting from gametic union, or *syngamy*) when fertilization occurs.

    c. The zygote typically develops mitotically into the embryo; thus, there is no further change in chromosome number.

    d. Because of meiosis and syngamy, the individual developing from the zygote receives one-half of its DNA from each parent; thus, the chromosome number for the species remains constant.

    e. Sexual reproduction allows the spread of changes through a population.

V. Growth and development allow for the characteristic size range of a species to be maintained and for the differentiation of organs and tissues to be accomplished.

  A. In multicellular organisms, growth may involve an increase in the number of cells, an increase in the size of cells, or both.

  B. The zygote develops mitotically into a multicellular organism. In man and other multicellular organisms, development, or differentiation, accompanies growth.

  C. In higher animals, such as man, the basic development patterns are similar.

    1. The zygote undergoes cleavage to produce a cluster of cells known as a *morula*.

    2. The morula develops into a *blastula* or *blastocyst*; this is a hollow ball of cells with a cavity known as a *blastocoel*.

    3. The blastula develops into a two-layered *gastrula* with a cavity known as a *gastrocoel* or *archenteron*.

a. The outer germ layer of the gastrula is the *ectoderm*.

b. The inner germ layer of the gastrula is the *endoderm*.

c. The third germ layer, *mesoderm*, develops between the ectoderm and the endoderm.

4. Each germ layer gives rise to definite body structures and tissues.

a. From the ectoderm develops the nervous system, some sense organs such as the eye, and the outer skin.

b. From the mesoderm develops the muscle system, skeletal system, muscle of the viscera, mesenteries, and circulatory system.

c. From the endoderm develops the lining of the digestive tract, the lungs, much of the liver and pancreas, the thyroid, parathyroid, and thymus glands.

VI. Nutritional processes, involving the obtaining and utilizing of food, are exhibited by all organisms.

A. Food may be defined as any substance which can be used by the organism as a source of energy and as a source of materials for growth and maintenance of the body.

1. Food is organic; the process involving the conversion of inorganic materials into organic foods is photosynthesis.

a. This process occurs only in green plants, in the presence of the chlorophylls and in the presence of light as an energy source.

(1) The chloroplast is the cellular organelle in which photosynthesis occurs.

b. All organisms (except for a few algae and prokaryotes which may exhibit similar processes) depend directly or indirectly on photosynthesis for food.

B. Organisms obtain food in some way.

1. Autotrophs, such as green plants, manufacture food within their bodies from inorganic environmental materials.

2. Heterotrophs receive organic food from the environment.

a. Saprotrophs digest food externally and absorb the digested food into the body; most bacteria and fungi are saprotrophs.

b. Parasites live on and at the expense of a host.

c. Phagotrophs, such as man and most animals, ingest solid food into a digestive cavity of some sort.

(1) The digestive cavity of phagotrophic protozoa may be a food vacuole; this is characteristic of the cellular level of organization.

(2) The digestive cavity of simple animals such as coelenterates and flatworms is a gastrovascular cavity with a mouth as its only opening; this is characteristic of the tissue level of organization or simpler versions of the system level.

(3) The digestive cavity of humans and most other animals is a complete digestive tract (digestive system) with a mouth at one end and an anus at the other end; this is characteristic of the system level of organization.

C. Food which has been obtained must be digested, changed into a usable, absorbable state. This occurs in the digestive system in humans.

1. In lower animals, digestion occurs in a food vacuole, (as in protozoa) a gastrovascular cavity, or a simple gut.

D. The digested food is distributed throughout the body to the cells.

1. In humans, the circulatory or vascular system distributes the food to the cells.

E. Utilization of food, or *metabolism*, occurs in the cells.

1. Oxidation of glucose within the cells, (in the mitochondria), yields energy for life and for life's activities.

a. Aerobic oxidation is most common, involving the use of free, molecular oxygen. Enzymes control each step of oxidation.

(1) Oxygen is made available by means of respiratory organs, or, in the case of humans, the respiratory system.

(2) Oxygen is absorbed from air inhaled into the lungs of man and transported to the cells by means of the circulatory system.

(a) In man, oxygen is transported in combination with hemoglobin of the red blood cells.

(3) Carbon dioxide resulting from the oxidation of glucose is transported by the blood stream to the lungs for elimination through exhalation.

(4) As a result of oxidation of glucose, the energy transporting substance, adenosine triphosphate (ATP) is formed. ATP transfers energy to the areas that need it or to specialized areas and compounds for energy storage.

(5) Liquid waste from metabolism is collected, concentrated, and eliminated by the excretory system.

2. The synthesis of other compounds, proteins, and secretory products occurs in the cell.

F. Solid indigestible wastes are eliminated from the digestive system; in humans, elimination occurs through the anus.

VII. Organisms must adapt to the environment in which they live in order to survive.

A. Organisms may possess or develop certain traits that enable them to live or thrive in a specific environment.

1. Changes in populations may originate and spread throughout the population, making survival and thriving a greater possibility.

a. Changes that are conducive to survival are conserved, accumulate, and may eventually lead to a new variety or race.

B. Organisms, by their presence and exploitation of an environment, may change the environment to the extent that it becomes suitable for a different group or species. Thus, succession occurs as the environment continues to change under the influence of different species, causing other species to adapt to or invade the environment.

VIII. Two types of nucleic acids are known; all organisms possess one or both types. Most organisms possess both.

A. Deoxyribonucleic acid (DNA) functions as the genetic information of an individual. Different parts of the genetic information contained in the structure of DNA can be used for the following purposes: day to day regulation of cellular processes (metabolism), development of a new individual (heredity), or manufacture of RNA. DNA is contained within the nucleus of eukaryotic cells and is attached to the inner side of the cell membrane in prokaryotic cells.

   1. DNA is a long, double-stranded, chain-like molecule that is twisted into the form of a helix (double helix). Each strand is a chain of "building units" which are smaller molecules called nucleotides.

      a. A nucleotide consists of a sugar, (deoxyribose), a phosphate, and a purine or pyrimidine base.

         (1) The purine bases are *guanine* and *adenine*.

         (2) The pyrimidine bases are *cytosine* and *thymine*.

   2. DNA is the pattern or template from which complementary RNA (ribonucleic acid) is synthesized.

      a. RNA is similar in structure to DNA except that it is much smaller and consists of only one strand. Like DNA, the single strand of RNA is a chain of nucleotides.

         (1) The purine bases of RNA nucleotides are *guanine* and *adenine*.

         (2) The pyrimidine bases of RNA nucleotides are *cytosine* and *uracil*.

      b. There are three types of RNA and all of them play essential roles in protein synthesis. Together, DNA and RNA form a system for the storage and use of information needed to make the proper structure of each of the many different types of proteins used by a individual organism.

         (1) Messenger RNA serves as the actual pattern or template for the sequential arrangement of amino acids into a chain to make a protein. The information in a molecule of messenger RNA is copied from part of a DNA molecule (transcription); this information is equivalent to a *gene* or a group of related genes.

         (2) Transfer RNA carries amino acids to specific complementary spots on the messenger RNA template, insuring that amino acids are placed in the correct sequence for a particular protein (translation).

         (3) Ribosomal RNA is the key component of ribosomes which are the cellular sites for the synthesis of proteins.

Of major concern in the health sciences is an understanding of how man functions biologically, psychologically, and socially. Man's behavior is influenced by his environment; thus, the "laws of nature" apply to man as well as to other organisms and to the matter making up his environment. It is necessary, therefore, for a person involved in the health sciences to have knowledge of the physical sciences as well as of the life sciences.

The following chart demonstrates the interrelationships between the sciences and man's existence.

CONCEPTS RELATED TO HEALTH SCIENCES

Concepts	Related Topics

I. Concepts about man
    A. Develops from a single cell (zygote).
        1. Reproduction is a basic function of life.
            a. Man reproduces by sexual reproduction (mating), the union of male and female sex cells.
            b. Man transmits like characteristics to offspring.
        2. Heredity, the transmission of traits, can be explained in terms of
            a. Mendel's Law
            b. Gene theory
            c. Blending
            d. Meiosis
            e. Chromosomal influence in sex determination.
        3. Deoxyribonucleic acid (DNA) is the only known type of self-duplicating molecule and plays a central role in heredity by ensuring the orderly development of offspring into a form similar to that of their parents.
        4. Fertilization produces a zygote which then begins to grow by mitosis, the first stage of life of the embryo.
        5. Mature cells group together in distinct patterns to form tissues. Tissues unite to form organs, and organs unite to form the lifesystems of the body.
    B. Life processes based on metabolism
        1. All human cells must utilize oxygen through respiration, receive nutrition through digestive processes, eliminate wastes, and grow to their potential stage of maturity.
        2. These life processes involve chemical changes (called *metabolism*) that are controlled by enzymes.
        3. The energy needed for life-processes in man cames from food: proteins, carbohydrates, and fats. Energy from food is used to make adenosine triphosphate (ATP), which is used as a universally available source of energy in all cells of the body.
        4. The cell constantly interacts with its environment through the processes of osmosis and diffusion.
	Cell structure
	Similarities and differences in animal and plant cellular activities
	
	Animal cell division
	
	Plant cell division
	Mutations
	
	Dominant and recessive genes
	Hybrids
	Punnett Square
	
	Role of RNA and DNA
	
	Fetal development
	
	Energy transfer mechanisms in living cells
	ATP cycle
	Aerobic and anaerobic respiration
	Oxidation of carbohydrates
	Photosynthesis
	
	Protein and lipid synthesis
	Classification systems for living organisms

Concepts	Related Topics
5. All cellular functions depend on specific types of proteins, especially enzymes. By controlling the manufacture of specific proteins, DNA (with the help of RNA) is able to control all cellular functions.	
6. The maintenance of internal balance (called *homeostasis*) is a major part of metabolism. Internal conditions such as concentrations of substances in cells or body fluids, pH, and temperature are kept within narrow ranges by constant regulation. These regulatory activities always require a major expenditure of energy by the organism. Much of homeostasis is done to satisfy the requirements of enzymes, which are always sensitive to physical conditions.	
C. Life processes conducted through bodily systems.	
1. The function of the respiratory system is to transport oxygen to the blood and eliminate carbon dioxide from the blood.	Gills, lungs, and tracheae Oxygen and carbon dioxide exchange
a. The quantity of available oxygen determines the effectiveness of respiration.	Positive and negative pressure breathing; basal metabolic rates
b. Oxygen consumption is directly proportional to the rate of bodily activity and energy use.	Energy production from metabolic processes
c. Metabolic processes of the body are directly affected by oxygen supply.	Factors affecting metabolic rate
d. Changes in oxygen consumption caused by an increase or decrease in activity temporarily affect the concentration of oxygen in the blood, which is then restored to normal by an increase or decrease in respiratory rate.	
2. The circulatory system transports all nutrients to the cells and wastes from the cells.	Rhythmic beating of heart Structure of arteries and veins Location of major blood vessels
a. The force of the circulatory flow (blood pressure) is created by the pumping of the heart. This force delivers blood to the capillaries where exchange of materials between the blood and tissues takes place.	
b. The stimulation of the heart comes from within the heart muscle, but the rate of beating is modified by chemicals (hormones) and nerve transmissions from the brain.	Capillary as medium for exchange
c. The rate of blood flow through the vessels is directly proportional to blood pressure and is partially maintained by the closed nature of the cardiovascular circuit.	Electrolytes Acids and bases

Concepts	Related Topics
d. The volume of blood pumped through the cardiovascular circuit per unit of time is directly proportional to blood pressure.	Hyper- and hypothermia Blood typing–Rh factor
e. Arteries are able to change their internal diameter by constriction or dilation; blood pressure is inversely proportional to the diameter of arteries.	Clotting mechanism
f. In capillaries, exchange of materials between the blood and tissues is accomplished by a combination of blood pressure, diffusion, and osmosis.	Body defenses in blood and lymph
g. Blood is returned to the heart through veins by the passive mechanisms of pushing from behind, squeezing of veins by skeletal muscles, and gravity.	Distribution of body fluids
3. The digestive system breaks down foods and delivers the nutrients to the circulatory system.	Solid and liquid components of blood
a. Food must be ingested into the system, mixed with digestive substances, broken down chemically (digestion), and selectively absorbed into the blood stream.	Materials required for plant growth (auxins, vitamins, etc.) Variations in digestive systems of living organisms.
b. The rate of digestion is directly related to the quantity of food.	a. Utilization of large quantities of food.
c. The lining of the alimentary tube provides mucus to lubricate the passage of food and protect the lining itself from enzymes or acid.	b. Utilization of fluids and soft tissues.
d. Chemical breakdown is the result of enzymes and activators.	Chemical digestion of carbohydrates, proteins, and fats
e. Nutrients are stored in the liver for reserve supply.	Role of vitamins and minerals Hydrolysis
f. Waste products are eliminated through the colon.	Structure formula and isomerism a. hydrocarbons b. halogen derivatives c. alcohols and phenols d. aldehydes and phenols e. amino acids f. heterocyclics g. lipids h. organometallics i. nucleic acid
4. The excretory (renal) system removes metabolic wastes and excess substances from the body.	Invertebrate mechanisms for excretion
a. The kidneys selectively absorb wastes and excess substances from the blood to form urine.	Role of nephron unit in homeostasis Filtration and dialysis Artificial kidney
b. The kidneys selectively reabsorb substances needed by the body and return them to the blood.	Excretion of wastes through skin

Concepts	Related Topics
c. Selective reabsorbtion conserves water and electrolytes, which balances their concentrations in the blood and tissues.	
d. The circulating volume of the blood has a direct affect on kidney activity.	
e. The ureters connect the kidneys to the bladder, a receptacle for holding urine.	
f. Micturition (urination) is a reflex action.	
5. The endocrine system regulates body activities.	Interrelationships of endocrine glands
a. Endocrine glands secrete hormones into the blood and tissues.	Function of insulin, thyroxin, parathyrin
b. Hormonal secretion is activated by chemical and neural factors.	Role of pituitary gland
	Sex hormones
c. Hormones regulate primary metabolic processes.	Steroids
	Release of energy by adrenalin
d. Hypo- or hyperactivity of endocrine glands results in disorders.	
6. The musculoskeletal system generates motion and maintains posture.	Location of bones in the skeleton and functional relationships of bones to one another
	Ligaments and joints
a. The bones and muscles are combined into individual lever systems to produce motion.	
b. In the human body, a lever system consists of a muscle (force), joint (fulcrum), and a bone (lever). The arrangement of a lever system permits movement with a minimal expenditure of energy.	Function of red and yellow marrow
c. Joints act as points of balance and are also sculptured to regulate the extent or direction of movement.	Smooth and striated muscles
d. Change in position is produced by a shift of weight accomplished by muscular force.	Major muscles of the body and functional relationships of muscles to bones
e. The longer the axis of the lever (bone) being moved, the greater the extent of movement.	Principles of energy and work
f. The use of muscular force consumes a large amount of energy and results in much waste heat, used to maintain body temperature, as a byproduct.	
7. The nervous system provides a means of internal communication that controls and coordinates all bodily activities in response to environmental stimuli.	Plant stimulus-response systems
	Responses to light, temperature, touch, and other physical conditions
a. Impulses travel along neurons (nerve cells).	Sensory and motor organs
b. Neurons are grouped together to form the central nervous system (brain and spinal cord) and nerves which connect the central nervous system to all parts of the body.	Brain centers
	Spinal nerves
c. Stimuli are changes in either the external or internal environment.	Cranial nerves

Concepts	Related Topics
d. The central nervous system receives stimuli and ensures that a proper response is given to each one.	Autonomic nervous system
e. Responses are initiated through the central nervous system and consist of either a muscular movement or secretion of a substance by a gland.	
II. Human potential for adaptation	Ecological balance
A. Interdependent relationships with other living forms	Producers, consumers, decomposers
1. Humans, like other living things, form complex relationships with the environment.	Movement of energy through ecosystems
2. The kinds and amount of life found in different environments is determined by temperature, moisture, sunlight, and soil.	Biomes
3. Humans, like other animals, depend on animal and plant sources of food (food chains).	Climatic effects on life processes
4. Only organisms with chlorophylls, such as plants, can make food.	Composition of sea water
5. Food chains exist because all living things need energy.	a. sodium chloride b. magnesium
6. The survival of humankind (and species in general) is influenced by other species in the same environment.	c. calcium d. sulfur e. oxygen
7. Living organisms in the same environment form an interrelated community in which many species out of the total number live in close associations with one another (symbiosis). Most of these symbiotic associations constitute mutualism (benefit to both partners) or parasitism (benefit to one partner at the expense of the other).	
B. Conservation of resources	Classification of matter
1. Supplies of natural resources are finite.	a. organic and inorganic
2. Population growth reduces the amount of resource available to individual humans.	b. elements, compounds, mixtures
3. Supplies of natural resources can be expanded to some extent, by new ways of increasing food production, development of new sources of energy, recycling of waste materials, conservation of natural habitats, and soil conservation.	Structure of matter a. atoms b. molecules Forms of matter a. liquid b. gas c. solid
4. Ultimately, population control is the only way to ensure adequate amounts of food, energy, and other resources for individual humans.	Changes in form a. physical b. chemical

Concepts	Related Topics
III. Human interaction with the environment 　　A. Environmental regulation of life processes 　　　1. Inorganic matter is synthesized into food for plants; plants provide food for animals 2. The physiological phenomena (assimilation, respiration, and growth) are controlled by temperature, light, moisture, nutrient supplies, and general atmospheric conditions. 　　B. Use and modification of the environment 　　　1. Humans must protect themselves from biological, physical, and radiological hazards. 　　　2. Humans must discover and develop new ways of using natural resources to minimize or reverse environmental destruction; conservation, recycling, and avoidance of "disposable" products are central elements in this strategy.	Physiology of plants Nitrogen cycle Photosynthesis Vaporization, distillation Carbon-oxygen cycle Magnetism Light, sound, electricity Pollution and pest control Gamma, Beta, Alpha rays Caustive organisms of disease Koch's postulates Natural and acquired immunity Antibiotics and disinfectants Sterilization, pasteurization, refrigeration Community characteristics, principle of succession Solar energy, heat production, transfer convection Nuclear fission

SCIENCE GLOSSARY

Items in capitals have a special entry in the glossary.

A

absolute zero
The lowest temperature which a gas can attain. This is 460 degrees below zero on the FAHRENHEIT scale and 273 degrees below zero on the CELSIUS scale.

absorption
The movement of water and/or dissolved substances into a cell, tissue, or organism.

acceleration
A change in the speed of an object. If the object speeds up, this is called *positive acceleration*. If the object goes slower, it is called *negative acceleration*.

acid
A compound with a pH less than 7, which means that it releases hydrogen ions when dissolved in water. An acid changes blue litmus paper to red.

acquired immunity
Immunity that is not natural or congenital; immunity obtained after birth.

active immunity
Immunity brought about by activity of certain cells of the body as a result of being exposed to an antigen.

active transport
An energy-requiring process by means of which materials are moved across a cell membrane.

adsorption
The gathering of molecules of a substance on a surface.

aerobe
Any organism living in the presence of and utilizing free, molecular oxygen (that is, oxygen not in chemical combination) in its oxidative processes.

alchemy
The science of transforming less valuable metals into gold or silver, and the philosophy behind this idea. The theories of the alchemists of the Middle Ages were false, but their experiments laid the foundation of modern chemistry.

alkali
A compound with a pH greater than 7. An alkaline substance changes red litmus paper to blue. It can combine with hydrogen. See BASE.

alkaline
A substance having the properties of an ALKALI.

allantois   One of four extraembryonic membranes attached to the body of the embryo or fetus of a land-dwelling vertebrate. In humans it is modified to form part of the placenta and umbilicus.

amino acid   An organic molecule containing an amino group (NH_2) and a carboxyl group (COOH) bonded to the same carbon atom; the "building blocks" of proteins.

amnion   The innermost of four extraembryonic membranes attached to the body of the embryo or fetus of a land-dwelling vertebrate. It forms a fluid-filled sac around the body that provides an aqueous environment and cushions the embryo from shocks.

ampere   A measurement of electric current, abbreviated *amp*. It was named after French scientist ANDRÉ MARIE AMPÈRE.

Ampère, André Marie   A French scientist (1775–1836) whose work and theory laid the foundation for the science of electrodynamics. His name lives on in the electrical measurement AMPERE.

amphipods   A crustacean group that includes sand fleas.

anaerobe   Any organism not requiring free, molecular oxygen for its cellular oxidative processes. Some anaerobes are *obligate*, and cannot survive in the presence of oxygen; others are *facultative*, and can survive with or without oxygen.

anatomy   The study of the structure of living things. Usually, "anatomy" refers to the structure of the human body.

anemone   A sea animal (a coelenterate) that resembles the flower of the same name.

antibiotic   A substance derived from lower organisms that can be used to prevent growth of certain pathogens, thus combating infection.

antibody   A specific type of protein molecule that is manufactured in the tissues, blood, or lymph in response to the presence of viruses or foreign cells. Each variety of antibody will attach to the surface of only one type of invader, enabling it to be recognized and marked for destruction by the immune system.

antigens   Protein molecules on the surface of viruses or foreign cells which provoke the manufacture of matching antibodies, enabling invaders to be recognized as such so they can be destroyed.

ATP   Adenosine triphosphate; the energy-transport compound of a cell.

atrium   The anterior chamber(s) of the heart of vertebrates.

attenuated   The state of being weakened, as in the case of pathogens used to induce active immunity.

auricle   The projecting outer portion, or pinna, of the ear.

autotroph   An organism, such as a green plant, capable of manufacturing its food from inorganic environmental materials.

B

bacteria   Unicellular, microscopic, PROKARYOTIC organisms, mostly SAPROTROPHIC or PARASITIC.

base   A compound with a pH greater than 7 that can react with an acid to form a salt. See ALKALI.

biochemistry   The study of the chemical makeup of organisms. This science is a branch of both chemistry and biology.

biology   The study of living things, a major science.

biome   A type of community recognized by certain characteristics of plants and climate, such as the plains of the Midwest.

bond   The force of attraction that holds two atoms together in a molecule. There are two major types of chemical bonds, COVALENT BONDS and IONIC BONDS.

botany   The study of plant life. Botany is a branch of BIOLOGY.

Brahe, Tycho   A Danish astronomer (1546–1601) who made a systematic study of the movement of celestial bodies. He is often referred to only as *Tycho*.

C

carbohydrate   A food substance made up of carbon, hydrogen, and oxygen.

carbon   An important chemical element that forms the basic skeleton of all ORGANIC compounds. Atoms of other elements are bonded to the carbon skeleton to form the many different varieties of organic compounds.

carbon dioxide   A compound made up of one atom of carbon and two atoms of oxygen. It exists in the form of a gas and is one of the principle waste byproducts resulting from CELLULAR RESPIRATION.

catalyst   A chemical substance which lowers the energy necessary for a chemical reaction to take place and makes the reaction proceed more rapidly. ENZYMES act as catalysts in living organisms.

celestial   An adjective referring to the sky.

cell   The basic structural and functional unit of organisms.

cellular respiration   The oxidation of glucose into carbon dioxide and water (or into other products, in the case of anaerobic respiration), leading to the release of energy.

Celsius   A system of measurement of temperature, often referred to as *centigrade*. On the Celsius scale the freezing point for water is 0 degrees and the boiling point is 100 degrees.

centriole   A cellular organelle characteristic of animal cells but not plant cells that migrates to the poles during mitosis; spindle fibers and astral rays arise from it.

centromere   The portion of the chromosome which holds the chromatids together and to which spindle fibers apparently attach.

chelicerae   The claw-like head appendages on certain arthropods, such as spiders.

chemistry   The science that studies the composition and transformation of matter; a major science.

Chlamydiae   Small intracellular obligate parasites closely related to the *Rickettsiae*.

chlorophylls   The green pigments of plants, produced in the presence of light and essential for photosynthesis.

chromosomes   Small cellular bodies containing tightly bound and packaged DNA that are formed during MITOSIS and MEIOSIS from loosely packaged DNA (chromatin). The hereditary determinants called GENES are carried on chromosomes.

colloid   A type of mixture intermediate between a SOLUTION and a SUSPENSION. It consists of liquid plus particles that are too small to settle out of the mixture and too large to dissolve. Colloids can exist in the form of a gel and pass through membranes either slowly or not at all.

commensalism   A symbiotic relationship in which one member is benefited, and the other member is neither benefited nor harmed.

compound The combination of two or more elements into a single unit.

condensation The transition of water vapor to liquid water due to a lowering of temperature.

conduction The transfer of heat from one object or physical medium to another by direct contact.

conservation of energy The principle that energy changes its form but cannot be created or destroyed.

conservation of matter The principle that matter can change its form but cannot be created or destroyed.

constellation A particular grouping of stars.

copepod A small aquatic crustacean.

Copernicus, Nicholas A Polish astronomer (1473–1543) who proposed the theory that the earth moves through space. It was generally believed up to that time that the earth was the immobile center of the universe.

cosmic year The time it takes the sun to go around its galaxy.

covalent bond A type of chemical bond created by the sharing of electrons between two atoms to achieve the maximum number of electrons in the outer electron orbit of each atom. Covalent bonds are the strongest type of chemical bonds.

crop rotation An agricultural method by which crops in an area are changed each year. This helps maintain the fertility of the soil.

crustaceans A group of aquatic animals with a hard outside covering. They are often included with mollusks in the group of "shellfish."

crystal A form of solid in which the constituent atoms or molecules are arranged in a very regular, repeating pattern.

cytoplasm In a prokaryotic cell, the entire contents of the cell contained within the plasma membrane. In a eukaryotic cell, the region of the cell lying within the plasma membrane but exterior to the nucleus.

D

Dalton, John An English chemist and physicist (1766–1844) who introduced the theory that matter is made up of atoms.

Darwin, Charles An English naturalist (1809–1883) who developed a theory of EVOLUTION.

deforestation The process by which land is cleared of forests.

density Mass per unit volume, often expressed as grams per milliliter.

dictyosome The *Golgi apparatus* of a cell, which serves as a collecting and packaging center for secretions.

diffusion The spontaneous movement of dissolved molecules from an area where they are in high concentration to an area where they are in lower concentration. This process requires no energy and, in living organisms, often takes place across semipermeable membranes.

distillation The purification of a liquid substance by heating it until it vaporizes and then cooling it to cause it to condense into liquid again.

DNA Deoxyribonucleic acid; a large, helical, double-stranded molecule in which the chromosomes code hereditary information.

dorso-ventral An adjective referring to a back-to-front plane.

E

eclipse The obscuring of a celestial body that takes place when one celestial object moves in front of another. When the moon comes between the earth and the sun, it casts a shadow, or *umbra*, on part of the earth. Since during this time the sun cannot be seen on that part of the earth, this is known as a *solar* eclipse. When the earth comes between the sun and the moon, it casts a shadow on the moon. Since the moon cannot be seen during this time, this is called a *lunar* eclipse.

Einstein, Albert A German physicist (1879–1955) who lived the last years of his life in the United States. His theories changed the field of PHYSICS. He, more than any other scientist, was responsible for nuclear fission.

electron A negatively charged particle in the atom that moves in an orbit around the NUCLEUS of the atom.

electronics   The study of the motion or movement of free electrons and ions, and the application of these phenomena to radio and television.

element   One of more than 100 known basic substances. These substances and their combinations make up all matter as far as is known.

embryology   The study of development of organisms from the time of conception.

energy   The capacity to do work.

enzyme   An organic CATALYST; specific types of proteins produced by cells that govern or otherwise affect all biological reactions. *Exoenzymes* act outside the cells that produce them, and *endoenzymes* act within the cells that produce them. Enzymes are sensitive to the pH and temperature of their environment, and deviations from the optimal pH and temperature for an enzyme will lessen its activity. The maintenance of optimal internal environments for enzymes is a major objective of HOMEOSTASIS.

erg   A unit of work or energy.

erythrocytes   Red blood cells.

eugenics   A science that deals with the improvement of hereditary qualities of a race or breed.

eukaryote   An organism characterized by cells containing a true or visible nucleus.

evaporation   The process by which liquids change to gases.

evolution, theory of   Usually refers to Darwin's theory that changes occur in populations because natural selection favors the survival of those organisms best fitted for their environment.

experiment   A test to see if an idea is true or false.

F

Fahrenheit   The system of measurement of temperature generally used in the United States. It was developed by Gabriel Fahrenheit (1686–1736), a German scientist. On the Fahrenheit scale, 32 degrees is the freezing point of water, 212 degrees is the boiling point of water, and 98.6 degrees is the average temperature of the human body. Another widely used temperature measurement is the CELSIUS scale.

Faraday, Michael   An English physicist and chemist (1791–1867) who developed the first dynamo and discovered that a magnet could induce an electric current in a conductor such as metal.

fertility   The ability to reproduce. *See* REPRODUCTION.

force   That which stops or creates motion, or changes the velocity of motion.

friction   The resistance created to the movement of an object when it rubs or collides with other objects.

fungi   A group of organisms, typically SAPROTROPHIC (or *parasitic*), many of which have a MYCELIUM. A few fungi, such as yeasts, do not have a mycelial body. *See* SAPROTROPH.

G

galaxy   A grouping of stars. Our sun is a star in the galaxy called the *Milky Way*.

Galileo   An Italian astronomer and physicist (1564–1642) who made many contributions to science. He discovered that objects of different weights and shapes fall to the ground at the same rate of speed, attracted by GRAVITY. He was a strong believer in COPERNICUS' theory that the earth moved in space and was persecuted for this belief.

gene   A hereditary determinant consisting of a segment of a DNA molecule that contains the coded information necessary for assembling a specific type of protein molecule. Each gene occupies a fixed locus on a specific CHROMOSOME, enabling the transmission of hereditary determinants from one generation to the next.

genetics   The study of HEREDITY, or the manner in which hereditary traits are passed on from one generation to the next.

genome   The genetic makeup of an individual; the genotype.

geology   The study of the formation, structure, and history of the earth.

geriatrics   The science of the diseases of aged persons.

gravitation   The tendency of objects in space to move towards each other.

gravity   The force of attraction between two bodies. It is the force that causes objects to fall to earth.

H

habitat The immediate surroundings or environment in which a particular species may live.

half-life The length of time required for the degradation to another substance of half the molecules in an amount of radioactive substance. The half-lives of radioactive ISOTOPES of elements can be used to date material containing radioactive substances. An example is the carbon-14 dating of living material.

Harvey, William An English physician and anatomist (1578–1657) who discovered how the blood moves through the body.

heat A form of energy.

hemoglobin A type of protein molecule that is bright red in color and binds reversibly to oxygen. It is carried within ERYTHROCYTES, enabling them to transport oxygen.

heredity The transmission of traits from generation to generation.

homeostasis The maintenance of internal balance by a living organism.

hormone A chemical regulator of many bodily activities. A hormone is produced by an endocrine gland.

hydrogen The chemical element with the smallest atom. It exists as a gas and is common in nature. Hydrogen is important to living organisms because it is a constituent of water and most organic compounds.

hypha A mycelial thread; one of the "strands" making up a MYCELIUM, which is a fungus body.

hypothesis An unproven explanation of something that has happened or might happen.

I

immunity Resistance to a particular disease or condition. (*See* ACTIVE, ACQUIRED, NATURAL, PASSIVE IMMUNITY).

immunization The process of making one immune, usually by the giving of antigens to induce active immunity via the production of antibodies.

immunoglobulins Antibodies.

indicator — A substance whose color is sensitive to the hydrogen-ion concentration of the solution to which it is added.

ion — An atom or radical that has acquired a positive charge by giving up or losing electron(s), or a negative charge by gaining electron(s).

ionic bond — A type of chemical bond created by one atom giving up an electron or electrons to another atom to achieve the maximum number of electrons in the electron orbit of each atom. Ionic compounds will separate in water to yield IONS. This process is called *dissociation*.

inorganic — An adjective meaning "not organic" and applying to any atom other than carbon or to a molecule not containing carbon. *See* ORGANIC.

insecticides — Chemical combinations used to destroy or control harmful insects.

interferon — An antiviral agent secreted by cells under attack from viruses.

interstellar — An adjective meaning "between stars."

isotopes — Atoms that belong to the same chemical element but have a different atomic mass.

K

Kepler, Johannes — A German astronomer (1571–1630) who made important discoveries about the orbits of planets.

kinetic energy — Energy that is in motion. The energy of a boulder tumbling down a mountainside is an example of kinetic energy. *See* POTENTIAL ENERGY.

Koch, Robert — A German doctor (1843–1910) who studied bacteria. He and LOUIS PASTEUR are considered the founders of the science of bacteriology.

L

Lamarck, Chevalier de — A French naturalist (1744–1829) who developed a theory of evolution. *See* DARWIN.

Lavoisier, Antoine — A French chemist (1743–1794) who made important discoveries concerning combustion, the conservation of matter, and the role of oxygen in respiration.

leukocytes   White corpuscles or blood cells.

lever system   An assemblage of parts for moving weight with the least amount of applied force. A lever system consists of a rigid rod *(lever)* applied to the weight, a point of balance *(fulcrum)* for the lever, and mechanical force applied to the lever. These parts can be arranged in different ways to accommodate different amounts of weight, but a common principle of all lever systems is that the greatest amount of lifting force is achieved when the point at which the force is applied is farthest from the fulcrum.

light year   The distance light travels in one year.

Linnaeus, Carolus   A Swedish botanist (1707–1778) best known for developing a system of nomenclature for animals and plants.

litmus   An indicator used to test for pH, or hydrogen-ion concentration. Litmus is red in acid solutions and blue in basic solutions.

litmus paper   A special paper containing LITMUS, used by chemists to test for acid and alkali.

lunar   An adjective referring to the moon. A lunar eclipse is an eclipse of the moon. *See* SOLAR; ECLIPSE.

lymph   A colorless fluid which has passed from the bloodstream through capillary walls into the intercellular spaces; lymph is collected by lymph ducts and returned to the bloodstream.

M

mandible   The lower jaw bone of vertebrates; the mouth part of arthropods that resembles a jaw and functions in biting.

marine   An adjective meaning "of or relating to the sea."

mechanics   The study of the effects of force on moving or motionless bodies; a branch of PHYSICS.

meiosis   A type of cellular division that results in gametes (sex cells) or gametic nuclei. It consists of two divisions resulting in four daughter cells, and the number of chromosomes in each daughter is reduced by half (haploid).

membrane   A thin sheet forming a semipermeable boundary, as in 1) a thin layer of soft tissue, 2) the outer boundary of a cell (see PLASMA MEMBRANE), or 3) the enclosing boundary of an intracellular structure (for example, the nucleus).

Mendel, Gregor Johann An Austrian monk and botanist (1822–1884) who made important discoveries concerning HEREDITY.

metabolism A cellular process by which food is oxidized for the release of energy and utilized for synthesis of cellular materials.

meteorology A science that studies the weather and the atmosphere.

mitochondrion The cellular organelle of EUKARYOTES in which cellular oxidation (*cellular respiration*) generates energy.

mitosis A type of cellular division that results in exact duplicates of the parent cell, as in asexual reproduction or growth. It consists of one division resulting in two daughter cells, and the number of chromosomes in each daughter is the same as in the parent (diploid).

molecule The smallest unit into which a compound can be divided and still retain its original properties. Molecules are made up of atoms.

mollusks Animals of the phylum *Mollusca*, characterized by a *mantle*, a *radula*, and a *muscular foot*. Some mollusks are aquatic, like the octopus, clam, and oyster. Others are terrestrial, like the snail and slug.

mutation A stable and abrupt change in a gene, and thus in the trait the gene determines, that is transmitted from generation to generation.

mutualism A symbiotic relationship of mutual benefit to its partners.

mycelium A mass of fungal threads or hyphae, composing the fungus body.

N

natural immunity Immunity or resistance to disease with which a person is born.

nebula A cloudy and gaseous mass found in INTERSTELLAR space.

nephron A functional unit of the kidney, consisting of Bowman's capsule with its glomerulus, and the associated ducts and convoluted tubules, with their capillaries.

neutron A small particle that is part of the atom and has no electrical charge. *See* ELECTRON and PROTON.

Newton, Isaac   An English mathematician and natural philosopher (1642–1727) who made major discoveries in astronomy and PHYSICS. His most important work was his study of GRAVITATION and OPTICS.

nonpolar compound   A substance in which the electromagnetic charge of each molecule is balanced so that there is no positively or negatively charged end to the molecule. Oils and fats are examples. *See* POLAR and SOLUBLE.

nuclear   An adjective referring to the NUCLEUS of the atom or of a cell.

nuclear fission   The splitting of an atom in order to produce energy.

nuclear fusion   The joining together of lightweight atoms resulting in the release of energy.

nucleic acid   DNA and RNA; the nucleic acids code and transcribe information about heredity.

nucleolus   A separate area within the NUCLEUS in which RNA is synthesized.

nucleotide   The "building unit" of NUCLEIC ACIDS, consisting of a sugar (ribose or deoxyribose), a phosphate, and a base (a purine or a pyrimidine).

nucleus   The center core of an object, as (1) the center of an atom, containing protons and neutrons; or (2) the regulatory center of a cell of an organism.

O

observatory   A specially constructed building containing one or more telescopes for observation of the heavens.

ohm   A unit for measuring electric resistance.

optics   The study of light and its effects, a branch of PHYSICS.

orbit   The route that an object in space (such as the moon) takes around another body (such as the earth).

organ   A structure consisting of several different types of TISSUE combined into a single unit. A single organ can perform one or more major functions and is usually linked with other organs to form a *system*.

organelle   An intracellular structure that performs a major function for the cell; the cellular equivalent of an organ.

organic   Characteristic of, pertaining to, or derived from organisms; an adjective referring to living things or organisms.

organism   A living thing, such as a human, a plant, or an animal.

oxide   A compound made of oxygen and another element.

P

parasitism   A symbiotic relationship in which one organism (*parasite*) lives on and at the expense of another (*host*).

passive immunity   Immunity (usually temporary) imparted without the person's body acting in its build-up; the immunity is imparted by the administration of foreign antibodies.

Pasteur, Louis   A French chemist (1822–1895) who made major discoveries in chemistry and biology, especially in the control of many diseases. He and ROBERT KOCH were the founders of the science of bacteriology.

pasteurization   The heating of milk, or some other beverage, to a certain temperature for a definite period of time to destroy certain pathogens without changing the flavor or quality of the beverage.

pH   A symbol used in expression of acidity or alkalinity. It denotes the negative logarithm of the concentration of hydrogen ions in gram atoms per liter.

phagotroph   An organism that feeds on other organisms, usually while they are still alive, by engulfing them to allow digestion and absorption to take place within the body.

physics   The study of matter and energy, and their interactions.

phytogeographic map A map showing plant life.

Planck, Max   A German physicist (1858–1947) who did notable work in thermodynamics; the "father of quantum physics."

planet   A large body that moves around the sun. The earth is a planet.

plankton   A group of sea life—both plant and animal—that drifts with tides and currents.

plasma   The liquid portion of the blood in which proteins and other substances are dissolved.

plasma membrane The cell membrane, the living covering of the cell.

plastids Cellular organelles that are found in plant cells and may contain pigments. The types of plastids are: 1) *chloroplasts*, which contain the chlorophyll and carotenoid pigments and which are green; 2) *chromoplasts*, which contain carotenoid pigments and range in color from yellow to brown; and 3) *leucoplasts*, which are colorless.

polar compound A substance in which the electromagnetic charge of each molecule is unevenly distributed so that the molecule is positively charged on one end and negatively charged on the other end. Water is an example. *See* NONPOLAR COMPOUND and SOLUBLE.

potential energy Energy that is available for use. The energy of a boulder balanced on a mountainside is an example of potential energy. It becomes *kinetic energy* when the boulder begins to roll.

precipitation The settling out of particles suspended in liquid. Precipitation can be the result of a chemical reaction in which dissolved reactants form an insoluble product. Material that settles out of a suspension is a *precipitate*.

Priestley, Joseph The English chemist (1738–1804) who discovered oxygen, though the element was named and its importance first recognized by LAVOISIER.

primeval An adjective meaning "the first" or "early."

prokaryote An organism characterized by cells not containing a true or definite NUCLEUS surrounded by a nuclear membrane.

protein A complex organic compound consisting of AMINO ACIDS.

proton A positively charged particle found in the nucleus of atoms.

protoplasm An outdated term for the living substance within a cell. Current terminology divides cellular content into CYTOPLASM and *nucleoplasm* (material within the nuclear membrane).

protoplast The entire cellular contents, surrounded by and including the cell membrane. The cell wall and/or capsule are not a part of the protoplast.

R

radical A group of atoms that carries a charge and stays together as a unit during chemical reactions or in solutions, such as the nitrate ion and the sulfate ion.

radio astronomy   The study of radio waves received from outer space.

regeneration   The ability of an organism to regrow parts of itself after an injury.

replication   The process by which DNA duplicates itself for distribution to daughter nuclei during mitosis and/or meiosis.

reproduction   The process by which organisms create offspring of their own species.

respiration   In cells, the oxidation of food for the release of energy; in aerobes, the intake of oxygen and the release of carbon dioxide.

ribosome   An intracellular structure consisting of RNA and protein whose function is to provide a site for the TRANSLATION phase of protein synthesis.

RNA   Ribonucleic acid; a large, helical, single-stranded molecule whose different types perform various tasks in the process of protein synthesis.

S

salinity   The degree of SALT present. Usually refers to the amount of salt in a fluid.

salt   A substance formed when an acid is mixed with a base.

saprotroph   An organism feeding on dead organic matter, usually digesting the food externally and absorbing the digested material into its body.

satellite   An object that orbits around a planet, such as a moon. In recent years, the earth has had several man-made satellites.

serum   The fluid portion of blood plasma after clotting.

slime mold   Large amoeboid protozoans which form spores similar to those of fungi.

solar   An adjective referring to the sun. A solar eclipse is an eclipse of the sun. *See* LUNAR; ECLIPSE.

solar system   The sun, planets, satellites, and asteroids.

soluble   The ability of a substance to mix completely with a liquid at the molecular level such that no particles of any kind are visible in the mixture. The substance must be compatible with the liquid; nonpolar substances will not dissolve in polar liquids or the reverse. Dissolved substances will often be able to pass through semipermeable membranes. *See* NONPOLAR COMPOUND, POLAR COMPOUND, SOLUTE, and SOLUTION.

solute   The substance dissolved in a fluid to form a solution. *See* SOLUTION, SOLUBLE, and SOLVENT.

solution   A solution is a type of mixture formed when one substance mixes completely with a liquid at the molecular level. For example, when sugar (POLAR COMPOUND) is mixed with hot water (also a POLAR COMPOUND), the result is a solution. *See* SOLUTE, SOLVENT, and SOLUBLE.

solvent   The fluid in which a solute is dissolved to form a SOLUTION. *See* SOLUBLE.

sonic   An adjective referring to sound.

spawn   Eggs of certain aquatic animals. Also used as a verb meaning "to lay eggs." Both forms are usually used in connection with fish.

stimulus   Any change in the external or internal environment of a living organism. Many stimuli cause a change in the organism's activity (response). For example, if a person has not eaten for some time, the smell of the food might make his mouth water. The stimulus is the sudden presence of food (detected by smell); the response is secretion of saliva.

sublimation   The transformation of a substance from a solid directly to a gaseous state without passing through a liquid state when warmed.

substratum   A layer lying beneath the top layer (geology); the surface of a medium on which microorganisms grow (biology); a material or compound on which enzymes act (biology). Also called the *substrate*.

supersonic   An adjective meaning "faster than sound."

suspension   A type of mixture in which large particles are mixed with a liquid and remain mixed only as long as they are agitated. The particles in a suspension will settle out if not continuously agitated. An example is the suspension of blood cells in the plasma of blood. Particles in suspension will not pass through a semipermeable membrane. *See* COLLOID and SOLUTION.

symbiosis A relationship between two different species living together. The relationship may be PARASITISM, MUTUALISM, or COMMENSALISM.

T

theory An explanation of natural events based on hypotheses confirmed by testing.

thermodynamics The study of heat and energy flow.

tissue A group of similar CELLS specialized to perform a single task. When different tissues are combined, they are arranged in sequential layers. *See* ORGAN.

transcription The formation of messenger RNA from the coded DNA.

transduction The passage of genetic material from one bacterial cell to another by means of viral parasites called *phages*.

transformation The passage of genetic material from one bacterium to another through the medium in which they are growing.

translation The formation of proteins from amino acids by the use of the coded information in the messenger RNA.

translocation The movement of materials throughout a plant.

U

unicellular An adjective meaning "one-celled." *See* CELL.

universe All things that exist in space, taken as a whole.

V

valence The number of electrons which can be accepted by, given up by, or shared by an atom or RADICAL. Positive valence numbers indicate electrons which can be given up to or shared with another atom or radical; negative valence numbers indicate electrons which can be accepted from another atom or radical. The positive and negative valences of reactants must balance for a chemical reaction to happen.

vapor The gaseous phase of a substance that is usually in a liquid state. Vaporization (*evaporation*) of water or another liquid is accomplished by heating the liquid.

vascular tissue   Tissue used to transport materials in multicellular organisms. In higher animals, blood is vascular tissue; in higher plants, xylem and phloem are vascular tissues.

vector   An organism, usually an arthropod, that carries and transmits pathogens from one animal to another.

velocity   The rate of motion of one object relative to another object.

Vesalius, Andreas   A Flemish anatomist (1514–1564) who studied the body. His discoveries were so important that he is often referred to as "the father of anatomy." *See* ANATOMY.

virus   An obligate intracellular parasite consisting essentially of a nucleic acid surrounded by a protein coat.

vitamin   An organic substance other than an ENZYME that is necessary for the proper maintenance of a metabolic process. A vitamin deficiency will cause metabolic dysfunction and an overall decline in health. Animals, including humans, must get their vitamins from the food they eat.

volt   The practical unit of measurement of electric potential and electromotive force.

W / X / Y / Z

water table   The level nearest to the surface of the ground where water is found.

work   The result of energy expenditure. Common example of work are movement, chemical reactions, and changes from one physical state to another.

yeast   A unicellular nonmycelial fungus. Some yeasts are of commercial importance in brewing and baking industries.

zoology   The study of animals. The science is a branch of BIOLOGY.

Answer Sheet
Science—Physical Sciences
TEST 1

1. Ⓐ Ⓑ Ⓒ Ⓓ	13. Ⓐ Ⓑ Ⓒ Ⓓ	25. Ⓐ Ⓑ Ⓒ Ⓓ	37. Ⓐ Ⓑ Ⓒ Ⓓ	49. Ⓐ Ⓑ Ⓒ Ⓓ
2. Ⓐ Ⓑ Ⓒ Ⓓ	14. Ⓐ Ⓑ Ⓒ Ⓓ	26. Ⓐ Ⓑ Ⓒ Ⓓ	38. Ⓐ Ⓑ Ⓒ Ⓓ	50. Ⓐ Ⓑ Ⓒ Ⓓ
3. Ⓐ Ⓑ Ⓒ Ⓓ	15. Ⓐ Ⓑ Ⓒ Ⓓ	27. Ⓐ Ⓑ Ⓒ Ⓓ	39. Ⓐ Ⓑ Ⓒ Ⓓ	51. Ⓐ Ⓑ Ⓒ Ⓓ
4. Ⓐ Ⓑ Ⓒ Ⓓ	16. Ⓐ Ⓑ Ⓒ Ⓓ	28. Ⓐ Ⓑ Ⓒ Ⓓ	40. Ⓐ Ⓑ Ⓒ Ⓓ	52. Ⓐ Ⓑ Ⓒ Ⓓ
5. Ⓐ Ⓑ Ⓒ Ⓓ	17. Ⓐ Ⓑ Ⓒ Ⓓ	29. Ⓐ Ⓑ Ⓒ Ⓓ	41. Ⓐ Ⓑ Ⓒ Ⓓ	53. Ⓐ Ⓑ Ⓒ Ⓓ
6. Ⓐ Ⓑ Ⓒ Ⓓ	18. Ⓐ Ⓑ Ⓒ Ⓓ	30. Ⓐ Ⓑ Ⓒ Ⓓ	42. Ⓐ Ⓑ Ⓒ Ⓓ	54. Ⓐ Ⓑ Ⓒ Ⓓ
7. Ⓐ Ⓑ Ⓒ Ⓓ	19. Ⓐ Ⓑ Ⓒ Ⓓ	31. Ⓐ Ⓑ Ⓒ Ⓓ	43. Ⓐ Ⓑ Ⓒ Ⓓ	55. Ⓐ Ⓑ Ⓒ Ⓓ
8. Ⓐ Ⓑ Ⓒ Ⓓ	20. Ⓐ Ⓑ Ⓒ Ⓓ	32. Ⓐ Ⓑ Ⓒ Ⓓ	44. Ⓐ Ⓑ Ⓒ Ⓓ	56. Ⓐ Ⓑ Ⓒ Ⓓ
9. Ⓐ Ⓑ Ⓒ Ⓓ	21. Ⓐ Ⓑ Ⓒ Ⓓ	33. Ⓐ Ⓑ Ⓒ Ⓓ	45. Ⓐ Ⓑ Ⓒ Ⓓ	57. Ⓐ Ⓑ Ⓒ Ⓓ
10. Ⓐ Ⓑ Ⓒ Ⓓ	22. Ⓐ Ⓑ Ⓒ Ⓓ	34. Ⓐ Ⓑ Ⓒ Ⓓ	46. Ⓐ Ⓑ Ⓒ Ⓓ	58. Ⓐ Ⓑ Ⓒ Ⓓ
11. Ⓐ Ⓑ Ⓒ Ⓓ	23. Ⓐ Ⓑ Ⓒ Ⓓ	35. Ⓐ Ⓑ Ⓒ Ⓓ	47. Ⓐ Ⓑ Ⓒ Ⓓ	59. Ⓐ Ⓑ Ⓒ Ⓓ
12. Ⓐ Ⓑ Ⓒ Ⓓ	24. Ⓐ Ⓑ Ⓒ Ⓓ	36. Ⓐ Ⓑ Ⓒ Ⓓ	48. Ⓐ Ⓑ Ⓒ Ⓓ	60. Ⓐ Ⓑ Ⓒ Ⓓ

TEST 2

1. Ⓐ Ⓑ Ⓒ Ⓓ   9. Ⓐ Ⓑ Ⓒ Ⓓ   17. Ⓐ Ⓑ Ⓒ Ⓓ   25. Ⓐ Ⓑ Ⓒ Ⓓ   33. Ⓐ Ⓑ Ⓒ Ⓓ

2. Ⓐ Ⓑ Ⓒ Ⓓ   10. Ⓐ Ⓑ Ⓒ Ⓓ   18. Ⓐ Ⓑ Ⓒ Ⓓ   26. Ⓐ Ⓑ Ⓒ Ⓓ   34. Ⓐ Ⓑ Ⓒ Ⓓ

3. Ⓐ Ⓑ Ⓒ Ⓓ   11. Ⓐ Ⓑ Ⓒ Ⓓ   19. Ⓐ Ⓑ Ⓒ Ⓓ   27. Ⓐ Ⓑ Ⓒ Ⓓ   35. Ⓐ Ⓑ Ⓒ Ⓓ

4. Ⓐ Ⓑ Ⓒ Ⓓ   12. Ⓐ Ⓑ Ⓒ Ⓓ   20. Ⓐ Ⓑ Ⓒ Ⓓ   28. Ⓐ Ⓑ Ⓒ Ⓓ   36. Ⓐ Ⓑ Ⓒ Ⓓ

5. Ⓐ Ⓑ Ⓒ Ⓓ   13. Ⓐ Ⓑ Ⓒ Ⓓ   21. Ⓐ Ⓑ Ⓒ Ⓓ   29. Ⓐ Ⓑ Ⓒ Ⓓ   37. Ⓐ Ⓑ Ⓒ Ⓓ

6. Ⓐ Ⓑ Ⓒ Ⓓ   14. Ⓐ Ⓑ Ⓒ Ⓓ   22. Ⓐ Ⓑ Ⓒ Ⓓ   30. Ⓐ Ⓑ Ⓒ Ⓓ   38. Ⓐ Ⓑ Ⓒ Ⓓ

7. Ⓐ Ⓑ Ⓒ Ⓓ   15. Ⓐ Ⓑ Ⓒ Ⓓ   23. Ⓐ Ⓑ Ⓒ Ⓓ   31. Ⓐ Ⓑ Ⓒ Ⓓ   39. Ⓐ Ⓑ Ⓒ Ⓓ

8. Ⓐ Ⓑ Ⓒ Ⓓ   16. Ⓐ Ⓑ Ⓒ Ⓓ   24. Ⓐ Ⓑ Ⓒ Ⓓ   32. Ⓐ Ⓑ Ⓒ Ⓓ   40. Ⓐ Ⓑ Ⓒ Ⓓ

SCIENCE TEST 1

Physical Sciences

45 Minutes   60 Questions

Directions: *Read each question carefully and consider all possible answers. When you have decided which choice is best, blacken the corresponding space on your answer sheet. There is only one best answer for each question.*

1. Oxygen gas can be obtained in appreciable quantities by heating all of the following *except*

    (A) H_2O
    (B) H_2O_2
    (C) HgO
    (D) PbO_2

2. All of the reactions between the following pairs will produce hydrogen *except*

    (A) copper and hydrochloric acid
    (B) iron and sulfuric acid
    (C) magnesium and steam
    (D) sodium and alcohol

3. When hydrochloric acid is added to sodium sulfite and the gas that is formed is bubbled through barium hydroxide, the salt formed is

    (A) $BaCl_2$
    (B) $BaSO_3$
    (C) $NaCl$
    (D) $NaOH$

4. When chlorine and carbon tetrachloride are added to a solution of an iodide and shaken, the color produced is

    (A) brown
    (B) orange
    (C) violet
    (D) yellow

5. An important use of silicon carbide is

    (A) as an abrasive
    (B) as a catalyst
    (C) as an explosive
    (D) in water purification

6. If an eudiometer tube was filled with 26 milliliters of hydrogen and 24 milliliters of oxygen and the mixture exploded, which of the following would remain uncombined?

    (A) 2 milliliters hydrogen
    (B) 14 milliliters hydrogen
    (C) 23 milliliters hydrogen
    (D) 11 milliliters oxygen

7. The gas resulting when hydrochloric acid is added to a mixture of iron filings and sulfur is

    (A) H_2S
    (B) SO_2
    (C) SO_3
    (D) H_2

8. When a colorless gas is dissolved in water and the resulting solution turns red litmus blue, the gas may be which of the following?

    (A) HCl
    (B) NH_3
    (C) H_2S
    (D) SO_2

9. Fluorine is the most active member of the halogen family because it

    (A) is a gas
    (B) has the smallest atomic radius
    (C) has no isotopes
    (D) combines with lithium

10. In sulfuric acid the valence number of sulfur is

    (A) plus 2
    (B) minus 2
    (C) minus 4
    (D) plus 6

11. The boiling points of the following gases are as follows: argon, $-185.7°C$.; helium, $-268.9°C$.; nitrogen, $-195.8°C$.; oxygen, $-183°C$. In the fractional distillation of liquid air, the gas that boils off last is

    (A) argon
    (B) helium
    (C) nitrogen
    (D) oxygen

12. The element selenium is most closely related to which of the following elements? (Refer to the periodic table on page 200.)

    (A) beryllium
    (B) oxygen
    (C) silicon
    (D) sulfur

13. Baking soda is also called

    (A) washing soda
    (B) caustic soda
    (C) soda ash
    (D) bicarbonate of soda

14. Solder is an alloy of

    (A) aluminum and copper
    (B) copper and tin
    (C) mercury and silver
    (D) tin and lead

15. Which of the following substances will raise the pH of a solution of hydrochloric acid?

    (A) NaCl
    (B) H_2CO_3
    (C) $NaHCO_3$
    (D) HNO_3

16. An oxide whose water solution will turn litmus red is

    (A) BaO
    (B) Na_2O
    (C) P_2O_3
    (D) CaO

17. A compound that has a high heat for formation is normally

    (A) easy to form from its elements and easy to decompose
    (B) easy to form from its elements and difficult to decompose

    (C) difficult to form from its elements and easy to decompose
    (D) difficult to form from its elements and difficult to decompose

18. A solution of zinc chloride should *not* be stored in a tank made of aluminum because

    (A) aluminum will displace the zinc in the zinc chloride solution
    (B) the zinc would become contaminated
    (C) the chloride ion will react with impurities in the solution
    (D) the two metals will react to produce an undesirable compound

19. The valence number of sulfur in the ion SO_4^{-2} is

    (A) -2
    (B) $+2$
    (C) $+6$
    (D) $+10$

20. The chemical name for sulfuric acid is

    (A) hydrogen sulfate
    (B) hydrogen sulfite
    (C) sulfur trioxide
    (D) hydrogen sulfide

21. The number of grams of hydrogen formed by the action of 6 grams of magnesium (atomic weight = 24) on an appropriate quantity of acid is

    (A) 0.5
    (B) 8
    (C) 22.4
    (D) 72

22. The symbol for two molecules of hydrogen is

    (A) H_2
    (B) $2H$
    (C) $2H+$
    (D) $2H_2$

23. The formula for sodium bisulfate is

    (A) $NaBiSO_4$
    (B) $NaHSO_4$
    (C) NaH_2SO_4
    (D) Na_2SO_4

24. The law of multiple proportions was first proposed by

    (A) Dalton
    (B) Davy
    (C) Priestley
    (D) Williams

25. One liter of a certain gas, under standard conditions, weighs 1.16 grams. A possible formula for the gas is

    (A) C_2H_2
    (B) CO
    (C) NH_3
    (D) O_2

26. Of the following acids, the one most commonly found in the home is

    (A) CH_3COOH
    (B) HNO_3
    (C) HCl
    (D) H_2SO_4

27. Of the following, which is an aromatic compound?

    (A) benzene
    (B) ethyl alcohol
    (C) iodoform
    (D) methane

28. Of the following, which is a monosaccharide?

    (A) dextrose
    (B) glycogen
    (C) lactose
    (D) sucrose

29. Fats belong to the class of organic compounds represented by the general formula, RCOOR´, where R and R´ represent hydrocarbon groups; therefore, fats are

    (A) ethers
    (B) soaps
    (C) esters
    (D) lipases

30. Of the following compounds, the one with the highest heat of formation is

    (A) NaCl
    (B) NaI
    (C) NaF
    (D) NaBr

31. A substance that will cause permanent hardness of water is

    (A) Na_2SO_4
    (B) H_2SO_4
    (C) $MgSO_4$
    (D) $Ca(HCO_3)_2$

32. Two atoms have the same atomic number but different atomic weights (masses); therefore, these atoms are

    (A) compounds
    (B) isotopes
    (C) neutrons
    (D) different elements

33. Bleaching powder has the formula

    (A) $CaCl_2$
    (B) CaOCL
    (C) $CaOCl_2$
    (D) $Ca(ClO_3)_2$

34. In forming an ionic bond with an atom of chlorine, a sodium atom will

    (A) receive one electron from the chlorine atom
    (B) receive two electrons from the chlorine atom
    (C) give up one electron to the chlorine atom
    (D) give up two electrons to the chlorine atom

35. Which of the following is an example of a transition element? (Refer to the periodic table on page 200.)

    (A) aluminum
    (B) astatine
    (C) nickel
    (D) rubidium

36. A gas lighter than air is

    (A) CH_4
    (B) C_6H_6
    (C) HCl
    (D) N_2O

37. Of the following gases, which is odorless and heavier than air?

    (A) CO
    (B) CO_2
    (C) H_2S
    (D) N_2

38. In a volume of air at a pressure of one atmosphere at sea level, the partial pressure of oxygen is equal to

    (A) 593 mm of mercury
    (B) 494 mm of mercury
    (C) 380 mm of mercury
    (D) 160 mm of mercury

39. The complete combustion of carbon disulfide would yield carbon dioxide and

    (A) sulfur
    (B) sulfur dioxide
    (C) sulfuric acid
    (D) water

40. Alcoholic beverages contain

    (A) wood alcohol
    (B) isopropyl alcohol
    (C) glyceryl alcohol
    (D) ethyl alcohol

41. Of the following compounds, which is more difficult to decompose than lithium fluoride?

    (A) lithium bromide
    (B) lithium chloride
    (C) lithium iodide
    (D) none of the above

42. All of the following terms are associated with the manufacture of gasoline *except*

    (A) alkylation
    (B) catalytic cracking
    (C) pickling
    (D) polymerization

43. The periodic table shows that the atomic number of fluorine is 9; this indicates that the fluoride atom contains

    (A) nine neutrons in its nucleus
    (B) nine protons in its nucleus and nine electrons in orbit around the nucleus
    (C) a total of nine protons and neutrons
    (D) a total of nine protons and electrons

44. In the electrolysis of brine, the element liberated at the cathode is

    (A) hydrogen
    (B) oxygen
    (C) chlorine
    (D) sodium

45. Of four copper wires with the following dimensions, which one would have the greatest resistance to electrical current?

    (A) length of one meter and diameter of 4 millimeters
    (B) length of two meters and diameter of 8 millimeters
    (C) length of one meter and diameter of 8 millimeters
    (D) length of two meters and diameter of 2 millimeters

46. The general formula for an organic acid is

    (A) RCOOR
    (B) ROH
    (C) ROR
    (D) RCOOH

47. An example of a strong electrolyte is

    (A) sugar
    (B) calcium chloride
    (C) glycerin
    (D) boric acid

48. A lead ball, a wooden ball, and a styrofoam ball, all with a mass of one kilogram, are thrown at a wall 16 meters away, and all of them hit the wall in two seconds. Which ball will strike the wall with the greatest force?

    (A) lead ball
    (B) wooden ball
    (C) styrofoam ball
    (D) all strike with the same force

49. The hydride ion H– has the same number of orbital electrons as an atom of

    (A) helium
    (B) lithium
    (C) beryllium
    (D) boron

50. When copper oxide is heated with charcoal, the reaction that occurs is an example of

    (A) reduction only
    (B) oxidation only
    (C) both oxidation and reduction
    (D) neither oxidation nor reduction

51. Nonmetal oxides, when dissolved in water, tend to form

    (A) acids
    (B) bases
    (C) salts
    (D) hydrides

52. Which substance is *not* used to soften hard water?

    (A) calcium hydroxide
    (B) sodium carbonate
    (C) calcium sulfate
    (D) permutit

53. The best reducing agent is

    (A) mercury
    (B) hydrogen
    (C) copper
    (D) carbon dioxide

54. The bonding of a water molecule is

    (A) electrovalent
    (B) covalent polar
    (C) coordinate covalent
    (D) covalent nonpolar

55. The test for a nitrate results in

    (A) a precipitate
    (B) a red flame
    (C) a brown ring
    (D) litmus turning blue

56. A solution that contains all the solute it can normally dissolve at a given temperature must be

    (A) concentrated
    (B) supersaturated
    (C) saturated
    (D) unsaturated

57. The oxides of barium and sulfur combine to form

    (A) a salt
    (B) a base
    (C) an acid
    (D) an anhydride

58. Chlorine gas is obtained commercially chiefly by the

    (A) replacement of chlorine from hydrochloric acid by use of a metal
    (B) replacement of chlorine by a more active halogen
    (C) electrolysis of hydrochloric acid
    (D) electrolysis of brine

59. The reason why concentrated H_2SO_4 is used extensively to prepare other acids is that concentrated sulfuric acid

    (A) is highly ionized
    (B) is an excellent dehydrating agent
    (C) has a high specific gravity
    (D) has a high boiling point

60. Which two liquids are immiscible?

    (A) ethyl alcohol and water
    (B) carbon tetrachloride and water
    (C) gasoline and kerosene
    (D) hydrochloric acid and water

Answer Key

1.	A	21.	A	41.	D
2.	A	22.	D	42.	C
3.	B	23.	B	43.	B
4.	C	24.	A	44.	A
5.	A	25.	A	45.	D
6.	D	26.	A	46.	D
7.	D	27.	A	47.	B
8.	B	28.	A	48.	D
9.	B	29.	C	49.	A
10.	D	30.	C	50.	C
11.	D	31.	C	51.	A
12.	D	32.	B	52.	C
13.	D	33.	C	53.	B
14.	D	34.	C	54.	B
15.	C	35.	C	55.	C
16.	C	36.	A	56.	C
17.	B	37.	B	57.	A
18.	A	38.	D	58.	D
19.	C	39.	B	59.	D
20.	A	40.	D	60.	B

Explanatory Answers

1. **(A)** Heating water to a very high temperature (about 2000 degrees C) will cause only about two percent of the water to dissociate into hydrogen and oxygen—a not very economical or efficient way of obtaining oxygen. Electrolysis will decompose water at a much lower temperature. Hydrogen peroxide and many oxides or metals can be decomposed more easily by heating alone.

2. **(A)** All acids contain hydrogen, which may be displaced by certain metals. However, copper ranks below hydrogen in the *electromotive* or *activity series. Activity* refers to the activity of a metal in displacing hydrogen in acids and in water. Metals ranked below hydrogen in the series do not displace hydrogen from acids.

3. **(B)** Hydrochloric acid can react with sodium hydrogen sulfite to produce sodium chloride, water, and sulfur dioxide. Sulfur dioxide can react with barium hydroxide to form barium sulfite and water.

4. **(C)** Iodine vapors are violet ; in many hydrocarbon solutions, iodine forms a violet color resembling the color of its vapors, while in alcohol, ether, and aqueous solutions, a brown color is produced. In the latter, iodine combines with the solvent, thereby producing the brown color. In the former (violet-colored solutions), iodine is uncombined and is in its free molecular state I_2.

5. **(A)** Silicon carbide (common name, carborundum) is a very hard substance and is used extensively as an abrasive in powders, hones, etc. It is made by heating sand and coke to a temperature of about 3500°C, causing chemical fusion.

6. **(D)** Since there is twice as much hydrogen as there is oxygen in a molecule of water (H_2O), the 26 milliliters of hydrogen could combine with only 13 milliliters of oxygen. This would leave 11 of the 24 milliliters of oxygen uncombined.

7. **(D)** Hydrochloric acid reacts with active metals, forming the chloride of that metal and releasing hydrogen.

8. **(B)** Litmus is an indicator that is blue in a basic solution. The colorless gas, then, would have to form a basic solution in water. Ammonia dissolves in water to form ammonium hydroxide, which is alkaline or basic.

9. **(B)** The halogens are similar in chemical behavior and in the compounds they form; but they are different in physical properties. Fluorine has the smallest atom of the halogens and the smallest atomic weight. The ease of combination with other elements decreases as the atomic weight increases; therefore, fluorine is the most active halogen.

10. **(D)** Sulfuric acid (H_2SO_4) contains four oxygens, each with a valence of minus 2; the total negative valence is 8. Each of the two hydrogens has a valence of plus 1; the total hydrogen valence equals plus 2. Therefore, sulfur would need a valence of plus 6 to equalize the positive and negative valences in the molecule.

11. **(D)** Fractional distillation can be used to separate the components of a mixture; the mixture is heated to boiling and the temperature is constantly raised. The component with the lowest boiling point vaporizes first; the component with the highest boiling point will vaporize last. Liquid oxygen has a boiling point of –183°C, which is higher than the boiling point of the other components. So oxygen will boil off last.

12. **(D)** Selenium often occurs in nature associated with sulfur, although it can be combined with copper and lead. Although less active than sulfur, its reactions are similar to those of sulfur. Both combine with metals and burn in air or oxygen (forming the dioxide that reacts with water to form acids); selenium reacts with hydrochloric acid to form H_2Se, just as sulfur reacts with hydrochloric acid to form H_2S. Both are in Group VI in the periodic table (see page 200).

13. **(D)** Chemically, baking soda is sodium hydrogen carbonate, or sodium bicarbonate ($NaHCO_3$). So it is sometimes called bicarbonate of soda.

14. **(D)** Solder is an alloy of tin and lead. An alloy is produced by mixing two or more metals in a molten condition, followed by solidification. The metals remain completely dissolved in each other in the solid state, forming a definite homogeneous substance. Lead is a soft dense metal; tin is less dense, but it is stronger and more pliable.

15. **(C)** $NaHCO_3$ will combine with HCl (hydrochloric acid) to form NaCL and H_2CO_3. H_2CO_3 is a weaker acid than HCl; therefore the net effect of replacing HCl molecules with H_2CO_3 molecules is to raise the pH of the solution. In causing this reaction, $NaHCO_3$ is acting as a *buffer*. NaCl is a salt that will have no effect on the pH of an HCl solution. The other two compounds are acids that would lower the pH of the solution further if added.

16. **(C)** Litmus turns red in acid solution. When phosphorus trioxide dissolves in water, phosphorus acid is formed. The other compounds named form alkaline solutions.

17. **(B)** The amount of heat absorbed or lost in a chemical reaction is the heat of reaction. It equals the heat content of the product(s) minus the heat content of the reactants. Heat is absorbed if more energy is stored in the products than in the reactants, and released if more energy is stored in the reactants than in the product(s). In the formation of a compound, the heat of reaction is called the heat of formation for that compound. A compound with more energy stored in it than is in the reactants (a compound with a high heat of formation) can be formed but is difficult to decompose.

18. **(A)** Zinc is ranked above the others but below aluminum in the activity series of metals. The higher the metal is ranked, the more energetic it is in its displacement ability. Therefore, aluminum could displace zinc in the zinc chloride solution, forming aluminum chloride. So one should not store zinc chloride in a tank made of aluminum because aluminum will displace the zinc in the zinc chloride.

19. **(C)** The four oxygen ions would have a total *valence* of negative 8 (each oxygen, minus 2); if the valence of the SO_4 ion is minus 2, the remaining valence of 6 would be matched to a positive valence. Therefore, sulfur must have a valence of plus 6.

20. **(A)** Sulfuric acid is composed of two hydrogen ions and one sulfate ion. The chemical formula is H_2SO_4; thus, its chemical name is hydrogen sulfate.

21. **(A)** Magnesium has an atomic weight of 24; hydrogen's atomic weight is approximately 1. As is true with many metals, magnesium can react with an acid, such as hydrochloric acid, to produce hydrogen ($Mg + 2HCl \rightarrow MgCl_2 + H_2$). The amount of hydrogen produced can be calculated by using the following equation:

$$\frac{\text{amount Mg}}{\text{atomic weight}} = \frac{\text{amount } H_2}{\text{atomic weight}}$$

Substituting in the equation, we get the following:

$$\frac{6 \text{ grams}}{24} = \frac{x \text{ grams}}{2} = 0.5 \text{ grams}$$

In working out problems in which one must determine the amount of a substance derived from a given reaction, the chemical equation must be balanced and molecular weight must be used. Thus, for diatomic gases, use twice the atomic weight.

22. **(D)** Hydrogen in molecular form is composed of two atoms; the formula for one molecule of hydrogen is H_2. Therefore, two molecules of hydrogen is $2H_2$.

23. **(B)** Sodium bisulfate differs from sodium sulfate in having hydrogen as a part of the molecule. Since the sulfate ion has a valence of minus 2, and hydrogen and sodium each have a valence of plus 1, then one sodium and one hydrogen must be in combination with the sulfate ion. ($NaHSO_4$)

24. **(A)** John Dalton discovered the facts concerning chemical combinations and suggested that materials are composed of atoms. He first proposed the law of multiple proportions in 1804. The law states that in a series of compounds formed by the same two or more elements, given a definite weight for one element, the different weights of the second element are in the ratio of small whole numbers to the weight of the first. For example, in sulfur dioxide (SO_2), the weight of oxygen is 32 (atomic weight = 16); in sulfur trioxide (SO_3), the weight of oxygen is 48. Therefore, the ratio is 2:3.

25. **(A)** One mole *(gram molecular weight)* of a gas occupies 22.4 liters under standard conditions. Since one liter of the gas in question is $\frac{1}{22.4}$ of one mole, it is $\frac{1}{22.4}$ of its gram molecular weight. Knowing this, the molecular weight of the gas can be determined. We can set up the equation as follows:

$$\frac{x \text{ (unknown gram mol. wt.)}}{22.4 \text{ liters}} = \frac{1.16 \text{ gram}}{1 \text{ liter}}$$

Solving the equation, we get 26 as one gram molecular weight. C_2H_2(ethane) fits this weight. (C = 12 ×2, H = 1 × 2)

26. **(A)** Nitric acid, hydrochloric acid, and sulfuric acid usually are not found in the home. Acetic acid is found in the home as vinegar.

27. **(A)** *Aromatic* compounds are so named because of their odors; they occur in ring structure (molecular structure) and include such compounds as benzene, tolulene, and xylene.

28. **(A)** Dextrose is a *monosaccharide*, in that its molecule is composed of one "sugar unit" and cannot be hydrolyzed into simpler sugars. Lactose and sucrose are *disaccharides*, each yielding two monosaccharides by hydrolysis. Glycogen is a *polysaccharide* composed of a large number of monosaccharide units.

29. **(C)** Fats are glyceryl esters that, when hydrolized, yield glycerol and fatty acids. The cleavage of the ester linkage upon hydrolysis can be achieved by saponification, acids, superheated steam, or lipase, which is an enzyme that hydrolyzes fats. This may be represented as follows:

$$RCOOR' + H_2O \longrightarrow RCOOH + R'OH$$

30. **(C)** Fluorine is the most active of the halogens, and the compounds formed from it cannot be decomposed easily. NaF, then, has the highest heat of formation.

31. **(C)** Both magnesium sulfate ($MgSO_4$) and calcium hydrogen carbonate ($Ca(HCO_3)_2$) cause hardness of water. However, water with hydrogen carbonates (bicarbonates) can be softened by boiling the water or by neutralizing the carbonate with a base. Therefore, carbonate hardness is temporary hardness. Permanent hardness, or noncarbonate hardness such as that caused by magnesium sulfate, requires other methods of softening. These often involve the addition of a substance that can yield a negative ion to replace the sulfate ion. Sulfuric acid and sodium sulfate are not compounds that cause hardness of water.

32. **(B)** The *atomic number* represents the number of protons within the nucleus of an atom; since an atom is electrically neutral, the atomic number also equals the number of electrons of the atom. The atomic weight *(mass number)* represents the total number of nuclear particles (protons plus neutrons). All atoms of the same element have the same number of protons and, thus, the same atomic number. If the number of neutrons differ, the mass number is different; these atoms, then, are *isotopes*.

33. **(C)** Calcium hypochlorite ($CaOCl_2$) is effective as a bleach due to the oxidizing activity of hypochlorous acid ($HClO$), which is produced from calcium hypochloride and from which chlorine gas can also be liberated.

34. **(C)** An ionic bond will form between two atoms if the loss of electrons from one to the other will result in both atoms having a completely filled outer electron orbit. A sodium atom has 11 electrons, two in its first electron orbit, eight in its second electron orbit, and one in its outer electron orbit. The loss of one electron from the sodium atom will eliminate its outer electron orbit, making the next orbit in toward the nucleus the new outer orbit with a full complement of eight electrons. A chlorine atom has 17 electrons, two in its first electron orbit, eight in its second, and seven in its outer electron orbit. The acceptance of one electron by the chlorine atom will fill its outer electron orbit with the full complement of eight electrons.

35. **(C)** Transition elements are characterized by atoms in which the two highest energy levels are incompletely filled. Consulting the periodic table indicates that of those listed, only nickel is a transition element (see the periodic table on page 200).

36. **(A)** Air is a mixture of gases; the gases present in greatest quantity are nitrogen and oxygen. The quantity of nitrogen in the air is almost four times that of oxygen. Of the compounds listed, methane (CH_4), with a molecular weight of 16, is lighter than air.

37. **(B)** Carbon dioxide is an odorless gas that is heavier than air. It is colorless, soluble in water, and about one and one-half times as heavy as air. It is a component of air, but comprises less than 0.05 percent of it.

38. **(D)** The pressure of a gas is measured by the distance in millimeters that it will lift a column of mercury in a barometer. The pressure of air is 760 mm of mercury at sea level. Air is a mixture of gases, and the pressure of each gas in such a mixture, referred to as its *partial pressure*, is equal to its concentration in the mixture. Oxygen constitutes 21% of air; therefore, its partial pressure at sea level would be 21% of 760 mm of mercury of pressure, or 160 mm of mercury.

39. **(B)** Carbon disulfide is highly inflammable; its complete combustion yields carbon dioxide and sulfur dioxide.

$$CS_2 + 3O_2 \longrightarrow CO_2 + 2SO_2$$

40. **(D)** The ethyl alcohol of alcoholic beverages is produced by fermentation of monosaccharides; usually yeast is used to supply the enzymes needed, and the fermentation process supplies the energy needed by the yeast.

$$C_6H_{12}O_6 \longrightarrow 2C_2H_5OH + 2CO_2$$

41. **(D)** Because fluorine is extremely active, it does not occur free in nature but combines naturally with all elements except the inert gases, forming very stable compounds. Because it is a vigorous oxidizing agent, it cannot be oxidized by other oxidizing agents. For these reasons, fluorides are more difficult to decompose than are compounds of the other halogens.

42. **(C)** Processes involved in the manufacture of gasoline include *catalytic cracking*, which is the decomposition of larger molecules into smaller ones with lower boiling points; *alkylation*, the changing of the molecules by the addition of other groups; and, eventually, *polymerization*, the rebuilding of larger molecules from the smaller ones. *Pickling* is a method used to clean iron in order to apply zinc to produce galvanized iron.

43. **(B)** The atomic number indicates the number of *protons*, positively charged particles, within the nucleus of an atom. Since an atom is electrically neutral, the number of protons is equal to the number of *electrons* (negatively charged particles) of the atom. Thus, the atomic number can indicate the number of electrons as well as the number of protons.

44. **(A)** Brine is a solution of salt; the solution can be decomposed by electrolysis. Hydrogen ions, with a positive charge, will collect at the negative cathode; chloride ions, with a negative charge, will collect at the positive anode. Unlike charges attract; like charges repel. Sodium will form sodium hydroxide.

45. **(D)** The resistance of a metal wire is directly proportional to its length and inversely proportional to its cross-sectional area. The longest wire with the smallest diameter will therefore have the greatest resistance.

46. **(D)** An *organic* acid is characterized by the presence of a carboxyl group (—COOH),

$$or - C \overset{\nearrow O}{\underset{\searrow OH}{}}$$

). R represents a hydrocarbon group or a radical derived from a hydro-carbon.

47. **(B)** An *electrolyte* is a substance that forms an electrically conducting solution when dissolved in water. This is caused by the dissociation of the compound into ions, or *ionization*. The greater the ionization, the stronger the electrolyte. Calcium chloride ionizes to a much greater degree than the others and is a strong electrolyte.

48. **(D)** Force is a function of mass, distance, and acceleration. Since all of these factors are equal in this example, all of the balls strike the wall with the same force. The force is calculated as $1 \text{ kg} \times 16 \text{ m}/ (2 \text{ sec})^2 = 4$ newtons.

49. **(A)** The helium atom has two electrons in the atom, both occupying the first orbit, the most stable state. The hydrogen ion has one electron in the first orbit. But hydrogen has the ability to combine directly with certain metallic elements to form hydrides, such as calcium hydride (CaH_2) and sodium hydride (NaH). The metallic element and the hydride probably share a pair of electrons, thus allowing hydrogen to have a second electron in its orbit as does helium.

50. **(C)** Charcoal is an amorphous form of carbon, and carbon can react with oxides of many metals and other substances to form CO, CO_2, and the carbides of the metals. Thus, the oxides would be reduced by the removal of oxygen, and carbon would be oxidized to carbon monoxide or carbon dioxide. So oxidation and reduction occur.

51. **(A)** Nonmetal oxides, such as oxides of sulfur, carbon, and nitrogen, can react with water to form acids. The equations below are examples:

$$CO_2 + H_2O \longrightarrow H_2CO_3$$
$$SO_2 + H_2O \longrightarrow H_2SO_3$$

52. **(C)** Permanent hardness of water is caused by sulfates, such as calcium sulfate or magesium sulfate. This hardness cannot be destroyed by boiling the water, as temporary hardness can be. Therefore, calcium sulfate cannot be used to soften water; rather, it will increase its hardness.

53. **(B)** Although hydrogen is relatively inert at ordinary temperatures, it can combine with free oxygen, with oxygen that is in chemical combination, with some metallic elements, and with many nonmetallic elements. The addition of hydrogen reduces a substance.

54. **(B)** A *covalent* bond is formed by the equal sharing of electrons; if half-filled orbitals of atoms overlap, the electrons are shared by the atoms in the overlap region. Bonding of a water molecule is covalent. In a water molecule, the positive and negative charges do not coincide; thus, water exhibits polarity. Therefore, the bonding of water is covalent, polar.

55. **(C)** The nitrate test involves the use of a sulfate, such as iron sulfate, and sulfuric acid. The nitrate and sulfate ions react, forming nitric oxide. Nitric oxide then combines with the ferrous ion to form a ferrous-nitrogen-oxygen complex, which produces a brown color.

56. **(C)** A *saturated* solution is one that is in equilibrium; a condition of equilibrium exists between the solvent and the solute, and no more of the solute can dissolve.

57. **(A)** Oxides of barium and sulfer can combine to produce barium sulfate, a salt.

$$BaO + SO_3 \longrightarrow BaSO_4$$

58. **(D)** Brine is a saturated salt solution; chlorine is prepared from a saturated sodium chloride solution by the oxidation of the chloride ion to chlorine. This is accomplished through electrolysis: the chloride ion loses an electron to become chlorine. The oxidation process occurs at the anode.

59. **(D)** Sulfuric acid has a high boiling point: 317°C. Because of this, it is not very volatile and can be used to prepare more volatile acids, such as hydrochloric and nitric acids.

$$NaCl + H_2SO_4 \longrightarrow NaHSO_4 + HCl$$

60. **(B)** In general, polar liquids mix with polar liquids; nonpolar liquids mix with nonpolar liquids; polar and nonpolar liquids will not mix well and are said to be *immiscible*. In other words, one will not dissolve in the other. The immiscibility can be explained on the basis of molecular shape and molecular dipole. Water is polar with the charges not coinciding on the molecule. Carbon tetrachloride is nonpolar, a regular tetrahedron. So water and carbon tetrachloride will not mix.

SCIENCE TEST 2

Physical Sciences

25 Minutes   **40 Questions**

Directions: *Read each question carefully and consider all possible answers. When you have decided which choice is best, blacken the corresponding space on your answer sheet. There is only one best answer for each question.*

1. Which of the following properties is considered a physical property?

    (A) flammability
    (B) boiling point
    (C) reactivity
    (D) osmolarity

2. Which one of the following substances is a chemical compound?

    (A) blood
    (B) water
    (C) oxygen
    (D) air

3. What are the differentiating factors for potential and kinetic energy?

    (A) properties—physical or chemical
    (B) state—solid or liquid
    (C) temperature—high or low
    (D) activity—in motion or in storage

4. How many calories are required to change the temperature of 2000 grams of H_2O from 20°C to 38°C?

    (A) 36 calories
    (B) 24 calories
    (C) 18 calories
    (D) 12 calories

5. The oxidation of one gram of CHO produces four calories. How much CHO must be oxidized in the body to produce 36 calories? (CHO is a carbohydrate.)

    (A) 4 grams
    (B) 7 grams
    (C) 9 grams
    (D) 12 grams

6. What is the atomic weight of the element in the figure below?

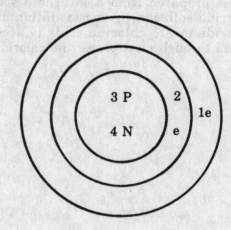

    (A) 2
    (B) 3
    (C) 4
    (D) 7

7. Which of the following kinds of radiation is most penetrating?

    (A) alpha
    (B) beta
    (C) gamma
    (D) X rays

8. I^{131} has a half-life of eight days. A 100-milligram sample of this radioactive element would decay to what amount after eight days?

    (A) 50 milligrams
    (B) 40 milligrams
    (C) 30 milligrams
    (D) 20 milligrams

9. A direct physiological effect of radiation on human tissues is

   (A) impairment of cellular metabolism
   (B) proliferation of white blood cells
   (C) formation of scar tissue
   (D) reduction of body fluids

10. What is the gram molecular weight of $C_6H_{12}O_6$? ($C = 12$, $H = 1$, $O = 16$)

   (A) 29 grams
   (B) 174 grams
   (C) 180 grams
   (D) 696 grams

11. Which one of the following equations is balanced?

   (A) $H_2O \rightarrow H_2 \uparrow + O_2 \uparrow$
   (B) $Al + H_2SO_4 \rightarrow Al_2(SO_4)_3 + H_2 \uparrow$
   (C) $S + O_2 \rightarrow SO_3$
   (D) $2HgO \rightarrow 2Hg + O_2 \uparrow$

12. A person with a fever would be expected to have

   (A) an increase in pulse rate
   (B) a decrease in pulse rate
   (C) no change in pulse rate
   (D) any one of the above

13. Which of the following bodily substances is a catalyst?

   (A) bile
   (B) hemoglobin
   (C) enzyme
   (D) mucus

14. In order to increase the temperature of a gas in a closed unit, it would be necessary to

   (A) increase the pressure
   (B) decrease the density
   (C) decrease the volume
   (D) increase the space

15. Which of the following equations represents an oxidation-reduction reaction?

   (A) $2Na + Cl_2 \rightarrow NaCl$
   (B) $CO_2 + H_2O \rightarrow H_2CO_3$
   (C) $HNO_3 + KOH \rightarrow KNO_3 + H_2O$
   (D) $CaO + H_2O \rightarrow Ca(OH)_2$

16. Which one of the following equations represents neutralization?

   (A) $2Na + Cl_2 \rightarrow 2NaCl$
   (B) $CO_2 + H_2O \rightarrow H_2CO_3$
   (C) $HNO_3 + KOH \rightarrow KNO_3 + H_2O$
   (D) $CaO + H_2O \rightarrow Ca(OH)_2$

17. What happens when a small amount of soap is added to hard water?

   (A) Copious suds are formed.
   (B) A scum is formed.
   (C) All sediments filter out.
   (D) Sediments diffuse equally throughout the solution.

18. A ten-percent solution of glucose will contain

   (A) 1 gram of glucose per 1000 milliliters of solution
   (B) 1 gram of glucose per 100 milliliters of solution
   (C) 10 grams of glucose per 10 milliliters of solution
   (D) 10 grams of glucose per 100 milliliters of solution

Questions 19–22 refer to the diagrams below. Each diagram represents one solution: One gram molecular weight of NaOH, one of KOH, and one of HCl, each dissolved in enough H_2O to make one liter.

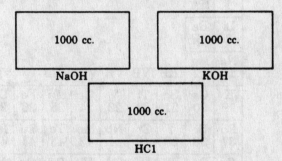

19. What is the molecular weight of NaOH? (Atomic weights: Na = 23; O = 16; H = 1)

   (A) 40×1
   (B) 40×10
   (C) 40×100
   (D) 40×1000

20. These are molar substances because

    (A) their molecular weights are equal to each other
    (B) the volume for each solution is the same
    (C) each solution contains one gram molecular weight
    (D) the percentage of solute to solvent is equal in each solution

21. Identify the products of the chemical reaction between 1 cubic centimeter of KOH and 1 cubic centimeter of HCl

    (A) $K^+ + Cl_2 + 2H + OH$
    (B) $KCl + H_2 + O_2$
    (C) $K + Cl + HOH$
    (D) $KCl + H_2O$

22. CA^{++} (atomic weight 40) is bivalent; hence, one gram equivalent weighs

    (A) 40 grams
    (B) 30 grams
    (C) 20 grams
    (D) 10 grams

23. A covalent bond between two amino acid molecules can be created by

    (A) inserting a water molecule between them
    (B) removing a water molecule from them
    (C) inserting a carbon atom between them
    (D) removing a carbon atom from one of them

24. Identify those elements in the periodic table at the bottom of the page that are inert gases (refer to columns).

    (A) IA
    (B) Zero
    (C) IIIB-VIIB
    (D) VIII

25. The basic inorganic raw materials for photosynthesis are

    (A) water and oxygen
    (B) water and carbon dioxide
    (C) oxygen and carbon dioxide
    (D) sugar and carbon dioxide

26. Production of Salk vaccine against polio depended upon discovery of a method for

    (A) growing the polio virus outside the human body
    (B) killing the polio virus
    (C) observing the polio virus in the human body
    (D) producing a polio antitoxin

27. Ringworm is caused by a(n)

    (A) alga
    (B) bacterium
    (C) fungus
    (D) protozoan

IA																VIIA	Zero
H 1	IIA											IIIA	IVA	VA	VIA	H 1	He 2
Li 3	Be 4											B 5	C 6	N 7	O 8	F 9	Ne 10
Na 11	Mg 12	IIIB	IVB	VB	VIB	VIIB		VIII		IB	IIB	Al 13	Si 14	P 15	S 16	Cl 17	Ar 18
K 19	Ca 20	Sc 21	Ti 22	V 23	Cr 24	Mn 25	Fe 26	Co 27	Ni 28	Cu 29	Zn 30	Ga 31	Ge 32	As 33	Se 34	Br 35	Kr 36
Rb 37	Sr 38	Y 39	Zr 40	Nb 41	Mo 42	Tc 43	Ru 44	Rh 45	Pd 46	Ag 47	Cd 48	In 49	Sn 50	Sb 51	Te 52	I 53	Xe 54
Cs 55	Ba 56	*La 57	Hf 72	Ta 73	W 74	Re 75	Os 76	Ir 77	Pt 78	Au 79	Hg 80	Tl 81	Pb 82	Bi 83	Po 84	At 85	Rn 86
Fr 87	Ra 88	#Ac 89															

*LANTHANIDE SERIES	Ce 58	Pr 59	Nd 60	Pm 61	Sm 62	Eu 63	Gd 64	Tb 65	Dy 66	Ho 67	Fr 68	Tm 69	Yb 70	Lu 71
#ACTINIDE SERIES	Th 90	Pa 91	U 92	Np 93	Pu 94	Am 95	Cm 96	Bk 97	Cf 98	Es 99	Fm 100	Md 101	No 102	Lr 103

28. The process responsible for the continuous removal of carbon dioxide from the atmosphere is

(A) respiration
(B) metabolism
(C) oxidation
(D) photosynthesis

29. All of the following concepts in genetics were first clearly stated by Gregor Mendel *except*

(A) dominance
(B) independent assortment
(C) segregation
(D) hybrid vigor

30. The relation between termites and their intestinal protozoa is an example of

(A) trophism
(B) parasitism
(C) mutualism
(D) commensalism

31. *Eugenics* is a program for improving a breed by controlling

(A) heredity
(B) environment
(C) both heredity and environment
(D) none of the above

32. The catalytic action of pancreatic juice affects

(A) minerals
(B) fats
(C) carbohydrates
(D) vitamins

33. The digestion of carbohydrates is initiated by

(A) ptyalin
(B) sucrose
(C) maltose
(D) lactose

34. One of the functions of bile in the digestive processes is to

(A) deaminize proteins
(B) hydrolyze starches and fats
(C) neutralize acidity of food from the stomach
(D) catalyze vitamin A and vitamin D

35. Which of the following substances is necessary for pepsinogen to be converted into pepsin?

(A) HCl
(B) CaCl
(C) vitamin B_{12}
(D) Fe

36. Glycogenesis occurs primarily in the

(A) blood cells and spleen
(B) pancreas and gallbladder
(C) small intestines and stomach
(D) liver and muscles

37. The end-products of the Krebs Cycle are

(A) carbon dioxide and water
(B) urea and bile pigments
(C) lactic acid and pyruvic acid
(D) ketones and acetones

38. The functional unit (or nephron) of the human kidney consists of

(A) Bowman's capsule and veins
(B) Bowman's capsule, the glomerulus, and renal tubule
(C) the ureter and renal tubule
(D) the ureter, urethra, and renal tubule

39. An organ that functions both as an endo-crine and an exocrine gland is the

    (A) salivary gland
    (B) gall bladder
    (C) thyroid gland
    (D) pancreas

40. Aerobic oxidation of glucose occurs in two major stages; these are

    (A) glycolysis and reduction
    (B) synthesis and the Krebs Cycle
    (C) glycolysis and the Krebs Cycle
    (D) degradation and hydrolysis

Answer Key

1.	**B**	21.	**D**
2.	**B**	22.	**C**
3.	**D**	23.	**B**
4.	**A**	24.	**B**
5.	**C**	25.	**B**
6.	**D**	26.	**A**
7.	**C**	27.	**C**
8.	**A**	28.	**D**
9.	**A**	29.	**D**
10.	**C**	30.	**C**
11.	**D**	31.	**A**
12.	**A**	32.	**B**
13.	**C**	33.	**A**
14.	**A**	34.	**C**
15.	**A**	35.	**A**
16.	**C**	36.	**D**
17.	**B**	37.	**A**
18.	**D**	38.	**B**
19.	**A**	39.	**D**
20.	**C**	40.	**C**

Explanatory Answers

1. **(B)** Physical properties are those that do not involve any change in the nature or chemical composition of the substance. Heating a substance to the temperature at which it boils (its *boiling point*) will change its physical state but will not alter its chemical state.

2. **(B)** Water is a compound formed by oxygen and hydrogen in chemical combination. Blood and air are mixtures, and oxygen is an element.

3. **(D)** *Potential energy* is, in effect, energy in storage, as energy that can be released when conditions are conducive. *Kinetic energy* is energy of activity; the energy is released as the activity occurs.

4. **(A)** One calorie (kilocalorie) will raise one kilogram (1000 grams) of water one degree Celsius. It would take 18 calories to raise 1000 grams of water 18 degrees (38°– 20°), or 36 calories to raise 2000 grams of water 18 degrees Celsius.

5. **(C)** If one gram of carbohydrate produces four calories, nine grams are required to produce 36 calories. 36 calories ÷ 4 calories/gram = 9 grams.

6. **(D)** The atomic weight (or mass number of an atom) equals the total of the number of protons and neutrons in the nucleus of the atom, or the total number of particles in the nucleus.

7. **(C)** Nearly every unstable nucleus of an atom gives off one or more of the three kinds of radiation: alpha, beta, and gamma. *Alpha* and *beta* radiation are particle emission; *gamma* rays are shortwave energy rays similar to X rays, but stronger and more penetrating. Both gamma rays and X rays are more penetrating than alpha and beta radiation.

8. **(A)** The *half-life period* can be defined as the time needed for half of a given amount of a substance to undergo spontaneous decomposition. This varies with different radioactive elements. There would be 50 milligrams left of a 100 milligram sample of material with a half-life of eight days after the eight days pass.

9. **(A)** Radiation can cause *mutations*, or genetic change. Any change in the genetic code would alter or destroy the trait associated with that particular gene. This could involve changes in enzyme produced and other factors associated with cellular metabolism.

10. **(C)** Gram molecular weight may be defined as the weight of the molecule expressed in grams. The molecular weight of glucose ($C_6H_{12}O_6$) is 180, as the following indicates: The weight of the six atoms of carbon equals 72 (6 × 12); twelve hydrogens weigh 12 (12 × 1); the weight of the six oxygens equals 96 (6 × 16). The total is 180; thus, the gram molecular weight of glucose is 180 grams.

11. **(D)** Equation (D) is balanced, because the amount of each substance is equal on both sides of the equation. There are two mercury atoms and two oxygen atoms on each side.

12. **(A)** A person with a fever has a higher temperature than normal. This reflects an increase in metabolic activities, since heat is given off as a waste product when energy in the form of ATP is used for metabolic purposes. Consequently, the pulse rate of a person with a fever is higher than normal because the heart is pumping blood at a greater rate so that the transport of materials like oxygen and glucose in the blood can accommodate this increased metabolic activity. Also, the circulatory system has to work harder to carry the greater amount of heat generated away from the tissues to be radiated from the surface of the body.

13. **(C)** Enzymes are called *organic catalysts*, in that they are produced by the organisms and catalyze reactions that occur within that organism. The other substances named do not function as catalysts.

14. **(A)** Gases are affected by temperature and pressure. If the gas is in a closed system, it cannot change its volume if temperature or pressure changes. Therefore, in a closed system, increasing the pressure would increase the temperature.

15. **(A)** For every oxidation, there must be a reduction. Oxidation can involve the removal of electrons, the removal of hydrogen, or the addition of oxygen; reduction, the opposite. In equation (A) metallic sodium loses an electron to become a positively charged ion; chlorine gains an electron to become a negatively charged chloride ion. Thus, sodium is oxidized and chlorine is reduced.

16. **(C)** Nitric acid reacts with the base potassium hydroxide to form potassium nitrate and water. For each hydrogen ion of the acid, there is a hydroxyl ion of the base to combine with it to form water. Therefore, neutralization occurs.

17. **(B)** Hard water contains calcium sulfate, calcium bicarbonate, or magnesium compounds. Soap is a mixture of sodium salts of organic acids that will react with these dissolved minerals. The insoluble calcium salt of the organic acid is precipitated out. This is the *scum*, or insoluble curdy material, that forms first. If enough soap is added, the soap acts as a cleansing agent after the first portion has precipitated the calcium ion.

18. **(D)** The concentration of a solution, on a percentage basis, contains a specific amount of solute in grams per 100 milliliters of solution. Thus, a ten-percent solution would have ten grams of solute per 100 milliliters of solution.

19. **(A)** The molecular weight of sodium hydroxide (NaOH) is 40 × 1, or 40. This can be calculated by adding the atomic weights of the atoms composing the molecule.

20. **(C)** A molar solution contains one gram molecular weight (the molecular weight of the molecule expressed in grams), or one mole per liter of solution. Therefore, each is a one-molar solution.

21. **(D)** Potassium hydroxide (KOH) and hydrochloric acid (HCl) react to form potassium chloride (KCl) and water. This is a double displacement.

$$KOH + HCl \longrightarrow K+Cl- + H_2O$$

22. **(C)** An *equivalent weight* of an element is that weight of the element that combines with or displaces one atomic weight of hydrogen. Since calcium has a valence of plus 2 while hydrogen has a valence of plus 1, one-half of the atomic weight of calcium will displace one atomic weight of hydrogen. Calcium has an atomic weight of 40; therefore, its equivalent weight is 20, or, expressed as grams, 20 grams The following equation can apply:

$$\text{equivalent weight} = \frac{\text{atomic weight}}{\text{valence}}$$

23. **(B)** Two amino acid molecules can be bonded together by removing a hydrogen atom from the amino group (NH_2) of one amino acid molecule and removing a hydroxyl ion (OH–) from the carboxyl group (COOH) of the other. The result is a molecule of water removed from the two amino acids and a covalent bond between the nitrogen atom in the amino group of one amino acid and the carbon atom in the carboxyl group of the other. This type of reaction is called *dehydration synthesis* and results in the production of water within cells that is called *metabolic water*. Creation of a bond between two amino acids can be illustrated as follows (R represents any of the 20 different side chains that can be included in amino acids):

Removing this water molecule will create a bond between the nitrogen and carbon.

24. **(B)** The periodic table places elements according to similarities in properties due to the number and arrangement of electrons in the atom. Group Zero is the inert gases. Metals and nonmetals are included in the remaining groups.

25. **(B)** Carbon dioxide and water, in the presence of light and the chlorophylls, yield glucose and oxygen. The water is absorbed by the root system of green plants and translocated through xylem to the leaves and other parts, which are the photosynthetic organs. Carbon dioxide enters the plants through epidermal stomates.

26. **(A)** Salk vaccine is prepared from inactivated polio virus. Viruses are obligate intracellular parasites; therefore, a method for growing viruses outside the human body had to be discovered and refined. Viruses typically are cultured in chick embryos.

27. **(C)** Ringworm is caused by fungi known as dermatophytes. These are sometimes known as the *Tineas*.

28. **(D)** *Photosynthesis* is the process characteristic of green plants by which carbon dioxide and water react to produce glucose and oxygen. The carbon dioxide used in the process enters the tissue from the air, passing in through stomata of the epidermis; oxygen produced by the reaction passes through the stomata into the air. This process occurs only in the presence of light, and therefore continuous carbon dioxide removal occurs only in the presence of light.

29. **(D)** Mendel's Laws clearly stated the concepts of dominance and segregation (first law–Law of Segregation) and of independent assortment (second law–Law of Independent Assortment), but did not deal with the concept of hybrid vigor.

30. **(C)** Any relationship between two individual species is *symbiosis*. The word *symbiosis* means "life together." There are several kinds of symbiotic relationships, including commensalism, parasitism, and mutualism. A *mutualistic* relationship is one in which strong bonds exist between the two species, and each member benefits from the relationship. This kind of symbiotic relationship exists between termites and the protozoans (flagellates) of their intestinal tract. There is evidence that some bacteria in the termite's intestinal tract also play a role in the relationship. The flagellates and bacteria digest the cellulose that the termites consume.

31. **(A)** *Eugenics* is a program for improving breeds by controlling heredity. The program would be based on selection of parents.

32. **(B)** Pancreatic juice, secreted by the pancreas through a duct into the small intestine, contains several enzymes. Among them is the enzyme lipase, which acts on fats, hydrolyzing them to glycerol and fatty acids.

33. **(A)** *Ptyalin* (amylase) is a salivary enzyme of the mouth that hydrolyzes starch, a carbohydrate, to maltose. Further digestion of carbohydrates occurs in the small intestine, where pancreatic amylase is added to the intestinal contents.

34. **(C)** Although bile, which is secreted by the liver into the small intestine, contains no enzymes, it emulsifies fats, breaking them up into smaller globules for easier digestion. Bile also serves to neutralize acidity. Bile, pancreatic juice, and intestinal juice have

high bicarbonate contents; therefore, the acidity that develops in the stomach because of the secretion of hydrochloric acid in the gastric juice is effectively neutralized.

35. **(A)** Pepsinogen is a precursor of the enzyme pepsin; this enzyme digests proteins to polypeptides. The enzyme is formed by hydrochloric acid and acts in an acid environment with a pH of about 1.6 to 2.5. This acid medium is produced by the hydrochloric acid, which is a part of the gastric juice secreted by the stomach lining.

36. **(D)** *Glycogenesis* is the formation of glycogen from glucose; glycogen is the form in which carbohydrates are stored in animals. Glycogen is stored in larger quantities and more permanently in the liver; some is produced and stored temporarily in muscle.

37. **(A)** Carbon dioxide and water are the end-products of the Krebs cycle, which is the second phase of aerobic cellular oxidation of glucose for the release of energy.

38. **(B)** The kidney has the function of filtering wastes from the blood. Each nephron performs this function; thus, it is the functional unit. Wastes and water are filtered out from the blood in the glomerulus, a mass of capillaries lying in Bowman's capsule; the water and wastes pass through the capsule wall into the renal tubule. Much of the water is reabsorbed into the bloodstream through the walls of the capillaries surrounding the loop of Henle of the renal tubule. The remaining liquid, or urine, passes into the renal pelvis, to the ureter and bladder, and is eventually eliminated through the urethra.

39. **(D)** An endocrine (or ductless) gland secretes hormone(s) directly into the bloodstream. The hormone is transported by the blood and will affect only the target tissue. An exocrine gland passes its secretion through a duct to a specific site. The pancreatic islet cells secrete the hormone, insulin; other cells of the pancreas secrete pancreatic juice, containing enzymes, through the pancreatic duct into the duodenum.

40. **(C)** In the first stage of aerobic oxidation, glucose is oxidized to pyruvic acid; this is known as glycolysis. The two pyruvates resulting from glycolysis of a molecule of glucose enter into the Krebs Cycle (Citric Acid Cycle) and are oxidized to carbon dioxide and water.

Answer Sheet
Life Sciences

TEST 3

1. Ⓐ Ⓑ Ⓒ Ⓓ   13. Ⓐ Ⓑ Ⓒ Ⓓ   25. Ⓐ Ⓑ Ⓒ Ⓓ   37. Ⓐ Ⓑ Ⓒ Ⓓ   49. Ⓐ Ⓑ Ⓒ Ⓓ

2. Ⓐ Ⓑ Ⓒ Ⓓ   14. Ⓐ Ⓑ Ⓒ Ⓓ   26. Ⓐ Ⓑ Ⓒ Ⓓ   38. Ⓐ Ⓑ Ⓒ Ⓓ   50. Ⓐ Ⓑ Ⓒ Ⓓ

3. Ⓐ Ⓑ Ⓒ Ⓓ   15. Ⓐ Ⓑ Ⓒ Ⓓ   27. Ⓐ Ⓑ Ⓒ Ⓓ   39. Ⓐ Ⓑ Ⓒ Ⓓ   51. Ⓐ Ⓑ Ⓒ Ⓓ

4. Ⓐ Ⓑ Ⓒ Ⓓ   16. Ⓐ Ⓑ Ⓒ Ⓓ   28. Ⓐ Ⓑ Ⓒ Ⓓ   40. Ⓐ Ⓑ Ⓒ Ⓓ   52. Ⓐ Ⓑ Ⓒ Ⓓ

5. Ⓐ Ⓑ Ⓒ Ⓓ   17. Ⓐ Ⓑ Ⓒ Ⓓ   29. Ⓐ Ⓑ Ⓒ Ⓓ   41. Ⓐ Ⓑ Ⓒ Ⓓ   53. Ⓐ Ⓑ Ⓒ Ⓓ

6. Ⓐ Ⓑ Ⓒ Ⓓ   18. Ⓐ Ⓑ Ⓒ Ⓓ   30. Ⓐ Ⓑ Ⓒ Ⓓ   42. Ⓐ Ⓑ Ⓒ Ⓓ   54. Ⓐ Ⓑ Ⓒ Ⓓ

7. Ⓐ Ⓑ Ⓒ Ⓓ   19. Ⓐ Ⓑ Ⓒ Ⓓ   31. Ⓐ Ⓑ Ⓒ Ⓓ   43. Ⓐ Ⓑ Ⓒ Ⓓ   55. Ⓐ Ⓑ Ⓒ Ⓓ

8. Ⓐ Ⓑ Ⓒ Ⓓ   20. Ⓐ Ⓑ Ⓒ Ⓓ   32. Ⓐ Ⓑ Ⓒ Ⓓ   44. Ⓐ Ⓑ Ⓒ Ⓓ   56. Ⓐ Ⓑ Ⓒ Ⓓ

9. Ⓐ Ⓑ Ⓒ Ⓓ   21. Ⓐ Ⓑ Ⓒ Ⓓ   33. Ⓐ Ⓑ Ⓒ Ⓓ   45. Ⓐ Ⓑ Ⓒ Ⓓ   57. Ⓐ Ⓑ Ⓒ Ⓓ

10. Ⓐ Ⓑ Ⓒ Ⓓ   22. Ⓐ Ⓑ Ⓒ Ⓓ   34. Ⓐ Ⓑ Ⓒ Ⓓ   46. Ⓐ Ⓑ Ⓒ Ⓓ   58. Ⓐ Ⓑ Ⓒ Ⓓ

11. Ⓐ Ⓑ Ⓒ Ⓓ   23. Ⓐ Ⓑ Ⓒ Ⓓ   35. Ⓐ Ⓑ Ⓒ Ⓓ   47. Ⓐ Ⓑ Ⓒ Ⓓ   59. Ⓐ Ⓑ Ⓒ Ⓓ

12. Ⓐ Ⓑ Ⓒ Ⓓ   24. Ⓐ Ⓑ Ⓒ Ⓓ   36. Ⓐ Ⓑ Ⓒ Ⓓ   48. Ⓐ Ⓑ Ⓒ Ⓓ   60. Ⓐ Ⓑ Ⓒ Ⓓ

TEST 4

1. Ⓐ Ⓑ Ⓒ Ⓓ	13. Ⓐ Ⓑ Ⓒ Ⓓ	25. Ⓐ Ⓑ Ⓒ Ⓓ	37. Ⓐ Ⓑ Ⓒ Ⓓ	49. Ⓐ Ⓑ Ⓒ Ⓓ
2. Ⓐ Ⓑ Ⓒ Ⓓ	14. Ⓐ Ⓑ Ⓒ Ⓓ	26. Ⓐ Ⓑ Ⓒ Ⓓ	38. Ⓐ Ⓑ Ⓒ Ⓓ	50. Ⓐ Ⓑ Ⓒ Ⓓ
3. Ⓐ Ⓑ Ⓒ Ⓓ	15. Ⓐ Ⓑ Ⓒ Ⓓ	27. Ⓐ Ⓑ Ⓒ Ⓓ	39. Ⓐ Ⓑ Ⓒ Ⓓ	51. Ⓐ Ⓑ Ⓒ Ⓓ
4. Ⓐ Ⓑ Ⓒ Ⓓ	16. Ⓐ Ⓑ Ⓒ Ⓓ	28. Ⓐ Ⓑ Ⓒ Ⓓ	40. Ⓐ Ⓑ Ⓒ Ⓓ	52. Ⓐ Ⓑ Ⓒ Ⓓ
5. Ⓐ Ⓑ Ⓒ Ⓓ	17. Ⓐ Ⓑ Ⓒ Ⓓ	29. Ⓐ Ⓑ Ⓒ Ⓓ	41. Ⓐ Ⓑ Ⓒ Ⓓ	53. Ⓐ Ⓑ Ⓒ Ⓓ
6. Ⓐ Ⓑ Ⓒ Ⓓ	18. Ⓐ Ⓑ Ⓒ Ⓓ	30. Ⓐ Ⓑ Ⓒ Ⓓ	42. Ⓐ Ⓑ Ⓒ Ⓓ	54. Ⓐ Ⓑ Ⓒ Ⓓ
7. Ⓐ Ⓑ Ⓒ Ⓓ	19. Ⓐ Ⓑ Ⓒ Ⓓ	31. Ⓐ Ⓑ Ⓒ Ⓓ	43. Ⓐ Ⓑ Ⓒ Ⓓ	55. Ⓐ Ⓑ Ⓒ Ⓓ
8. Ⓐ Ⓑ Ⓒ Ⓓ	20. Ⓐ Ⓑ Ⓒ Ⓓ	32. Ⓐ Ⓑ Ⓒ Ⓓ	44. Ⓐ Ⓑ Ⓒ Ⓓ	56. Ⓐ Ⓑ Ⓒ Ⓓ
9. Ⓐ Ⓑ Ⓒ Ⓓ	21. Ⓐ Ⓑ Ⓒ Ⓓ	33. Ⓐ Ⓑ Ⓒ Ⓓ	45. Ⓐ Ⓑ Ⓒ Ⓓ	57. Ⓐ Ⓑ Ⓒ Ⓓ
10. Ⓐ Ⓑ Ⓒ Ⓓ	22. Ⓐ Ⓑ Ⓒ Ⓓ	34. Ⓐ Ⓑ Ⓒ Ⓓ	46. Ⓐ Ⓑ Ⓒ Ⓓ	58. Ⓐ Ⓑ Ⓒ Ⓓ
11. Ⓐ Ⓑ Ⓒ Ⓓ	23. Ⓐ Ⓑ Ⓒ Ⓓ	35. Ⓐ Ⓑ Ⓒ Ⓓ	47. Ⓐ Ⓑ Ⓒ Ⓓ	59. Ⓐ Ⓑ Ⓒ Ⓓ
12. Ⓐ Ⓑ Ⓒ Ⓓ	24. Ⓐ Ⓑ Ⓒ Ⓓ	36. Ⓐ Ⓑ Ⓒ Ⓓ	48. Ⓐ Ⓑ Ⓒ Ⓓ	60. Ⓐ Ⓑ Ⓒ Ⓓ

SCIENCE TEST 3

Life Sciences

45 Minutes   60 Questions

Directions: *Read each question carefully and consider all possible answers. When you have decided which choice is best, blacken the corresponding space on your answer sheet. There is only one best answer for each question.*

1. Diabetes mellitus initially results from

    (A) oversecretion of pancreatin
    (B) undersecretion of insulin
    (C) excessive intake of sugar
    (D) inadequate intake of fats

2. The so-called "bag of water," which breaks during labor in the pregnant female, is the

    (A) amniotic sac
    (B) yolk sac
    (C) placenta
    (D) chorionic membrane

3. Sebaceous glands are most numerous in areas where

    (A) there are small amounts of hair
    (B) there are large amounts of hair
    (C) the skin is thin
    (D) sweat glands are located

4. Hereditary determiners are found in

    (A) PKU
    (B) RNA
    (C) DNA
    (D) SMA

5. Skin color varies with the amount of

    (A) melanin
    (B) matrix
    (C) hair
    (D) keratin

6. The deciduous teeth contain no

    (A) cuspids
    (B) bicuspids
    (C) canines
    (D) incisors

7. The material covering the surface of the tooth below the gum line is

    (A) cementum
    (B) dentine
    (C) enamel
    (D) pulp

8. Before the body can use oxygen, it must be combined with

    (A) thyroxin
    (B) hemoglobin
    (C) bilirubin
    (D) water

9. The sex of the new individual is determined by

    (A) the female
    (B) the male
    (C) either the female or the male
    (D) neither the female or male

10. The umbilical cord is cut immediately after a baby is born because

    (A) of the need to stop circulation between the fetus and the placenta
    (B) the mother's blood will contaminate the baby's blood
    (C) the baby has less need for blood
    (D) the mother will hemorrhage

11. The major difference between plasma and blood is

    (A) cellular content
    (B) acid–base balance
    (C) anion–cation placement
    (D) solute–solvent concentrations

12. The blood cells that cause blood clotting are called

    (A) leucocytes
    (B) erythrocytes
    (C) thrombocytes
    (D) lymphocytes

13. The longest, strongest, and heaviest bone in the body is the

    (A) tibia
    (B) spinal column
    (C) femur
    (D) radius

14. Iron is needed for

    (A) development of nervous tissue
    (B) formation of red blood cells
    (C) growth of hair and nails
    (D) utilization of vitamins

15. Which of the following is necessary for digestion?

    (A) transamination
    (B) glucogenolysis
    (C) Krebs cycle
    (D) peristalsis

16. Which of the following organs is vital to life?

    (A) adrenal glands
    (B) thymus
    (C) liver
    (D) spleen

17. Which of the following body wastes is normally removed by the lungs?

    (A) carbon dioxide
    (B) urea
    (C) acetone
    (D) creatinine

18. Three-dimensional vision is related to which of the following structures?

    (A) iris
    (B) pupil
    (C) optic chiasma
    (D) retina

19. Reflex muscular action is produced by an external stimulus through a circuit consisting of

    (A) dendrite→cyton→axon
    (B) axon→cyton→dendrite
    (C) dendrite→axon→cyton
    (D) axon→dendrite→cyton

20. Which of the following hormones is predominant in females?

    (A) androgen
    (B) testosterone
    (C) gonadotrophin
    (D) estrogen

21. Proteins have the chemical structure of

    (A) hydrocarbons
    (B) amino acids
    (C) heterocyclics
    (D) alcohols

22. Which one of the following statements is true?

    (A) Bone marrow produces red blood cells in the adult.
    (B) The spleen synthesizes vitamins in the child.
    (C) The liver manufactures glucose and stores bile.
    (D) The lymphatic system refines fats and stores water.

23. The most widely distributed of all tissues is

    (A) epithelial
    (B) osseous
    (C) connective
    (D) nervous

24. The chemical reaction that supplies immediate energy for muscular contractions can be summarized as

    (A) $ATP \rightarrow ADP + P$
    (B) lactic acid$\rightarrow CO_2 + H_2O$
    (C) lactic acid$\rightarrow$glycogen
    (D) glycogen$\rightarrow ATP$

25. The body's reaction to stress includes which of the following mechanisms?

    (A) conversion of carbohydrates into glycogen
    (B) decreased pumping action of the heart
    (C) secretion of adrenalin
    (D) pooling of blood in the veins

26. After rigorous exercise, the body is depleted of

    (A) Na and H_2O
    (B) Glucose and H_2O
    (C) H_2O and K
    (D) H_2O and colloids

27. Which of the following is related to the cause of heart disease?

    (A) absence of serum transaminase
    (B) accumulation of urea nitrogen
    (C) decreased levels of bilirubin
    (D) increased levels of blood cholesterol

28. The endocrine glands in the body have the function of

    (A) purifying the blood
    (B) regulating bodily activities
    (C) controlling the blood distribution
    (D) preventing antigenic action

29. Persons with overactive thyroids have which of the following changes in body functions?

    (A) decrease in metabolic rate
    (B) increase in metabolic rate
    (C) loss of appetite
    (D) gain in weight

30. The basic unit of the lung tissue is

    (A) lacunae
    (B) nephron
    (C) alveolus
    (D) cyton

31. Hemorrhoids, commonly called piles, affect which of the following structures?

    (A) pyloric sphincter
    (B) rectal sphincter
    (C) urethral orifice
    (D) mitral orifice

32. Which of the following substances produces the most calories per gram when oxidized?

    (A) nucleic acids
    (B) proteins
    (C) fats
    (D) carbohydrates

33. CO_2 would be produced from which of the following processes?

    (A) deaminization
    (B) fermentation
    (C) hydrolysis
    (D) anabolism

34. The speech processes are primarily controlled by which area of the brain?

    (A) frontal
    (B) cerebellum
    (C) parietal
    (D) occipital

35. In the circulating system, oxygenated blood is pumped out of the heart from the

    (A) right ventricle
    (B) left ventricle
    (C) right atrium
    (D) left atrium

36. The chest is separated from the abdomen by the

    (A) diaphragm
    (B) carina
    (C) mediastinum
    (D) pectoralis

37. Smooth muscle tissue is found in the

    (A) heart
    (B) kidneys
    (C) intestines
    (D) skeletal muscles

38. The exchange of gases between the respiratory system and the circulating system is by means of the pulmonary

    (A) arteries
    (B) veins
    (C) capillaries
    (D) venules

39. The digestive tract receives blood from which of the following vessels?

    (A) celiac axis
    (B) profunda
    (C) phrenic superior
    (D) vesicle inferior

40. In systemic circulation, venous blood is different from arterial blood in that the

    (A) CO_2 concentration is lower than the O_2 concentration
    (B) CO_2 concentration is higher than the O_2 concentration
    (C) overall concentration is high and the rate of flow is low
    (D) overall concentration is low and the rate of flow is high

41. Sperm and egg cells have the haploid number of chromosomes as a result of

    (A) meiosis
    (B) cleavage
    (C) mitosis
    (D) fertilization

42. Fraternal twins develop from

    (A) one fertilized egg
    (B) two fertilized eggs
    (C) one egg fertilized by two sperms
    (D) two eggs fertilized by the same sperm

43. Blood in the adult human body makes a complete circulation in about

    (A) 10 seconds
    (B) 30 seconds
    (C) 1 minute
    (D) 3 minutes

44. The "pacemaker" of the heart is located in the

    (A) left atrium
    (B) left ventricle
    (C) right atrium
    (D) right ventricle

45. Which generalization concerning sex determination is true?

    (A) The female determines the sex of the offspring
    (B) The XY chromosomes are found in the male
    (C) The sex of the offspring is first determined during maturation
    (D) There is a greater chance of getting female offspring than male offspring

46. A decrease in the number of red corpuscles would result in a corresponding decrease in the blood's ability to

    (A) transport oxygen
    (B) destroy disease germs
    (C) form fibrinogen
    (D) absorb glucose

47. After being in a small, poorly ventilated room for an hour with eleven other persons, a student noticed that his rate of breathing had increased. The most probable reason for this increase is that the

    (A) air in the room had become hot
    (B) carbon dioxide concentration in his blood had increased
    (C) oxygen concentration in his blood had increased
    (D) excess water in his body needed to be eliminated

48. In a normal person the largest part of the central nervous system is the

    (A) cerebrum
    (B) cerebellum
    (C) medulla
    (D) spinal cord

49. Which one of the following terms is *not* directly associated with the same sense organ as the three others?

    (A) stapes
    (B) cochlea
    (C) tympanic membrane
    (D) cornea

50. Carbohydrates are the main source of energy because they

    (A) produce more calories than other foods
    (B) rapidly oxidize
    (C) produce fat through synthesis
    (D) stimulate metabolism

51. When citrus fruits are not included in a person's diet, one should increase the amount of

    (A) cabbage
    (B) dates
    (C) apples
    (D) cereals

52. A good substitute for milk would be

    (A) meat, fish, poultry
    (B) cheese, ice cream, pudding
    (C) orange, grapefruit, tangerine
    (D) carrots, sweet potatoes, peaches

53. Milk is called the almost perfect food because it

    (A) supplies essential nutrients and is easily digested
    (B) is a liquid, therefore high in calories, and is easily digested
    (C) contains little fat and is low in carbohydrates
    (D) supplies water for metabolism

54. An important contribution of fresh, green leafy vegetables to the diet is

    (A) protein
    (B) carbohydrate
    (C) vitamin C
    (D) sodium

55. If you are presently consuming 3000 calories daily (and maintaining constant weight), and you reduce your intake to 2000 calories a day, you should lose approximately

    (A) 1 pound per day
    (B) 1 pound per week
    (C) 2 pounds per week
    (D) 5 pounds per week

56. Protein is catabolized to meet energy needs when the diet is inadequate in

    (A) carbohydrate
    (B) fat
    (C) minerals and vitamins
    (D) calories

57. Which of the following statements is correct?

    (A) Folic acid is required for nucleic acid synthesis.
    (B) Vitamin C aids in biosynthesis of cholesterol.
    (C) Vitamin E aids in absorption of iron.
    (D) Vitamin E protects vitamin A from oxidation.

58. The major contributions of whole wheat or enriched bread or cereal to the diet are

    (A) carbohydrate and vitamin B complex
    (B) protein and iron
    (C) calcium and riboflavin
    (D) protein and vitamin B complex

59. A good label for canned goods always includes

    (A) picture of product to give idea of color, size, and appearance
    (B) net contents, number of portions, and quality of product
    (C) brief but specific instructions or directions for use
    (D) brand name

60. Caloric needs are highest during

    (A) infancy
    (B) childhood
    (C) adulthood
    (D) middle age

Answer Key

1.	B	21.	B	41.	A
2.	A	22.	A	42.	B
3.	B	23.	C	43.	B
4.	C	24.	A	44.	C
5.	A	25.	C	45.	B
6.	B	26.	A	46.	A
7.	A	27.	D	47.	B
8.	B	28.	B	48.	A
9.	B	29.	B	49.	D
10.	A	30.	C	50.	B
11.	A	31.	B	51.	A
12.	C	32.	C	52.	B
13.	C	33.	B	53.	A
14.	B	34.	A	54.	C
15.	D	35.	B	55.	C
16.	C	36.	A	56.	D
17.	A	37.	C	57.	A
18.	C	38.	C	58.	A
19.	A	39.	A	59.	B
20.	D	40.	B	60.	A

Explanatory Answers

1. **(B)** Insulin increases the permeability of the cell membrane to glucose, thus enhancing the uptake of glucose from the blood by the cells. If insulin is deficient, glucose is not removed from the blood and utilized by the cells, resulting in an excess of glucose in the blood and leading to other symptoms of diabetes.

2. **(A)** The amnion is one of the extraembryonic structures formed during embryonic development. It surrounds the embryo and becomes filled with fluid in which the embryo floats. The amniotic fluid probably provides protection from mechanical shock for the embryo.

3. **(B)** Sebaceous glands are associated with hair follicles: the cells lining the glands form the secretion, and the entire cellular lining, plus the fatty secretion, form sebum, which is expelled into the hair follicle. Sebum serves to keep the hair and skin pliable.

4. **(C)** DNA (deoxyribonucleic acid) is found in the nucleus of each cell and "stores" genetic information, or the genetic code. DNA replicates itself before mitosis or meiosis begins, and genetic information is distributed equally to the daughter nuclei. RNA (ribonucleic acid), transcribed on DNA, translates the genetic or hereditary information.

5. **(A)** Melanin is a dark pigment found in the cells of the basal layers of the skin. Skin color varies with the size and density of the melanin particles: the more melanin present, the darker the skin.

6. **(B)** Each person has a set of 20 deciduous teeth, as contrasted to 32 permanent or nondeciduous teeth. The set of deciduous teeth contains no bicuspids, and only two molars per quadrant rather than three molars. A set per quadrant of deciduous teeth includes two incisors, one canine, and two molars; a set per quadrant of nondeciduous teeth includes two incisors, one canine, two premolars (bicuspids), and three molars.

7. **(A)** Cementum covers the surface of roots of teeth; enamel covers the surface of the crowns of teeth.

8. **(B)** Oxygen must combine with hemoglobin found in red blood cells to form oxyhemoglobin. In this form, oxygen is transported by the bloodstream to the cells of the body, where it is used in cellular respiration, or metabolism, for the release of energy.

9. **(B)** The XY chromosomes are found in the male, while the female carries XX. As a result of meiosis, a sperm will carry either an X or Y chromosome; all eggs will carry one X. Fertilization of an X-bearing egg by a Y-bearing sperm produces an XY zygote, which develops into a male. Fertilization of an X-bearing egg by an X-bearing sperm produces an XX zygote, which develops into a female.

10. **(A)** The fetus and the mother have independent circulatory systems. Fetal blood passing to and from the placenta by way of the umbilical blood vessels is separated from the mother's blood in the placenta by thin tissues; food, gases, and metabolic wastes can diffuse through these tissues between the two bloodstreams. After birth, the placenta's function has ended and as the baby's systems become "active," there is no longer an exchange of materials between the two bloodstreams.

11. **(A)** *Plasma* is the liquid portion of the blood. *Whole blood* consists of plasma with its dissolved materials, and the blood cells.

12. **(C)** Thrombocytes disintegrate when blood flows from a blood vessel, releasing a phospholipid, thrombokinase, that acts to convert prothrombin in the plasma to thrombin. Thrombin acts enzymatically on fibrinogen in the plasma, converting it to fibrin, which is insoluble and forms a mesh trapping blood cells. This mesh is the blood clot.

13. **(C)** The femur is the thigh bone of the leg. It is the longest, strongest, and heaviest bone of the body.

14. **(B)** Iron is a part of the hemoglobin molecule, the red, oxygen-carrying pigment of red blood cells. If iron is deficient, hemoglobin cannot be produced, and the formation of red blood cells is inhibited.

15. **(D)** *Peristalsis* is the wave of muscular contractions that pushes food through the esophagus into the stomach and through the intestine. Food must reach the digestive sites, the stomach and small intestine, for digestion to occur. The other possible answers are involved in metabolic processes, not in digestion.

16. **(C)** The liver is the largest glandular organ of vertebrates and has the important function of regulating organic materials such as wastes, glucose, and proteins in the blood. It can also perform other essential functions, such as detoxifying blood by converting toxic substances into harmless wastes, fat digestion and storage functions, immune responses, and protein metabolism. It is essential for life.

17. **(A)** Carbon dioxide resulting from cellular metabolism is passed into the blood from cells and thus transported to the lungs. It diffuses through capillary walls into the alveoli of the lungs and is eliminated by exhalation.

18. **(C)** Nerve fibers from the retina of the eye form the optic nerve of the eye; at the crossover point (*optic chiasma*), fibers from the nasal halves (inner halves) of each retina cross to the opposite side of the brain, while fibers of the temporal halves (outer halves) of each retina remain uncrossed. Thus, each optic nerve, after the chiasma, contains fibers from both retinas. This means that objects in one field of vision (either left or right) produce effects in two eyes that are transmitted to one side of the brain. In other words, the two halves of the retina of each eye are represented on opposite sides of the brain, producing a stereoscopic effect and permitting perception of depth.

19. **(A)** *Dendrites* are nerve fibers that transmit impulses from a stimulus site (where the stimulus is received) to the nerve cell body, the *cyton*. An axon will carry an impulse from the nerve-cell body to the reacting muscle.

20. **(D)** *Estrogen* is a complex of female sex hormones that is responsible for the appearance of secondary sex characteristics, such as widening of the pelvis, breasts, etc. Estrogen also functions in the menstrual cycle, preparing the uterus for implantation of the embryo.

21. **(B)** A protein consists of numerous amino acids joined through peptide linkages. The amino acids present and their sequence determines the primary structure of a protein molecule.

22. **(A)** Red blood cells are produced in the bone marrow in the adult. The other statements are incorrect as follows: vitamins typically are consumed with food (two possible exceptions); glucose is a product of digestion, and bile is stored in the gallbladder; water is a part of almost all tissues, and fats are refined by the bile from the liver.

23. **(C)** *Connective tissues* are those whose cells are not contiguous but scattered throughout a noncellular matrix. Connective tissues can bind and support other tissues; therefore, they are widely distributed. Some examples of connective tissues are blood, bone, cartilage, adipose, tissues composing tendons, and ligaments.

24. **(A)** The limited amount of ATP stored in muscle tissue supplies immediate energy for contraction when the ATP is converted to ADP. When the ATP is used up, it is recreated by energy from a reserve, creatine phosphate. When the creatine phosphate is consumed, oxidation of glucose to CO_2 and water provides energy for muscle contraction and for the resynthesis of creatine phosphate. Lactic acid can form anaerobically during severe muscle exertion, and its accumulation is partly responsible for the feeling of fatigue. Lactic acid diffuses out of the muscle tissue into the bloodstream and thus to the liver, where some of it is oxidized to produce further energy, and some can be converted to glycogen for carbohydrate storage.

25. **(C)** Adrenalin, or epinephrine, secreted by the adrenal medulla, is normally released in small quantities and helps to regulate blood circulation and carbohydrate metabolism. Under stressful conditions, the adrenal medulla is stimulated to release larger amounts of adrenalin, which increases blood pressure, heart rate, carbohydrate metabolism, and conversion of glycogen to sugar, thus raising the blood sugar level, etc. This prepares the body to cope with the stressful situation. Hence, the "flight or fight" response.

26. **(A)** Exercise will cause perspiration, which evaporates from the skin. *Perspiration* is a liquid composed of water, salt, and a small amount of urea and is drawn from the bloodstream (from capillaries in the sweat glands) and released to the body surface through pores. Thus, rigorous exercise will cause the body to lose sodium (salt) and water.

27. **(D)** Cholesterol is a lipid that is insoluble in fluids such as blood; therefore, it is bound to proteinaceous carriers for transport. Evidence indicates that cholesterol is involved in the fatty deposits in arteries, even infiltrating cells and the intercellular spaces of arterial walls, if carried by certain carriers. This can lead to plaque

and clot formation, blocking off the arteries and interfering with blood circulation. This same plaque and clot formation can occur in the coronary artery supplying heart muscle, causing a heart attack.

28. **(B)** The endocrine glands secrete hormones directly into the bloodstream; the hormones are transported throughout the body, but only specific "target" cells or tissues can pick up a specific hormone. Thus, the hormone may regulate cellular activities in tissues some distance from the cells that secreted it. By regulating cellular activities of tissues, hormones regulate body activities.

29. **(B)** The thyroid hormone controls the rate of cellular metabolism for the release of energy. An overactive gland secretes an excess of hormone, which will increase the metabolic rate. A deficiency of thyroid hormone causes the rate of metabolism to be lowered.

30. **(C)** The *alveolus* is a small, thin-walled sac of the lung; it is the blind end of the smallest bronchioles. Each alveolus (approximately 300 million are present in human lungs) is surrounded by, or adjacent to, small capillaries. It is here that gaseous exchange between the blood and lungs occur. Carbon dioxide passes into the alveolus from the blood, and oxygen passes from the alveolus into the bloodstream through the capillary walls.

31. **(B)** A *hemorrhoid* is a dilation of veins in the anal region. This can lead to a enlargement of tissue, especially the rectal sphincter, which is a ring-shaped muscle controlling the anal opening.

32. **(C)** A *calorie*, a unit for measuring the heat energy value of food, can be defined as the amount of heat needed to raise one kilogram of water one degree Celsius. More energy per gram is released by the oxidation of fats than by oxidation of proteins or of carbohydrates. Fat is the most concentrated body fuel.

33. **(B)** Fermentation is one of the kinds of cellular respiratory or metabolic processes that result in the release of energy. Fermentation is an *anaerobic* process in that molecular or gaseous oxygen is not involved. As a result of fermentation, carbon dioxide and either an alcohol or an organic acid are produced. Probably the best known of fermentation processes is that in which carbon dioxide and ethyl alcohol are released.

$$C_6H_{12}O_6 \rightarrow 2C_2H_5OH + 2CO_2$$

34. **(A)** The *cerebrum* is the largest part of the human brain; it is here that thought, memory, learning, and the various senses (taste, smell, etc.) are controlled. Located in the frontal lobe of the cerebrum is Broca's speech area, which controls the muscles associated with speech.

35. **(B)** Oxygenated blood passes from the lungs to the left atrium of the heart by way of the pulmonary veins. From the left atrium blood moves to the left ventricle, from which it is pumped through the aorta to the arterial system of the body, and thus throughout the body, where oxygen is diffused into the cells and carbon dioxide is picked up by the blood. The carbon-dioxide-laden blood is returned to the heart, entering the right atrium, and passing to the right ventricle. From the right ventricle, it is pumped to the lungs through the pulmonary arteries, where it becomes oxygenated again.

36. **(A)** The *diaphragm* is a horizontal muscular sheet found in mammals, separating the thoracic cavity from the abdominal cavity. Its muscular action functions in breathing.

37. **(C)** The three basic kinds of muscle tissue are *smooth, skeletal,* and *cardiac.* Smooth muscle is characteristic of the digestive tract and arteries, organs not under voluntary control. Cardiac muscle is found in the heart. Skeletal muscle (striated) makes up the muscles associated with voluntary movement. The kidney is nonmuscular.

38. **(C)** Gaseous exchange between the respiratory system and the circulatory system occurs by means of the capillaries present in the lungs surrounding alveoli. These are referred to as the *pulmonary capillaries.*

39. **(A)** The *celiac axis* is an artery that originates from the dorsal aorta and branches to supply the digestive tract.

40. **(B)** Blood in systemic veins is returning to the right atrium of the heart from the cells of the body. Therefore, it is high in concentrations of carbon dioxide and metabolic wastes that were received from the cells as a result of cellular metabolism. Venous blood of the pulmonary system is returning to the left atrium of the heart from the lungs, where it gave up carbon dioxide to be expelled from body and acquired oxygen. Therefore, it has a higher concentration of oxygen.

41. **(A)** The first division of *meiosis* results in a reduction of the number of chromosomes because the members of each pair of chromosomes are separated from one another. Each daughter nucleus resulting from meiosis receives only one chromosome of each pair present in the parent nucleus, or one-half the number of chromosomes of the parent nucleus. Nuclei resulting from meiosis are *haploid*, as contrasted to the *diploid* condition of the parent nucleus.

42. **(B)** *Fraternal*, or nonidentical, twins result from two fertilized eggs, or *zygotes*. If two eggs are released during ovulation and both are fertilized (one sperm per egg), fraternal twins result. These twins are like ordinary siblings, whereas identical twins resulting from a single *zygote* are genetically identical.

43. **(B)** Higher vertebrates are characterized by a double circulation. This means that the blood passes through the heart twice on one complete circuit, from the left side of the heart to the body and back to the right side of the heart, and from the right side of the heart to the lungs and back to the left side of the heart. Blood is pumped through the blood vessels at a very rapid rate; it takes only about twenty seconds for blood to pass from the heart to a part of the body and back, and about thirty seconds for blood to make the complete circuit, passing through the heart twice.

44. **(C)** Specialized muscle cells, known as the "pacemaker" of the heart, make up a region of the right atrium. When these cells are excited, the atria are stimulated to contract, emptying the blood into the ventricles. Certain muscle fibers then carry the excitation stimulus, by way of the atrio-ventricular node, to muscles of the ventricles, stimulating them to contract and force blood from the heart.

45. **(B)** The XY chromosomes are found in the male, while the female carries XX. As a result of meiosis, a sperm will carry either an X or a Y chromosome; all eggs will carry an X. Fertilization of an X-bearing egg by a Y-bearing sperm produces an XY zygote, which develops into a male. Fertilization of an X-bearing egg by an X-bearing sperm produces an XX zygote, which develops into a female.

46. **(A)** Red blood cells contain the pigment hemoglobin, which has as its function the transport of oxygen. If the number of red blood cells is decreased, the ability of the blood to transport oxygen is decreased.

47. **(B)** In a small, poorly ventilated room, the concentration of carbon dioxide will increase and that of oxygen will decrease because of people breathing. Exhalation would put more carbon dioxide into the air, and inhalation would remove oxygen from the air. Poor circulation would prevent the "freshening" of the air. Eventually, persons would be inhaling air with high concentrations of carbon dioxide, raising the carbon dioxide level of the blood; this higher level of blood carbon dioxide stimulates more rapid breathing in an effort to get more oxygen into the blood and to the tissues.

48. **(A)** The cerebrum is the largest division of the central nervous system of man. It is the origin of thinking, controls learning, memory, thought, some voluntary movements, and the senses. In the animal kingdom, observations indicate that intelligence increases with cerebrum size. Man has the largest cerebrum, in proportion to body size, in the animal kingdom.

49. **(D)** The stapes, cochlea, and tympanic membrane are all parts of the ear: The *stapes* is one of the vibrating bones of the middle ear, the *cochlea* is the receptor portion of the inner ear from which electrical impulses ("messages") are transmitted to the brain through the auditory nerve, and the *tympanic membrane* is the eardrum. The *cornea*, on the other hand, is the transparent covering over the front of the lens of the eye.

50. **(B)** Carbohydrates metabolize (oxidize) rapidly and readily within cells, producing energy. Although they do not produce as many calories per gram as do fats, fats and proteins have to undergo conversion processes to carbohydrate forms before they can enter into the energy-producing oxidative processes. Thus, obtaining energy from fats and proteins is a slower process than obtaining energy from carbohydrates.

51. **(A)** Citrus fruits, tomatoes, potatoes, and green vegetables, including cabbage, contain vitamin C. Of the answers listed, cabbage would provide vitamin C in the absence of citrus fruits. The lack of vitamin C in the diet causes a disease known as *scurvy*.

52. **(B)** Cheese, ice cream, and pudding are dairy products and have nutritive values similar to those of milk, since they are made from milk.

53. **(A)** Milk supplies essential nutrients, including minerals, vitamins carbohydrates, fats, and proteins. The foods in milk, especially the carbohydrates, are easily digested and metabolized.

54. **(C)** Green, leafy vegetables are rich in vitamin C and could be substituted for citrus fruits in the diet. They are poor in the other nutrients named.

55. **(C)** There are about 4000 calories in a pound of fat, and fat will be digested first in a weight-loss program. Consuming 1000 fewer calories per day will cause the loss of about one-quarter pound per day, nearly two pounds per week.

56. **(D)** If a person consumes fewer calories than needed, stored foods will be broken down and oxidized to meet energy needs. Proteins and fats will then be oxidized or catabolized.

57. **(A)** Folic acid, found in green, leafy vegetables, egg yolks, soybeans, etc., is required for the synthesis of adenine and thymine; both of these are components of DNA (deoxyribonucleic acid). Folic acid also is essential for growth and blood-cell formation; a deficiency of folic acid causes anemia and kidney hemorrhage.

58. **(A)** Cereals (grains) are rich in certain of the vitamin B complex: because of the starchy endosperm in seeds, cereals also are high in carbohydrates.

59. **(B)** Labels on canned goods may include a variety of information about the product, but the net contents by weight or volume and the quality should always be included. The number of portions may vary per net contents, according to the nature of the product; so knowledge of the number of servings is useful information. Other information may also be included on the label.

60. **(A)** Caloric needs vary with age as well as with physiological state, activity, and the size of the individual. Both physical and mental growth and development are more rapid during infancy and early childhood than at any other time in one's life. Therefore, more food is needed in proportion to size to provide the needed calories of energy and to provide the materials for growth. A proper diet is essential for normal development.

SCIENCE TEST 4

Life Sciences

45 Minutes   60 Questions

Directions: *For each of the following items, select the choice which best answers the question or completes the statement. Blacken the corresponding space on your answer sheet.*

1. Passage of water through the membrane of a cell is called

   (A) assimilation
   (B) osmosis
   (C) circulation
   (D) transpiration

2. The largest portion of the iron supplied to the body by foods is used by the body for the

   (A) growth of hard bones and teeth
   (B) manufacture of insulin
   (C) development of respiratory enzymes
   (D) formation of hemoglobin

3. The small structures growing on the roots of a legume are called

   (A) lenticels
   (B) nodules
   (C) bulbs
   (D) tubers

4. A new drug for treatment of tuberculosis was being tested in a hospital. Patients in group A actually received doses of the new drug; those in group B were given only sugar pills. Group B represents a(n)

   (A) scientific experiment
   (B) scientific method
   (C) experimental error
   (D) experimental control

5. Which is most closely associated with the process of transpiration?

   (A) spiracles of a grasshopper
   (B) root of a geranium
   (C) leaf of a maple
   (D) gills of a fish

6. Which term includes all the others?

   (A) organ
   (B) tissue
   (C) system
   (D) organism

7. When several drops of pasteurized milk were placed in a petri dish containing sterilized nutrient agar, many colonies developed. This experiment shows the milk

   (A) contained some bacteria
   (B) contained harmful bacteria
   (C) should have been sterilized
   (D) was incorrectly stamped "pasteurized"

8. The growth of green plants toward light is related most specifically to the distribution in the plant of

   (A) minerals
   (B) enzymes
   (C) auxins
   (D) amino acids

9. The four-chambered heart is found in

   (A) fish and mammals
   (B) birds and mammals
   (C) amphibia and birds
   (D) amphibia and reptiles

10. To determine whether an unknown black guinea pig is pure or hybrid black, it should be crossed with

    (A) a white
    (B) a hybrid black
    (C) a pure black
    (D) another unknown

11. In a series of rock layers arranged one on top of another, fossils found in the lowest layers are

(A) completely different from fossils found in the upper layers
(B) older than the fossils found in the upper layers
(C) of organisms simpler than organisms fossilized in the upper layers
(D) of organisms more complex than organisms fossilized in the upper layers

12. The principal way in which forests help to prevent soil erosion is that the

(A) trees provide homes for wildlife
(B) leaves of the trees manufacture food
(C) forest floors absorb water
(D) forest shields the soil from the sun's heat

13. Which factor in the environment of an organism causes it to react?

(A) a stimulus
(B) a response
(C) a reflex
(D) an impulse

14. A breeder wanted to develop a strain of beef cattle with good meat and the ability to thrive in a hot, dry climate. How can she best accomplish this?

(A) continued selection among the members of a prize herd
(B) crossbreeding followed by selection
(C) inbreeding to bring out desirable hidden traits
(D) inbreeding followed by selection

15. If many tall pea plants were crossed, which result would be the *least* probable?

(A) 100% pure tall
(B) 50% pure tall, 50% hybrid tall
(C) 50% tall, 50% short
(D) 75% tall, 25% short

16. Which plant tissues are mostly concerned with storage?

(A) phloem and xylem
(B) phloem and cambium
(C) palisade cells and epidermis
(D) pith and spongy cells

17. Amphibians, which usually hibernate during the winter by burying themselves in the mud at the bottom of a pond or stream, are able to survive because

(A) the temperature of the mud is always above their body temperature
(B) sufficient oxygen can be absorbed through their moist skin
(C) they do not need energy during this time
(D) the mud serves as insulation to protect them from the cold

18. Which reagent should be used in the urine test for diabetes?

(A) iodine
(B) nitric acid
(C) ammonia
(D) Benedict's solution

19. The great fear of snakes that many humans have is an illustration of

(A) instinct
(B) inherited behavior
(C) conditioned behavior
(D) simple reflex

20. What was the weak point in Darwin's theory that De Vries' discovery of mutations helped to explain?

(A) overproduction
(B) natural selection
(C) survival of the fittest
(D) variations

21. The removal for microscopic examination of a small bit of living tissue from a patient is called

(A) biopsy
(B) surgery
(C) dissection
(D) therapy

22. The presence of which substance is most important for all cell activity?

    (A) light
    (B) carbon dioxide
    (C) water
    (D) chlorophyll

23. The end-products of digestion that enter the lacteals are

    (A) glucose
    (B) amino acids
    (C) minerals
    (D) fatty acids

24. A student in the laboratory tossed two pennies from a container one hundred times and recorded these results: both heads, 25; one head and one tail, 47; both tails, 28. Which cross between plants would result in approximately the same ratio?

    (A) Aa × AA
    (B) Aa × Aa
    (C) AA × aa
    (D) Aa × aa

25. Mutants would occur most commonly in

    (A) cattle
    (B) garden peas
    (C) fruit flies
    (D) guinea pigs

26. Tissue culture has been extensively used as a research method in all of the following fields of biological investigation *except*

    (A) photosynthesis
    (B) virology
    (C) development of nerve cells
    (D) experimental embryology

27. After each transfer of a culture of bacteria, the wire loop should be

    (A) dipped into alcohol
    (B) held in a flame
    (C) dipped into liquid soap
    (D) washed repeatedly in water

28. *Transduction* is a term applied to a method of

    (A) liquid transfer in vascular plants
    (B) electrolyte diffusion through a cell membrane
    (C) oxygen absorption of a red corpuscle
    (D) genetic transmission in bacteria

29. In which one of the following ways does combustion differ from cellular respiration?

    (A) More heat is produced.
    (B) More energy is wasted.
    (C) It is less rapid.
    (D) It occurs at a higher temperature.

30. Of the following, an enzyme responsible for the digestion of proteins is

    (A) maltase
    (B) trypsin
    (C) ptyalin
    (D) steapsin

31. Failure of blood to clot readily when exposed to air may be due to a(n)

    (A) oversupply of erythrocytes
    (B) deficiency of leucocytes
    (C) overabundance of fibrin
    (D) inadequacy of thrombokinase

32. Cone cells are most closely associated with the function of

    (A) digestion
    (B) absorption
    (C) vision
    (D) secretion

33. Semicircular canals are thought to be most sensitive to which of the following?

    (A) light
    (B) odor
    (C) gravity
    (D) sound

34. Most of the carbon dioxide in the blood is carried in the

    (A) liquid portion
    (B) leucocytes
    (C) erythrocytes
    (D) platelets

35. Increased blood pressure may be brought about by excess secretion of

    (A) thyroxin
    (B) insulin
    (C) ACTH
    (D) adrenalin

36. Of the following, the plant hormone concerned with growth is

    (A) auxin
    (B) estrogen
    (C) testosterone
    (D) ATP

37. Bread mold resembles ferns in that both develop

    (A) mycelia
    (B) hyphae
    (C) pinnules
    (D) spores

38. Sap rises in woody stems because of root pressure and

    (A) transpiration pull
    (B) enzyme action
    (C) molecular adhesion
    (D) photosynthesis

39. Vascular plants contain tissues called xylem and

    (A) cambium
    (B) phloem
    (C) meristem
    (D) lenticels

40. Stored food for the embryo of a bean seed is found in the

    (A) plumule
    (B) hypocotyl
    (C) cotyledons
    (D) testa

41. Of the following, an example of a carnivorous plant is

    (A) sundew
    (B) mandrake
    (C) cowslip
    (D) jewelweed

42. In the structure of a flower, the stigma is most closely positioned to the

    (A) style
    (B) ovary
    (C) sepal
    (D) ovule

43. Of the following taxonomic groups, the one that is most varied and abundant at the present time is the

    (A) Protista
    (B) Bryzoa
    (C) Brachiopoda
    (D) Vertebrata

44. Of the following organisms, the one that is *not* in the same taxonomic class as the others is the

    (A) salamander
    (B) mud puppy
    (C) newt
    (D) lizard

45. The vocal organ of birds is the

    (A) trachea
    (B) larynx
    (C) syrinx
    (D) air sac

46. In a demonstration of a test for vitamin C, one might effectively use

    (A) acetic acid
    (B) bromthymol blue
    (C) congo red
    (D) indophenol

47. Rod-shaped bacteria are classified as

    (A) bacilli
    (B) cocci
    (C) vibrios
    (D) spirilla

48. A stain used in classifying bacteria is

    (A) Gram's
    (B) Wright's
    (C) Loeffler's
    (D) Giemsa

49. A bacteriophage is a kind of

    (A) enzyme
    (B) toxin
    (C) bacterium
    (D) virus

50. Of the following, the marsupial native to the United States is the

    (A) raccoon
    (B) wombat
    (C) opossum
    (D) armadillo

51. The first fully terrestrial vertebrates were the

    (A) amphibians
    (B) reptiles
    (C) birds
    (D) mammals

52. A cartilaginous vertebrate that parasitizes fish is the

    (A) pilot fish
    (B) lamprey
    (C) barracuda
    (D) moray eel

53. Of the following, the one to which the horseshoe crab is most closely related is the

    (A) blue crab
    (B) lobster
    (C) garden spider
    (D) chambered nautilus

54. The *titanotheres* were a group of fossil

    (A) fish
    (B) amphibians
    (C) reptiles
    (D) mammals

55. Of the following, a crustacean that lives on land is the

    (A) centipede
    (B) millipede
    (C) sow bug
    (D) tick

56. Of the following, the one that is *not* an animal is the

    (A) sea lily
    (B) sea cucumber
    (C) sand dollar
    (D) diatom

57. Of the following, the hydra is most closely related to

    (A) coral
    (B) flatworm
    (C) sponge
    (D) roundworm

58. An unforeseen result of the widespread use of DDT is the

    (A) control of mosquitoes
    (B) development of insects immune to DDT
    (C) development of fishes immune to DDT
    (D) destruction of harmful birds

59. Oxygen enters protistans chiefly through the

    (A) cell membrane
    (B) vacuoles
    (C) oral grooves
    (D) pseudopodia

60. Air passes into and out of the insect body by way of

    (A) gills
    (B) lungs
    (C) skin
    (D) tracheae

Answer Key

1.	**B**	21.	**A**	41.	**A**
2.	**D**	22.	**C**	42.	**A**
3.	**B**	23.	**D**	43.	**A**
4.	**D**	24.	**B**	44.	**D**
5.	**C**	25.	**C**	45.	**C**
6.	**D**	26.	**A**	46.	**D**
7.	**A**	27.	**B**	47.	**A**
8.	**C**	28.	**D**	48.	**A**
9.	**B**	29.	**D**	49.	**D**
10.	**A**	30.	**B**	50.	**C**
11.	**B**	31.	**D**	51.	**B**
12.	**C**	32.	**C**	52.	**B**
13.	**A**	33.	**C**	53.	**C**
14.	**B**	34.	**A**	54.	**D**
15.	**C**	35.	**D**	55.	**C**
16.	**D**	36.	**A**	56.	**D**
17.	**B**	37.	**D**	57.	**A**
18.	**D**	38.	**A**	58.	**B**
19.	**C**	39.	**B**	59.	**A**
20.	**D**	40.	**C**	60.	**D**

Explanatory Answers

1. **(B)** Although other mechanisms may be involved in passage of materials through a cell membrane, the passage of some materials, especially water, occurs by diffusion; *diffusion* occurs from regions of higher concentrations of the substance to regions of lower concentration. Diffusion through a membrane, such as the cell membrane, is known as *osmosis*.

2. **(D)** Iron is a part of the hemoglobin molecule, and, as such, is essential for its formation. Hemoglobin is the oxygen-carrying pigment found in red corpuscles.

3. **(B)** Nodules on the roots of legumes contain nitrogen-fixing bacteria that convert gaseous atmospheric nitrogen to nitrates that can be utilized by plants. *Bulbs* and *tubers* are specialized stems; *lenticels* are openings or pores in the bark of woody plants.

4. **(D)** A *control* is used with experiments for comparison. The control is treated in the same manner as is the experimental group except for one variable. In this case, the variable would be the administering of the drug or sugar pills. Thus, any differences between the groups in experimental results could be attributed to this one variable.

5. **(C)** *Transpiration* is the loss of water in a gaseous state, through epidermal stomata, from the aerial parts of a plant. Most transpiration occurs through the leaf epidermis. Stomata are not found in root epidermis.

6. **(D)** An organism is a living thing or individual. An organism consists of "systems," which consist of organs, which consist of tissues, especially in the case of higher organisms. This statement would not apply to lower organisms that have not reached the system level of phylogenetic development.

7. **(A)** Milk is not sterile; it contains numerous bacteria. Pasteurization does not sterilize milk, but does destroy certain harmful bacteria that can be carried in milk.

8. **(C)** *Auxins* are growth hormones found in plants; in stems, auxins stimulate growth. If a plant is unevenly illuminated, auxins are more concentrated on the side of the stem that is more poorly illuminated, stimulating growth on that side. This will cause the stem to bend toward the light.

9. **(B)** Birds and mammals have four-chambered hearts consisting of two atria and two ventricles. A fish has a two-chambered heart, one atrium and one ventricle; the hearts of amphibians and reptiles contain three chambers, two atria and one ventricle.

10. **(A)** Black is dominant over white in this case; therefore, the white guinea pig carries only white genes and is *homozygous* or pure recessive. When such a test backcross is made, the offspring will indicate the genotype of the black guinea pig. If the black guinea pig is hybrid or *heterozygous* black (carrying one white gene), black and white offspring will result in a theoretical ratio of 1:1; if the black guinea pig is pure or homozygous black, all offspring will be black because of dominance, although all of the offspring will be hybrid because they carry a white gene.

11. **(B)** Fossils found in the lowest rock layers are the oldest because these layers were deposited before the ones that lie above them. Fossils in upper layers are not always different from the lower layers. Some species have very long histories and leave fossils in more than one layer. Conversely, fossils in upper layers are never completely the same as fossils in lower layers. At least some species of organisms whose fossils lie in lower layers would have become extinct and been replaced by fossils of different organisms by the time upper layers were deposited. Older organisms were not always simpler than modern organisms and were certainly not more complex.

12. **(C)** The roots of plants help to hold the soil in place and prevent soil erosion; the ground can absorb water. Eroded lands do not absorb water readily. Water may run off, carrying with it some of the topsoil; and this reduces the quality of the land. Where plants are present, the run-off is reduced or diminished, and the ground absorbs water.

13. **(A)** A *stimulus* is anything that can cause a *reaction* or response by the organism. The reaction may be involuntary, such as batting the eye when an object approaches, or voluntary, such as moving from an area of discomfort.

14. **(B)** Crossbreeding between strains with the desired traits, followed by selection of the offspring for future breeding and establishing the herd, is the best way to accomplish the breeder's

goal. Inbreeding is just as likely to bring out undesirable hidden traits.

15. **(C)** In pea plants, tall is dominant over short. It is possible that some of the tall plants used in the cross are hybrid, but the maximum number of short individuals from a *monohybrid* cross (both parents hybrid tall) would be 25 percent, a 3:1 ratio. If all tall parents are *homozygous*, or pure tall, all offspring would be pure tall. If one parent is pure tall, and the other hybrid tall, the offspring would occur in a 1:1 ratio of pure tall to hybrid tall. Only a cross between a hybrid tall and a pure short (Tt × tt) would give a ratio of one tall to one short. So C is the least probable.

16. **(D)** Pith typically consists of *parenchyma* cells, which store starch in typical green plants. Spongy cells, characteristic of dicot leaves, also store starch, but temporarily.

17. **(B)** Amphibians are cold-blooded animals; therefore, they would not be affected significantly by lowered temperatures. Because they need less oxygen during hibernation, due to decreased metabolic activity, they can absorb sufficient oxygen through their skin. During the active periods, both the respiratory organs and the moist skin are needed to supply oxygen.

18. **(D)** A symptom of diabetes is sugar (glucose) in the urine. *Benedict's solution* is a reagent used to test for the presence of reducing sugars such as glucose.

19. **(C)** Human fears are learned through experience or teaching. Therefore, this is *conditioned* behavior.

20. **(D)** Darwin recognized the fact that variations could be seen and traced in populations, and proposed the theory that those individuals with changes that best fitted them for the environment would survive. However, Darwin could offer no explanation as to how these variations came about. De Vries' discovery of mutations offered a possible explanation for the variations Darwin had observed.

21. **(A)** A small amount of living tissue can be removed from a specific organ of a patient and examined by a pathologist to give the attending physician information needed for diagnosis. This excision and diagnostic study of living tissue is a *biopsy*, a useful diagnostic tool especially for diseases of a cancerous nature.

22. **(C)** Water constitutes about 75–85 percent of the typical living cell. No activities associated with life can occur without water.

23. **(D)** Fats are *emulsified*, or broken up into small droplets, by bile secreted from the liver into the small intestine. The enzyme lipase then digests the fat droplets into fatty acids and glycerin. These products are not absorbed through capillary walls directly into the bloodstream, but enter the small lymph vessels, or *lacteals*, located in the villi of the intestine.

24. **(B)** The results of the penny toss approximate a 1:2:1 ratio, which is the same ratio that is obtained from a monohybrid cross:
$$Aa \times Aa \rightarrow 1AA:2Aa:1aa.$$

25. **(C)** Fruit flies have a brief reproductive and life cycle, compared to the others. Because of this, and the large number of offspring produced, more and larger generations can be studied in a given period of time. Thus, the chances of finding a mutant among the large numbers of organisms is increased.

26. **(A)** Tissue culture is the technique of growing tissues or cells in solutions of water and nutrients. This technique is especially useful in studying growth, differentiation, and morphology.

27. **(B)** Incineration is an effective method of sterilization; holding a loop in a flame sterilizes the loop, preventing contamination of surfaces on work areas, etc., and the possible spread of infectious bacteria.

28. **(D)** Genetic material can be transmitted from one bacterium to another by conjugation, transduction, or transformation. *Transduction* involves transmission by the use of a virus. The virus, formed in the bacterial cell, can pick up some bacterial-cell DNA and, when the bacterium is disrupted by the viral infection, carry the bacterial DNA with it when it invades a new bacterial cell. Thus, the virus transmits a bit of bacterial DNA along with its own.

29. **(D)** *Combustion*, or burning, is a rapid reaction giving off much heat and light in short period of time. The energy is expended more rapidly; thus, the reaction occurs at a higher temperature since the temperature of the combustible material must be raised to a combustion point. Cellular respiration occurs more slowly, at lower temperatures, and is controlled by enzymes. If cellular

respiration occurred at combustion temperatures, cells would be destroyed.

30. **(B)** *Trypsin,* an enzyme found in pancreatic juice, digests proteins, peptones, and proteoses to peptides. The digestion of peptides to amino acids also occurs in the small intestine under the control of the enzyme erepsin. Some protein digestion (to peptones and proteoses) occurs in the stomach, under the control of the enzyme pepsin. Ptyalin and maltase act on carbohy-drates; steapsin, on fats.

31. **(D)** Thrombocytes disintegrate when ruptured, as when blood flows from an injured blood vessel, releasing thrombokinase (thromboplastin), which acts to convert prothrombin to thrombin. Thrombin acts on fibrinogen in the plasma, converting it to insoluble fibrin, the material that forms the clot. Inadequacy of thrombokinase would prevent the first step of clotting, the formation of thrombin from prothrombin.

32. **(C)** *Cone cells* are photoreceptor cells found in the retina of the eye. They are responsible for color vision. Cone cells are functional only in bright light; therefore, color is not perceived in dim light.

33. **(C)** *Semicircular canals* compose that portion of the inner ear responsible for the maintenance of balance or equilibrium. The movement of fluids within the canals in response to gravity, caused by a change in head position, stimulates the receptors in the canals; thus, one is aware of the position of the head.

34. **(A)** Most of the carbon dioxide is transported in the blood plasma in the form of sodium bicarbonate ($NaHCO_3$). *Erythrocytes, leucocytes,* and *platelets* (thrombocytes) are blood cells suspended in the plasma.

35. **(D)** *Adrenalin,* a hormone secreted by the adrenal glands, causes increases in blood pressure, heart rate, breathing, glucose blood levels, etc., preparing the body for stressful situations.

36. **(A)** *Auxins* are plant growth hormones; *testosterone* and *estrogen* are animal sex hormones. *ATP* (adenosine triphosphate) is an energy-transport compound found in cells.

37. **(D)** Bread mold is a fungus, while ferns are vascular plants. Both bread mold and ferns, however, produce spores as asexual reproductive cells. A *mycelium* is a mass of fungal hyphae and is not a part of the fern-plant body. *Pinnules* are the "leaflets" of a fern frond and are not part of a fungus.

38. **(A)** *Transpiration* is the loss of gaseous water from a plant through epidermal stomata of the aerial parts of the plant, especially the leaves. Water forms a continuous column in the xylem tissue. The pull of water effected by transpiration is a factor in the rise of *sap* (water plus dissolved materials). The process is much the same as drinking liquid through a straw.

39. **(B)** Xylem and phloem serve the purpose of transporting materials in vascular tissues. Upward translocation of plant sap is accomplished mainly through vessels (in angiosperms) and tracheids of xylem. Downward translocation is accomplished through the sieve tubes of phloem.

40. **(C)** The cotyledons of dicotyledonous plants (such as beans) store food for use by the plant embryo as it develops into a seedling that can carry on photosynthesis. The *plumule* is composed of the embryonic or first leaves of the embryo; the *hypocotyl* is the lower embryonic stem, and the *testa* is the seed coat.

41. **(A)** The sundew is a plant with special structures capable of capturing insects that land on it and digesting the insects' tissues. *Carnivorous* plants ("meat eaters") can obtain some essential nutrients, such as nitrogen, in this manner.

42. **(A)** The *stigma* is the top portion of the pistil on which pollen lands in pollination. The *style* is the neck-like portion of the pistil, located between the stigma and the ovary, the basal part. *Ovules* are potential seeds.

43. **(A)** The Kingdom Protista is a very diverse group of mostly unicellular eukaryotes that includes many phyla that are as different from one another as those of animals or plants. Protistans are extremely abundant in terms of individuals because of their usually small size and their ability to reproduce rapidly. The Bryzoa and Brachiopoda are two phyla of animals with relatively few species, restricted distribution, and modest abundance. The Vertebrata is the largest subphylum of the animal phylum Chordata and is ranked second to the Protista in this list in terms of variety and abundance.

44. **(D)** The salamander, newt, and mud puppy, which is also a salamander, are amphibians; they spend the early or developmental part of their lives in water and the adult stages on land. Lizards are reptiles, developing completely on land.

45. **(C)** The *syrinx* is the vocal organ of birds; it is situated at the bifurcation of the trachea into bronchi. The *larynx* is the area at the upper end of the trachea of higher animals (such as primates); vocal cords are contained in the larynx. An *air sac* is the alveolus of the lung.

46. **(D)** *Indophenol* is one of the quinonimine compounds, which are amines of quinone. Some are chemical indicators of acidity and alkalinity, and can be used to determine the hydrogen ion concentration of unknown solutions.

47. **(A)** There are three morphological types, or shapes, of bacteria: spherical-shaped bacteria are called *cocci*; rod-shaped bacteria are called *bacilli*; curved or spiral-shaped bacteria are usually known as *spirilla*.

48. **(A)** Bacteria are classified as gram positive or gram negative; this depends on their ability to retain crystal violet, the primary stain of the gram stain. Those bacteria that cannot be decolorized with ethanol but retain crystal violet are classified as gram positive. Those that can be decolorized are gram negative. The difference is due to the chemical composition of the cell wall.

49. **(D)** A *bacteriophage* is a kind of virus that attacks and destroys the bacterial cell. The viruses can pass their DNA into the bacterial cells and cause the cells to manufacture viral DNA and viral protein.

50. **(C)** A *marsupial* is a viviparous mammal that gives birth to immature embryos; the development of the young is completed in the female's pouch, located on her ventral side. Nourishment for the embryo is from the mammary glands, the nipples of which are located in the pouch.

51. **(B)** Reptiles are the first vertebrates in evolutionary development that spend the early or developmental part of their lives, as well as adult stages, on land. They do not possess gills for breathing in water as do the larval stages of amphibians.

52. **(B)** The lamprey is an eel-shaped fish with a sucker-like mouth containing strong teeth. It attaches itself to the host-fish with its mouth, and rasps a hole in the host's skin with its strong teeth; thus, it can suck blood from its host.

53. **(C)** The horseshoe crab, lobster, blue crab, and spider are members of the phylum Arthropoda; the chambered nautilus, because of its mantle and lack of jointed appendages, is placed in the phylum Mollusca. All arthropods are characterized by jointed appendages, a well-developed exoskeleton containing chitin, and an annelid-type nervous system. On the basis of certain characteristics, such as the presence or absence of antennae and mandibles, the phylum is divided into four subphyla. Of these subphyla, Trolobita consists of only extinct forms. Among extant arthropods, the subphylum Chelicerata is characterized by a lack of antennae and mandibles, the presence of chelicerae, and an unsegmented cephalothroax and abdomen; spiders and the horseshoe crab are placed in this subphylum. The Subphylum Crustacea includes arthropods, such as the blue crab and lobster, which have mandibles, branched appendages, and two pairs of antennae. The Subphylum Uniramia includes insects and related arthropods, all of which have mandibles, unbranched appendages, and one pair of antennae.

54. **(D)** The *titanotheres* are a large group of extinct mammals of the Eocene and Oligocene epochs; they were large-hoofed, horned herbivores.

55. **(C)** All named are members of the phylum Arthropoda, but only the sowbug is a crustacean. The characteristics of the class Crustacea are two pairs of antennae, three pairs of mouth parts, and a three-part body. Most crustaceans are aquatic, gilled animals, but a few live on land. The sowbug is one of these.

56. **(D)** A *diatom* is a unicellular golden alga characterized by possession of carotenoid pigments and a siliceous (glass-like) cell wall. It belongs to the Kingdom Protista. The sand dollar, sea lily, and sea cucumber are all echinoderms in the Kingdom Animalia.

57. **(A)** The hydra and corals are coelenterates, diploblastic animals characterized by a gastrovascular cavity.

58. **(B)** Many insects have developed an immunity to or tolerance of DDT, so it does not kill them. However, DDT can accumulate in the bodies of insects and then be transferred to the tissues of birds, fishes, and other insect predators. These predators can accumulate DDT and, when consumed by their predators, pass on the DDT. Thus, this harmful insecticide can be passed up the food chain with the concentration in animal tissues increasing at each level, and it can have harmful effects on higher animals that consume the lower DDT-containing animals.

59. **(A)** Oxygen is absorbed from the water or medium in which the protozoan lives through the cell membrane. Carbon dioxide is eliminated by passing through the membrane into the medium.

60. **(D)** The insect respiratory system consists of a complex system of tubules ramifying throughout the insect's body. These tubules anastomose to form the *tracheae*, tubules leading to *spiracles*. The spiracles are openings on the body through which air is pumped into and out of the tracheae by action of the wings and abdominal movements.

60. **(D)** The insect respiratory system consists of a complex system of tubules ramifying throughout the insect's body. These tubules anastomose to form the *tracheae*, tubules leading to *spiracles*.

The spiracles are openings on the body through which air is pumped into and out of the tracheae by action of the wings and abdominal movements.

Answer Sheet
General Science
TEST 5

1. Ⓐ Ⓑ Ⓒ Ⓓ   13. Ⓐ Ⓑ Ⓒ Ⓓ   25. Ⓐ Ⓑ Ⓒ Ⓓ   37. Ⓐ Ⓑ Ⓒ Ⓓ   49. Ⓐ Ⓑ Ⓒ Ⓓ

2. Ⓐ Ⓑ Ⓒ Ⓓ   14. Ⓐ Ⓑ Ⓒ Ⓓ   26. Ⓐ Ⓑ Ⓒ Ⓓ   38. Ⓐ Ⓑ Ⓒ Ⓓ   50. Ⓐ Ⓑ Ⓒ Ⓓ

3. Ⓐ Ⓑ Ⓒ Ⓓ   15. Ⓐ Ⓑ Ⓒ Ⓓ   27. Ⓐ Ⓑ Ⓒ Ⓓ   39. Ⓐ Ⓑ Ⓒ Ⓓ   51. Ⓐ Ⓑ Ⓒ Ⓓ

4. Ⓐ Ⓑ Ⓒ Ⓓ   16. Ⓐ Ⓑ Ⓒ Ⓓ   28. Ⓐ Ⓑ Ⓒ Ⓓ   40. Ⓐ Ⓑ Ⓒ Ⓓ   52. Ⓐ Ⓑ Ⓒ Ⓓ

5. Ⓐ Ⓑ Ⓒ Ⓓ   17. Ⓐ Ⓑ Ⓒ Ⓓ   29. Ⓐ Ⓑ Ⓒ Ⓓ   41. Ⓐ Ⓑ Ⓒ Ⓓ   53. Ⓐ Ⓑ Ⓒ Ⓓ

6. Ⓐ Ⓑ Ⓒ Ⓓ   18. Ⓐ Ⓑ Ⓒ Ⓓ   30. Ⓐ Ⓑ Ⓒ Ⓓ   42. Ⓐ Ⓑ Ⓒ Ⓓ   54. Ⓐ Ⓑ Ⓒ Ⓓ

7. Ⓐ Ⓑ Ⓒ Ⓓ   19. Ⓐ Ⓑ Ⓒ Ⓓ   31. Ⓐ Ⓑ Ⓒ Ⓓ   43. Ⓐ Ⓑ Ⓒ Ⓓ   55. Ⓐ Ⓑ Ⓒ Ⓓ

8. Ⓐ Ⓑ Ⓒ Ⓓ   20. Ⓐ Ⓑ Ⓒ Ⓓ   32. Ⓐ Ⓑ Ⓒ Ⓓ   44. Ⓐ Ⓑ Ⓒ Ⓓ   56. Ⓐ Ⓑ Ⓒ Ⓓ

9. Ⓐ Ⓑ Ⓒ Ⓓ   21. Ⓐ Ⓑ Ⓒ Ⓓ   33. Ⓐ Ⓑ Ⓒ Ⓓ   45. Ⓐ Ⓑ Ⓒ Ⓓ   57. Ⓐ Ⓑ Ⓒ Ⓓ

10. Ⓐ Ⓑ Ⓒ Ⓓ   22. Ⓐ Ⓑ Ⓒ Ⓓ   34. Ⓐ Ⓑ Ⓒ Ⓓ   46. Ⓐ Ⓑ Ⓒ Ⓓ   58. Ⓐ Ⓑ Ⓒ Ⓓ

11. Ⓐ Ⓑ Ⓒ Ⓓ   23. Ⓐ Ⓑ Ⓒ Ⓓ   35. Ⓐ Ⓑ Ⓒ Ⓓ   47. Ⓐ Ⓑ Ⓒ Ⓓ   59. Ⓐ Ⓑ Ⓒ Ⓓ

12. Ⓐ Ⓑ Ⓒ Ⓓ   24. Ⓐ Ⓑ Ⓒ Ⓓ   36. Ⓐ Ⓑ Ⓒ Ⓓ   48. Ⓐ Ⓑ Ⓒ Ⓓ   60. Ⓐ Ⓑ Ⓒ Ⓓ

GENERAL SCIENCE TEST

45 Minutes   60 Questions

Directions: *For each of the following items, select the choice that best answers the question or completes the statement. Blacken the corresponding space on your answer sheet.*

1. A tree native to China and *not* to the United States is the

    (A) silvery maple
    (B) chestnut
    (C) gingko
    (D) tulip tree

2. Mammals are believed to have evolved directly from

    (A) fish
    (B) amphibians
    (C) reptiles
    (D) birds

3. Sphenodon is the sole surviving species of an otherwise extinct group of

    (A) fish
    (B) amphibians
    (C) reptiles
    (D) mammals

4. Which of the following groups, in primate phylogeny, includes the primate most closely related to man?

    (A) Old World monkeys
    (B) great apes
    (C) New World monkeys
    (D) lemurs

5. Stanley Miller recently obtained evidence supporting the possibility of spontaneous generation by achieving laboratory synthesis of

    (A) amino acids
    (B) DNA
    (C) RNA
    (D) glucose

6. The principal prey of the chicken hawk or red-shouldered hawk is

    (A) poultry
    (B) songbirds
    (C) frogs
    (D) rodents

7. During what season is hail most likely to occur during thunderstorms?

    (A) fall
    (B) winter
    (C) spring
    (D) summer

8. We can see only one side of the moon because the

    (A) earth rotates on its own axis
    (B) moon makes one rotation as it makes one revolution around the earth
    (C) moon has no refractive atmosphere
    (D) sun does not shine on the moon's unseen side

9. Which of the following birds would most probably *not* be found in a wooded area?

    (A) thrush
    (B) barred owl
    (C) green heron
    (D) towhee

10. The reason for the red appearance of the setting sun is also the reason why

    (A) a red barn looks redder at sunset than at noon
    (B) red is a better color than blue for the navigation lights on top of radio-transmission towers
    (C) a blue object looks black in red light
    (D) the flame from burning calcium is red

11. Of the following, vitamin B$_{12}$ is most useful in combating

    (A) pernicious anemia
    (B) night blindness
    (C) rickets
    (D) goiter

12. Both malaria and yellow fever are

    (A) caused by protistans
    (B) cured with antibiotics
    (C) prevented by vaccination
    (D) controllable by swamp drainage or hormonal insecticides

13. The tassel of a corn plant

    (A) produces pollen
    (B) provides protection
    (C) forms the pistil
    (D) produces ovules

14. Of the following electrical devices found in the home, the one that develops the highest voltage is the

    (A) electric broiler
    (B) radio tube
    (C) television picture tube
    (D) electric steam-iron

15. Most soluble food substances enter the blood stream through the

    (A) small intestine
    (B) duodenum
    (C) capillaries in the stomach
    (D) hepatic vein

16. Of the following, the animal that is *not* a rodent is the

    (A) beaver
    (B) guinea pig
    (C) squirrel
    (D) skunk

17. The "dark" side of the moon refers to the

    (A) craters, into which no sunlight has ever reached
    (B) south pole of the moon's axis
    (C) hemisphere that has never reflected the sun's rays on the earth
    (D) moon itself in the early phases of the month

18. Of the following, the one *not* characteristic of poison ivy is

    (A) milky juice
    (B) shiny leaves
    (C) three-leaflet clusters
    (D) white berries

19. *Cholesterol* is

    (A) a basic part of bone structure
    (B) an alcohol formed in the body
    (C) a substance found in blood
    (D) the cause of colitis

20. The diameter of the moon is approximately

    (A) 2000 miles
    (B) 8000 miles
    (C) 186,000 miles
    (D) 240,000 miles

21. Of the following, the one present in greatest amounts in dry air is

    (A) carbon dioxide
    (B) oxygen
    (C) water vapor
    (D) nitrogen

22. Of the following groups of animals, the one in which alternation of generations occurs is the

    (A) coelenterates
    (B) sponges
    (C) annelids
    (D) molluscs

23. A ventral nerve cord is found in which of the following?

    (A) earthworm
    (B) frog
    (C) amphioxus
    (D) lamprey eel

24. Of the following materials, the one *not* found in the supporting structure of sponges is

    (A) lime
    (B) silica
    (C) cartilage
    (D) spongin

25. It is believed by scientists that worker bees indicate to their hive-mates the direction and distance of a supply of food by

    (A) strokes of their antennae
    (B) buzzing of sounds
    (C) an oriented dance in front of the hive
    (D) none of the above

26. The normal height of a mercury barometer at sea level is

    (A) 15 inches
    (B) 30 inches
    (C) 32 feet
    (D) 34 feet

27. Of the following phases of the moon, the invisible one is called

    (A) crescent
    (B) full moon
    (C) new moon
    (D) waxing and waning

28. Of the following, the statement that best describes a "high" on a weather map is that the air

    (A) extends farther up than normal
    (B) pressure is greater than normal
    (C) temperature is higher than normal
    (D) moves faster than normal

29. The nerve endings for the sense of sight are located in the part of the eye called the

    (A) cornea
    (B) sclera
    (C) iris
    (D) retina

30. Malaria is caused by

    (A) bacteria
    (B) mosquitoes
    (C) protistans
    (D) bad air

31. A 1000-ton ship must displace a weight of water equal to

    (A) 500 tons
    (B) 1000 tons
    (C) 1500 tons
    (D) 2000 tons

32. Of the following instruments, the one that can convert light into an electric current is the

    (A) radiometer
    (B) dry cell
    (C) electrolysis apparatus
    (D) photoelectric cell

33. On the film in a camera, the lens forms an image that by comparison with the original subject, is

    (A) right side up and reversed from left to right
    (B) upside down and reversed from left to right
    (C) right side up and not reversed from left to right
    (D) upside down and not reversed from left to right

34. Of the following, the plant whose seeds are *not* spread by wind is the

    (A) cocklebur
    (B) maple
    (C) dandelion
    (D) milkweed

35. Of the following, the insect harmful to man's food supply is the

    (A) dragonfly
    (B) grasshopper
    (C) ladybug
    (D) praying mantis

36. Of the following, the one that is generally fall-blooming is the

    (A) azalea
    (B) hickory
    (C) tulip
    (D) witch hazel

37. Flagellated male gametes may be found in the cells of

    (A) bread mold
    (B) gingko
    (C) protococcus
    (D) slime mold

38. One-celled eukaryotes belong to the group of living things known as

    (A) protistans
    (B) poriferans
    (C) annelids
    (D) arthropods

39. Spiders can be distinguished from insects because spiders have

    (A) hard outer coverings
    (B) large abdomens
    (C) four pairs of legs
    (D) biting mouth parts

40. An important ore of uranium is called

    (A) hematite
    (B) bauxite
    (C) chalcopyrite
    (D) pitchblende

41. The lightest element known on earth is

    (A) hydrogen
    (B) helium
    (C) oxygen
    (D) air

42. Of the following gases in the air, the most plentiful is

    (A) argon
    (B) nitrogen
    (C) oxygen
    (D) carbon dioxide

43. The time it takes for light from the sun to reach the earth is approximately

    (A) four years
    (B) four months
    (C) eight minutes
    (D) sixteen years

44. Of the following kinds of clouds, the kind the occurs at the greatest height is called

    (A) cirrus
    (B) cumulus
    (C) nimbus
    (D) stratus

45. The time it takes for the earth to rotate 45 degrees is

    (A) one hour
    (B) three hours
    (C) four hours
    (D) ten hours

46. Of the following glands, the one that regulates the metabolic rate is the

    (A) adrenal
    (B) salivary
    (C) thyroid
    (D) thymus

47. In the small intestine, a digestive enzyme can break the peptide bond between two amino acids in a protein molecule by

    (A) removing a water molecule from them
    (B) inserting a water molecule between them
    (C) removing a carbon atom from one of them
    (D) inserting a carbon atom between them

48. The usual vector in the transmission to humans of rickettsial diseases is

    (A) birds
    (B) rodents
    (C) arthropods
    (D) snails

49. Passive immunity to diptheria may be achieved by taking an injection of a(n)

    (A) vaccine
    (B) toxin
    (C) toxoid
    (D) antitoxin

50. Of the following, the only safe blood transfusion would be

    (A) group A blood into a group O person
    (B) group B blood into a group A person
    (C) group O blood into a group AB person
    (D) group AB blood into a group B person

51. Of the following groups of plants, the one from which coal was largely formed is the

    (A) thallophytes
    (B) bryophytes
    (C) pteridophytes
    (D) spermatophytes

52. The water-conducting tissue in an angio-sperm is

    (A) phloem
    (B) xylem
    (C) pith
    (D) cambium

53. The time that it takes the earth to complete a 60-degree rotation is

    (A) 1 hour
    (B) 4 hours
    (C) 6 hours
    (D) 24 hours

54. Of the following, the most common metal found in the earth's crust is

    (A) iron
    (B) copper
    (C) aluminum
    (D) tin

55. Of the following, the gas needed for burning is

    (A) carbon dioxide
    (B) oxygen
    (C) nitrogen
    (D) argon

56. Of the following, the process that will result in water most nearly chemically pure is

    (A) aeration
    (B) chlorination
    (C) distillation
    (D) filtration

57. The number of degrees on the Fahrenheit thermometer between the freezing point and the boiling point of water is

    (A) 100 degrees
    (B) 180 degrees
    (C) 212 degrees
    (D) 273 degrees

58. One is most likely to feel the effects of static electricity on a

    (A) cold, damp day
    (B) cold, dry day
    (C) warm, humid day
    (D) warm, dry day

59. Of the following planets, the one that has the largest number of satellites is

    (A) Jupiter
    (B) Mercury
    (C) Neptune
    (D) Pluto

60. The Beaufort Scale indicates

    (A) temperature
    (B) air pressure
    (C) wind force
    (D) wind direction

Answer Key

1.	C	21.	D	41.	A
2.	C	22.	A	42.	B
3.	C	23.	A	43.	C
4.	B	24.	C	44.	A
5.	A	25.	C	45.	B
6.	D	26.	B	46.	C
7.	D	27.	C	47.	B
8.	B	28.	B	48.	C
9.	C	29.	D	49.	D
10.	B	30.	C	50.	C
11.	A	31.	B	51.	C
12.	D	32.	D	52.	B
13.	A	33.	B	53.	B
14.	C	34.	A	54.	C
15.	A	35.	B	55.	B
16.	D	36.	D	56.	C
17.	C	37.	B	57.	B
18.	A	38.	A	58.	B
19.	C	39.	C	59.	A
20.	A	40.	D	60.	C

Explanatory Answers

1. **(C)** The gingko is native to the Orient but has been imported into the United States and now is in widespread use as an ornamental tree.

2. **(C)** Evidence indicates that a primitive reptile known as a therapsid is the ancestor of mammals. These early reptiles of the Triassic period had acquired some mammalian characteristics such as warm bloodedness, hair, and mammary glands. They are sometimes referred to as "premammals."

3. **(C)** The sphenodon is the only living representative of an otherwise extinct order of reptiles. It is a primitive lizard with simple sac-like lungs found only in New Zealand. It is sometimes referred to as a "living fossil."

4. **(B)** Fossil evidence indicates that there was an isolation of ape-like forms, including hominids (man-like creatures), during the Pliocene period. These seemingly originated from the same "branch" of the evolutionary "tree." Lemurs, New World monkeys, and Old World monkeys apparently evolved earlier.

5. **(A)** It was found that if a mixture of methane, ammonia, and hydrogen is continuously bombarded with spark discharges as an energy source, amino acids are formed. If inorganic phosphate is added to the mixture, ATP, the energy compound of cells, is formed also. The earth, at its very early age, had the inorganic substances, and the sun could have provided the energy source.

6. **(D)** Hawks in general prey on small rodents such as rats, mice, and rabbits. Only rarely will a hawk prey on other birds or on cold-blooded animals.

7. **(D)** Thunderstorms, caused by a clash between warm and cold air masses, are more common in the summer because the reflection of heat from the earth warms the air of the lower atmosphere. The air of the upper atmosphere is much colder. Hail consists of pellets of ice and snow combined in alternating layers. Raindrops formed in the warm portions of the clouds are swept upward by air currents into the colder air masses, where the drops freeze into ice and collect a layer of snow. As they descend, they are coated with moisture and swept upward to freeze again. This up and down movement continues until the pellets are too heavy to be supported by the air. They then fall to earth as hail.

8. **(B)** As the moon revolves around the earth, it rotates on its axis so that only one side of the moon faces earth. Because the moon makes one rotation with one revolution around the earth, one side of the moon never faces the earth.

9. **(C)** The heron is a bird found in wet, marshy, or swampy habitats. It is a wading bird, feeding mostly on fish and amphibians, but will also eat rodents and small snakes. The other birds are found in wooded habitats.

10. **(B)** Red light has the longest wavelength of light of the visible spectrum; in a vacuum, all light of all wavelengths travels at the same speed. However, light of longer wavelengths travels slightly faster in air than light of shorter wavelengths. Light travels in a straight line, but when light passes from one medium to another, it is *refracted* (bent); shorter wavelengths are refracted at a sharper angle than longer wavelengths. When the sun is setting, the longer wavelengths of red are not refracted as sharply by air and the particles it contains, thus more red light can be seen, making the sun appear red. The greater speed and less refraction of red light make red light more visible and useful as a navigation light, especially when the air contains many particles as on a foggy, smoggy, or rainy night. Blue light has shorter wavelengths, travels slightly more slowly in air, and is refracted at a greater angle than is red light.

11. **(A)** A deficiency of vitamin B_{12} leads to *pernicious anemia*, a condition in which red blood cells fail to mature. Vitamin B_{12} is essential for the formation of red blood cells.

12. **(D)** Both the virus that causes yellow fever and the protistan that causes malaria are transmitted by mosquitoes. Since mosquito eggs are laid and larvae develop in water, swamp drainage would reduce the breeding areas, thereby reducing mosquito populations and hence the incidence of the diseases. However, swamp drainage destroys the ecosystem of an area and is, therefore, undesirable. A juvenile hormone has been discovered in larvae that promotes the retention of larval characteristics and inhibits the molting hormone. Chemical analogs of the molting hormone have been used as insecticides; these produce abnormal final molts of the larva or block larval development, thus preventing the larva from becoming an adult. These insecticides are very promising, and they are highly specific;

they act only on the targeted insect and do not cause great changes in the environment.

13. **(A)** The tassel at the top of a corn plant is a cluster of imperfect male flowers. Each flower contains the male reproductive part, the stamen, which produces pollen.

14. **(C)** In a cathode-ray tube, such as is found in televison sets (picture tube), a *cathode* (negative terminal) and an *anode* (positive terminal) are present. There is no material between the two through which electricity (electrons) can flow from one terminal to another: a vacuum exists in the tube. A heated cathode generates electrons, which become excited by heat and can acquire enough energy to leave the cathode. Once they do, they are attracted to the anode because of the difference in charges (electrons have a negative charge) and flow across the gap toward the anode. In other appliances, the material through which the electricity flows may produce some resistance; in a picture tube, the electrons are flowing across a space in a vacuum and encounter no resistance.

15. **(A)** The small-intestine lining is characterized by millions of *villi*, small, thin-walled projections into the lumen. Each villus is supplied with capillaries and a lacteal. The large number of villi greatly increase the absorptive area of the small intestine, and the blood vessels and lacteal are close to the food supply. Thus, digested foods are absorbed with ease through the thin-walled villus and thin capillary walls into the bloodstream or, in the case of fats, into the opened ends of the lacteals.

16. **(D)** One characteristic of rodents is their long, sharp incisors, which enable them to gnaw on and through hard materials. The skunk is not a gnawing animal.

17. **(C)** The moon shines by the reflected light of the sun. Because the moon rotates on its axis as it revolves around the earth, one side of the moon never faces the earth. This side, the dark side of the moon, can never reflect the sun's light onto the earth.

18. **(A)** Poison ivy has a clear juice rather than a milky sap. Three-leaflet clusters, white berries, and shiny leaves are all characteristic of poison ivy.

19. **(C)** *Cholesterol* is a fatty substance found in animal fats. It can enter the bloodstream and become involved in the buildup of fatty deposits on the walls of capillaries and other blood vessels.

20. **(A)** The moon is a spherical body with a diameter of about 2000 miles, revolving around the earth in an orbit approximately 240,000 miles distant from the earth.

21. **(D)** Air is a mixture of gases; dry air consists of about 78 percent nitrogen and 21 percent oxygen. The remaining one percent consists of other gases, including carbon dioxide.

22. **(A)** Some coelenterates (phylum *Coelenterata*) exhibit a life cycle in which a sexually reproducing medusa alternates with an asexually reproducing polyp; this is *alternation of generations*.

23. **(A)** The earthworm (and any other annelids) is characterized by a ventral nerve cord; this is true of arthropods as well. Members of the phylum *Chordata*, to which the lancelet amphioxus, the eel, and the frog belong, have a dorsal nerve cord.

24. **(C)** The supporting structures of sponges, *spicules*, can be made up of lime (calcium carbonate) silicon, or a proteinaceous material called spongin. Cartilage is found in vertebrates.

25. **(C)** Bee behavior has been studied, and scientists can interpret some of the movements of the worker bees' dance. The movements are known to give information as to the location of the pollen or nectar they have discovered. The angle of the tail-wag, direction and pattern of movement, sound and duration of sound, and the duration of the dance are ways of giving information as to distance and direction to the food supply. Floral odors on the dancers' bodies indicate the correct flowers in the area.

26. **(B)** Air pressure at sea level is 14.7 pounds/square inch. This pressure, at 0 degrees C supports a barometer mercury column of 76 centimeters, or 30 inches. This is equivalent to one atmosphere of pressure.

27. **(C)** The moon phases occur because the moon shines only by the reflected light of the sun and because only one hemisphere is seen from the earth. The four phases, as seen from the northern hemisphere, are 1) the new moon, in which the face is completely in the shadow, the "invisible phase"; 2) the first quarter, with the eastern half illuminated; 3) the full moon, with the entire face illuminated; and 4) the last quarter, with the western half illuminated.

28. **(B)** A *high* indicates an area of high air pressure, while a *low* indicates an area of low air pressure. Weather can be predicted by measuring differences between pressures. A high usually indicates fair weather, whereas low pressure areas indicate storms and bad weather.

29. **(D)** The retina of the eye contains rods and cones; these are the photoreceptors of the eye, so named because of their shape. Rods are concerned with perception of gray to black in dim light, while cones respond to light of high intensity and are concerned with color perception. Nerve fibers from these receptors eventually converge to form the optic nerves leading to the brain.

30. **(C)** Malaria is a parasitic disease caused by protistans in the genus *Plasmodium*. Some of the life cycle stages of *Plasmodium* are passed in mosquitoes of the genus *Anopheles*, which transmit the disease.

31. **(B)** Archimedes' Principle indicates that an object will displace its weight in water. Thus, a 1000-ton ship would displace 1000 tons of water.

32. **(D)** A photoelectric cell works on the principle that light can be used to produce electric currents in some metals. When light energy strikes the metal (usually cesium) in the photoelectric cell, it is converted into electric energy. The cesium emits electrons. The greater the amount of light striking the metal, the more electric energy produced.

33. **(B)** A camera lens is convex; light passing through such a lens is bent toward the center of the lens. Light reflected near the object and passing through the thinner outer edges of a convex lens bends more than light passing through the thicker areas, and light passing through the exact center of the lens does not bend at all. Because light reflected from an object is focused through such a lens and bent, rather than passing in a straight line, as it would if passing through plain glass, the image formed is reversed and is smaller than the original object.

34. **(A)** The dandelion and maple fruits, containing seed(s), have modifications that enable them to be dispersed easily by air currents and stronger winds. These modifications are the "wings" of the maple fruit and the "hairs" of the dandelion fruit. Milkweed seeds also have such appendages for wind dispersal. The cocklebur fruit is spiny, which causes it to attach to animals for dispersal.

35. **(B)** Grasshoppers feed on plants, including those used by man as food. A swarm of grasshoppers can strip all the plants of an area of leaves and tender green parts in a very short time. The dragonfly, ladybug, and praying mantis are predatory insects, feeding on other insects.

36. **(D)** Azaleas, tulips, and hickory trees flower in the spring; witch hazel typically flowers in the fall. Flowering is usually in response to the length of daylight received during a twenty-four hour period. This response is known as *photoperiodism*. Long-day plants flower in the spring and early summer when days are long, while short-day plants flower in the fall, when days are growing shorter. Some indeterminate, or day-neutral, plants do not flower in response to the relative length of day.

37. **(B)** Sperm, which are produced in the pollen tube of the gingko, contain many probasal bodies that arrange themselves spirally in the sperm. Each probasal body becomes a basal body, from which emerges a short flagellum.

38. **(A)** Unicellular eukaryotes, including colonial forms, belong to the Kingdom *Protista*. The other organisms in this question belong to phyla in the Kingdom *Animalia*, all members of which are multicellular. Phylum *Annelida* includes segmented worms, such as the earthworm. Phylum *Porifera* includes sponges. Phylum *Arthropoda* includes animals such as insects, spiders, crabs, crayfish, and millipeds that have a chitinous exoskeleton and jointed appendages.

39. **(C)** Spiders are characterized by a two-part body and four pairs of legs, while insects have a three-part body and three pairs of legs.

40. **(D)** *Pitchblende* is a natural mineral that contains uranium and radium, as well as many other substances. Uranium also occurs in other minerals, such as carnotite.

41. **(A)** Hydrogen is the lightest element known, having an atomic weight of 1.008. The atom contains one proton, no neutrons, and one electron.

42. **(B)** Nitrogen composes nearly four-fifths of the air; oxygen nearly one-fifth. The remainder of air consists of other gases.

43. **(C)** Light travels at a speed of about 186,000 miles per second; the sun is approximately 93,000,000 miles from the earth. Thus, calculations (93,000,000 miles divided by 186,000 miles per second) show that it takes about 500 seconds, or a bit more than eight minutes, for light from the sun to reach the earth.

44. **(A)** Cirrus clouds are feathery, finely textured clouds occurring in feathery bands across the sky; these occur at the greatest heights and usually are the fastest moving. Nimbus, cumulus and stratus clouds are lower and slower.

45. **(B)** The earth makes one complete rotation on its axis (360 degrees) in 24 hours; 45 degrees is one-eighth of 360 degrees. Therefore, it would take one-eighth of 24 hours, or three hours, for the earth to rotate 45 degrees.

46. **(C)** The thyroid regulates metabolic rate under normal conditions. A deficiency of thyroid hormone will cause a low basal metabolism, while an excess of the hormone will increase the metabolic rate.

47. **(B)** A *peptide bond* is the covalent bond that links the nitrogen atom on the end of one amino acid molecule with the carbon atom on the opposite end of another amino acid molecule. A peptide bond is formed by removing a molecule of water from the two amino acid molecules (see the explanatory answer for question 23 in Science Test 2 for an explanation of dehydration synthesis). Therefore, inserting a water molecule between two amino acids linked by a peptide bond will break the bond by putting a hydrogen atom back onto the nitrogen atom of one amino acid and a hydroxyl ion (OH−) back onto the terminal carbon atom of the other amino acid. Breaking a bond between two molecules by inserting a water molecule between them is called *hydrolysis* and is a common way of digesting large organic molecules such as starches and proteins.

48. **(C)** Rickettsial diseases, such as Rocky Mountain spotted fever and typhus, are transmitted by arthropod vectors, such as ticks and fleas. The rickettsial pathogen, an obligate intracellular parasite, can be acquired by the vector when it bites an animal or human harboring or infected with the pathogen; the pathogen is then transmitted to a healthy person when bitten by the vector. With some of rickettsial diseases, a warm blooded animal, such as a rodent, can act as a reservoir from which the vector may acquire the pathogen and then transmit it to humans.

49. **(D)** Passive immunity involves administering an antibody (an antitoxin, in the case of diptheria) to the patient. This immunity is temporary, since the patient's body is not stimulated to form antibodies, as it would be if an antigen were administered. The temporary immunity is considered *passive* because the body is not active in forming antibodies. If an antigen stimulates the body to form its own antibodies against it, the immunity produced is *active*. Passive immunity provides temporary protection to one who has been exposed to a disease, or a method of treatment until the patient's body has started producing its own antibodies if the disease has been contracted. Active immunity imparts more lasting protection.

50. **(C)** Group O blood lacks antigen A and antigen B. Although it can form antibodies against both A and B, it cannot stimulate the formation of antibodies against A and B. Persons of group O are known as *universal donors*. Group AB blood has both antigens A and B but cannot form antibodies against either. Persons of group AB are known as *universal recipients*. Since group O has neither antigen, and AB cannot form either antibody, the only safe transfusion of those listed is choice (C). Persons of group A contain antigen A and can form antibodies against antigen B; blood group B contains antigen B and can form antibodies against A.

51. **(C)** *Pteridophytes*, vascular plants that do not produce seeds, were among the predominant plants during the Carboniferous era. Primitive gymnosperms were also present. These plants formed great forests, which were compressed by flooding and changes in the earth's land masses into the coal deposits and oil pools we use as fuel today.

52. **(B)** Xylem, characterized in angiosperms by vessels, conducts material upward in the plant. Most of the material conducted upward is water that has been absorbed from the soil by the root system. The water contains dissolved minerals and may contain, especially in deciduous perennials in the spring, sugar that has been formed by the digestion of starch stored in the lower plant parts.

53. **(B)** The earth rotates 360 degrees on its axis every 24 hours. 60 degrees is one-sixth of 360 degrees; therefore, it would take one-sixth of 24 hours, or four hours, for the earth to rotate 60 degrees.

54. **(C)** The rocks of the *lithosphere*, the earth's crust, are made up mostly of eleven elements, plus trace amounts of others. These eleven elements occur almost entirely in the form of compounds rather than in the free state. Aluminum is the third most abundant element; only oxygen and silicon occur in greater quantities.

55. **(B)** Oxygen is the gas that supports combustion, or burning. Materials will not burn in an oxygen-free environment.

56. **(C)** Distillation involves *evaporation*, or changing the water from a liquid to a gaseous state (usually by heating), and collecting and *condensing* the gaseous water back to a liquid. The water, because it is in a gaseous state, is separated from any impurities since they cannot evaporate with the water.

57. **(B)** On the Fahrenheit scale, the boiling point of water is 212 degrees; the freezing point is 32 degrees. Subtracting 32 degrees from 212 degrees results in a difference of 180 degrees, the number of degrees between the boiling and the freezing points of water.

58. **(B)** *Static electricity* is a non-moving electrical charge that accumulates on the surface of an object. A substance that contains an equal number of *protons* (positively charged particles) and *electrons* (negatively charged particles) is electrically neutral. If electrons are gained or lost, the substance becomes charged. When one object loses electrons and becomes positively charged, another must gain electrons and become negatively charged. If electrons are not in motion, the electricity is static. However, warm, moist air is a good conductor of electricity; moisture collects on the surfaces of objects and conducts electrons away from the surface, preventing the object from becoming charged. Cold air acts as a good insulator, preventing the movement of electrons away from the object. Therefore, static electricity can best be felt on a cold, dry day, when the electrons can accumulate on an object or surface.

59. **(A)** Jupiter is the largest planet known in our solar system, and is known to have twelve moons, or satellites, revolving around it. Neptune and Pluto are the greatest distance from the earth: two moons are identified for Neptune, and knowledge about Pluto, the most distant planet, is incomplete. Mercury is difficult to study because of its closeness to the sun. The glare of the sun makes observations difficult during the day, and the planet is very low in the sky at night. However, with present explorations and studies of our solar system resulting in the accumulation of more knowledge, changes in previously held concepts are taking place.

60. **(C)** The force and speed of wind are measured by an instrument called an *anemometer*; these factors are indicated by a number on the Beaufort Scale of the anemometer. The numbers range from 0 for winds below one mile per hour, up to 12 for winds above 75 miles per hour.

Answer Sheet
Final Science Examinations
TEST 6

1. Ⓐ Ⓑ Ⓒ Ⓓ   15. Ⓐ Ⓑ Ⓒ Ⓓ   29. Ⓐ Ⓑ Ⓒ Ⓓ   43. Ⓐ Ⓑ Ⓒ Ⓓ   57. Ⓐ Ⓑ Ⓒ Ⓓ

2. Ⓐ Ⓑ Ⓒ Ⓓ   16. Ⓐ Ⓑ Ⓒ Ⓓ   30. Ⓐ Ⓑ Ⓒ Ⓓ   44. Ⓐ Ⓑ Ⓒ Ⓓ   58. Ⓐ Ⓑ Ⓒ Ⓓ

3. Ⓐ Ⓑ Ⓒ Ⓓ   17. Ⓐ Ⓑ Ⓒ Ⓓ   31. Ⓐ Ⓑ Ⓒ Ⓓ   45. Ⓐ Ⓑ Ⓒ Ⓓ   59. Ⓐ Ⓑ Ⓒ Ⓓ

4. Ⓐ Ⓑ Ⓒ Ⓓ   18. Ⓐ Ⓑ Ⓒ Ⓓ   32. Ⓐ Ⓑ Ⓒ Ⓓ   46. Ⓐ Ⓑ Ⓒ Ⓓ   60. Ⓐ Ⓑ Ⓒ Ⓓ

5. Ⓐ Ⓑ Ⓒ Ⓓ   19. Ⓐ Ⓑ Ⓒ Ⓓ   33. Ⓐ Ⓑ Ⓒ Ⓓ   47. Ⓐ Ⓑ Ⓒ Ⓓ   61. Ⓐ Ⓑ Ⓒ Ⓓ

6. Ⓐ Ⓑ Ⓒ Ⓓ   20. Ⓐ Ⓑ Ⓒ Ⓓ   34. Ⓐ Ⓑ Ⓒ Ⓓ   48. Ⓐ Ⓑ Ⓒ Ⓓ   62. Ⓐ Ⓑ Ⓒ Ⓓ

7. Ⓐ Ⓑ Ⓒ Ⓓ   21. Ⓐ Ⓑ Ⓒ Ⓓ   35. Ⓐ Ⓑ Ⓒ Ⓓ   49. Ⓐ Ⓑ Ⓒ Ⓓ   63. Ⓐ Ⓑ Ⓒ Ⓓ

8. Ⓐ Ⓑ Ⓒ Ⓓ   22. Ⓐ Ⓑ Ⓒ Ⓓ   36. Ⓐ Ⓑ Ⓒ Ⓓ   50. Ⓐ Ⓑ Ⓒ Ⓓ   64. Ⓐ Ⓑ Ⓒ Ⓓ

9. Ⓐ Ⓑ Ⓒ Ⓓ   23. Ⓐ Ⓑ Ⓒ Ⓓ   37. Ⓐ Ⓑ Ⓒ Ⓓ   51. Ⓐ Ⓑ Ⓒ Ⓓ   65. Ⓐ Ⓑ Ⓒ Ⓓ

10. Ⓐ Ⓑ Ⓒ Ⓓ   24. Ⓐ Ⓑ Ⓒ Ⓓ   38. Ⓐ Ⓑ Ⓒ Ⓓ   52. Ⓐ Ⓑ Ⓒ Ⓓ   66. Ⓐ Ⓑ Ⓒ Ⓓ

11. Ⓐ Ⓑ Ⓒ Ⓓ   25. Ⓐ Ⓑ Ⓒ Ⓓ   39. Ⓐ Ⓑ Ⓒ Ⓓ   53. Ⓐ Ⓑ Ⓒ Ⓓ   67. Ⓐ Ⓑ Ⓒ Ⓓ

12. Ⓐ Ⓑ Ⓒ Ⓓ   26. Ⓐ Ⓑ Ⓒ Ⓓ   40. Ⓐ Ⓑ Ⓒ Ⓓ   54. Ⓐ Ⓑ Ⓒ Ⓓ   68. Ⓐ Ⓑ Ⓒ Ⓓ

13. Ⓐ Ⓑ Ⓒ Ⓓ   27. Ⓐ Ⓑ Ⓒ Ⓓ   41. Ⓐ Ⓑ Ⓒ Ⓓ   55. Ⓐ Ⓑ Ⓒ Ⓓ   69. Ⓐ Ⓑ Ⓒ Ⓓ

14. Ⓐ Ⓑ Ⓒ Ⓓ   28. Ⓐ Ⓑ Ⓒ Ⓓ   42. Ⓐ Ⓑ Ⓒ Ⓓ   56. Ⓐ Ⓑ Ⓒ Ⓓ   70. Ⓐ Ⓑ Ⓒ Ⓓ

FINAL SCIENCE EXAMINATION

60 Minutes   70 Questions

Directions: *After carefully reading each test item, select the best answer. Blacken the corresponding space on your answer sheet.*

1. Of the following human traits, the one under both genetic and hormonal control is

   (A) hemophilia
   (B) color blindness
   (C) baldness
   (D) blood type

2. When a solution has a pH value of 9.2

   (A) a drop of phenolphthalein indicator will redden it
   (B) magnesium will replace its hydrogen
   (C) litmus paper will turn red in it
   (D) the addition of calcium hydroxide will lower the pH value

3. The tissue to which gland cells belong is

   (A) connective
   (B) epithelial
   (C) secretory
   (D) nerve

4. Of the following, which is closest to the speed of sound in air at sea level?

   (A) one-fifth mile per second
   (B) one-half mile per second
   (C) one mile per second
   (D) five miles per second

5. The general formula for the acetylene series of hydrocarbons is

   (A) $C_nH_{2n} + 2$
   (B) C_nH_{2n}
   (C) $C_nH_{2n} - 2$
   (D) none of the above

6. Which of the following parts of the ear is partly responsible for maintaining body balance?

   (A) middle-ear
   (B) semi-circular canals
   (C) semi-lunar valves
   (D) cochlea

7. The vitamin that helps clotting of the blood is

   (A) C
   (B) D
   (C) E
   (D) K

8. The nuclei of pollen grains are similar in chromosome number to all except

   (A) egg
   (B) sperm
   (C) cell of a plant embryo
   (D) spore

9. *Cocci* are bacteria that are shaped like

   (A) chains of beads
   (B) rods
   (C) isolated spheres
   (D) spirals

10. A person is more buoyant when swimming in salt water than in fresh water because

    (A) the person keeps his or her head out of salt water
    (B) salt water has greater tensile strength
    (C) salt coats the person's body with a floating membrane
    (D) salt water is denser than an equal volume of fresh water

11. The main reason why a new antibiotic is thoroughly tested on rats before it is used by doctors is that

    (A) anything that will kill a human will kill a rat
    (B) anything that is harmful to rats is harmful to humans
    (C) a drug that injures one animal is likely to injure other animals
    (D) a drug that cannot cure a rat cannot cure people

12. The pH of a solution formed as the result of neutralization of nitric acid by sodium hydroxide is closest to

    (A) 1

    (B) 10

    (C) 7

    (D) 4

13. All of the following mechanisms affect the amount of glucose in the blood *except*

    (A) adrenalin secretion

    (B) insulin secretion

    (C) level of oxygen intake

    (D) level of physical activity

14. The most active mixing of many digestive juices occurs in the

    (A) stomach

    (B) duodenum

    (C) ileum

    (D) jejunum

15. A *cold-blooded* animal is one that

    (A) lacks red corpuscles

    (B) lacks white corpuscles

    (C) has a variable temperature

    (D) lives in arctic regions

16. The basic mechanism of hereditary transmission is

    (A) sexual reproduction

    (B) polyploidy

    (C) separation of chromosomes

    (D) the mitotic mechanism

17. If the electrical voice waves produced by a whistle are formed in one second, what is the wave frequency demonstrated in the following figure?

    (A) 4 hertz

    (B) 8 hertz

    (C) 12 hertz

    (D) 16 hertz

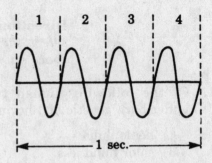

18. Of the following, the highest bactericidal activity of light occurs at a wavelength in angstrom units of

    (A) 2536

    (B) 3256

    (C) 5236

    (D) 6532

19. In the diagram below, the refraction of the light rays indicates that the lens is

    (A) thicker in center than edges

    (B) thinner at center than edges

    (C) uniform in thickness

    (D) consistent in dimensions

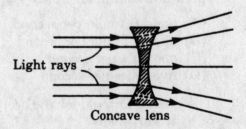

Light rays

Concave lens

20. A man hears the echo from a mountain wall five seconds after he has shouted. Of the following, the figure most nearly expressing the distance of the man from the mountain is

    (A) five miles

    (B) one mile

    (C) 900 yards

    (D) 1100 feet

21. Which of the following statements about wavelengths is true?

    (A) Visible wavelengths vary in lengths.
    (B) The wavelength of green is the longest.
    (C) Radio waves are electromagnetic waves shorter than infrared.
    (D) Infrared ray are shorter than red light rays.

22. An object appears white, or colorless, when it

    (A) absorbs the light reaching it
    (B) transmits only blue light
    (C) rejects all colors
    (D) reflects all colors at the same time

23. Of the following methods, the one that should be used to convert a steel knitting needle into a permanent magnet is

    (A) heating
    (B) jarring
    (C) stroking with a magnet
    (D) passing electricity through it

24. Of the following, a human blood disease that has been definitely shown to be due to a hereditary factor or factors is

    (A) pernicious anemia
    (B) sickle cell anemia
    (C) polycythemia
    (D) leukemia

25. All of the following elements are major constituents of a cell *except.*

    (A) carbon
    (B) potassium
    (C) hydrogen
    (D) phosphorus

26. If a machine listed for 1800 watts is plugged into a 110-volt system, approximately how many amps will it use?

    (A) 6.6
    (B) 13.0
    (C) 16.0
    (D) 19.8

27. The selection of algae as a possible source of additional food for man is based primarily on their ability to carry on

    (A) fermentation
    (B) digestion
    (C) photosynthesis
    (D) oxidation

28. Birds and bats are both flying, warm blooded vertebrates. Yet they are *not* considered closely related because of the difference in their

    (A) brain structure
    (B) manner of feeding their young
    (C) ability to see
    (D) ability to hear

29. At the beginning of a community succession, the first of the following living things to get a foothold on bare rocks, other things being equal, are

    (A) mosses
    (B) ferns
    (C) algae
    (D) lichens

30. Of the following, one difference between frog and man is that the frog has no

    (A) salivary glands
    (B) thyroid gland
    (C) pancreas
    (D) adrenal gland

31. Of the following, the part of the ship that gives it stability by lowering the center of gravity is the

    (A) bulkhead
    (B) anchor
    (C) keel
    (D) prow

32. Of the following, the one most likely to speed soil erosion is

    (A) planting trees
    (B) removing trees
    (C) contour plowing
    (D) terracing

33. Of the following nutrients, the one normally deficient in milk is

    (A) fat
    (B) minerals
    (C) protein
    (D) vitamin D

34. Exophthalmic goiter is caused by

    (A) hypoactivity of the thyroid
    (B) hyperactivity of the thyroid
    (C) deficiency of vitamin A
    (D) radioactive iodine

35. If other factors are compatible, a person who can most safely receive blood from any donor belongs to the basic blood group

    (A) O
    (B) A
    (C) B
    (D) AB

36. The Schick test indicates whether or not a person is probably immune to

    (A) tuberculosis
    (B) diptheria
    (C) poliomyelitis
    (D) scarlet fever

37. Evaporation of water is likely to be greatest on days of

    (A) high humidity
    (B) low humidity
    (C) little or no wind
    (D) low pressure

38. Of the following, the substance whose water solution will change the color of litmus from red to blue is

    (A) $CuSO_4$
    (B) K_2CO_3
    (C) NaNO
    (D) $Zn(NO_3)_2$

39. The percentage of oxygen by weight in $Al_2(SO_4)_3$ (atomic weights: Al = 27, S = 32, O = 16) is approximately

    (A) 19
    (B) 21
    (C) 56
    (D) 92

40. In backcrossing, a hybrid is always mated with

    (A) its own parent
    (B) another hybrid
    (C) a pure dominant
    (D) a pure recessive

41. Of the following processes, the one carried on exclusively by bacteria is

    (A) maturing of cheese
    (B) synthesis of antibiotics
    (C) formation of humus
    (D) synthesis of vitamin K in the intestines

42. Of the following, a structure found in mammals but *not* in reptiles is the

    (A) lung
    (B) brain
    (C) diaphragm
    (D) ventricle

43. The specific function of light energy in the process of photosynthesis is to

    (A) activate chlorophyll
    (B) split water
    (C) reduce carbon dioxide
    (D) form carbohydrates

44. The shape of which of the following does the vibrio shape of certain bacteria most closely resemble?

    (A) bacilli
    (B) spirilla
    (C) cocci
    (D) rickettsia

45. Coral is formed by

    (A) fresh-water algae
    (B) a mollusc found in the Caribbean
    (C) an animal related to the sea anemone
    (D) a seed plant

46. Which sequence correctly illustrates a food chain?

    (A) algae—insect larvae—fish—man
    (B) algae—fish—insect larvae—man
    (C) insect larvae—algae—fish—man
    (D) fish—insect larvae—algae—man

47. Grasses are usually pollinated by

    (A) wind
    (B) water
    (C) birds
    (D) insects

48. Among vertebrates the embryonic ecto-derm gives rise to which of the following?

    (A) nervous system
    (B) digestive system
    (C) skeletal system
    (D) respiratory system

49. Generally, life depends directly or indi-rectly for food, energy, and oxygen upon

    (A) parasitic organisms
    (B) green plants
    (C) fungi
    (D) animals

50. The functions of plant roots may normally include all of the following *except*

    (A) photosynthesis
    (B) food storage
    (C) absorption
    (D) support

51. The weight in grams of 22.4 liters of nitro-gen (atomic weight = 14) is

    (A) 3
    (B) 7
    (C) 14
    (D) 28

52. In the production of sounds, the greater the number of vibrations per second, the

    (A) greater the volume
    (B) higher the tone
    (C) lower the volume
    (D) lower the tone

53. Nitrogen-fixing bacteria are found in nod-ules on the roots of the

    (A) beet
    (B) carrot
    (C) potato
    (D) clover

54. Two areas in plants where growth occurs most rapidly by mitosis are the

    (A) root tip and cambium
    (B) cortex and cambium
    (C) cortex and pith
    (D) epidermis and fibrovascular bundle

55. Which one of the following characteristics represents a difference between plants and animals?

    (A) organ systems
    (B) specialization
    (C) sexual reproduction
    (D) cellular adaptation

56. Which one of the following graphs repre-sents Boyle's Law?

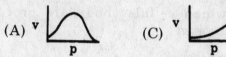
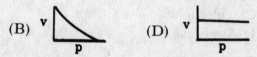

57. Which of the following minerals is restored to the soil by plants of the pea and bean family?

    (A) sulfates
    (B) nitrates
    (C) carbonates
    (D) phosphates

58. In humans, any hereditary defect caused by a gene on the Y chromosome would occur

    (A) only in males
    (B) only in females
    (C) only if the gene were recessive
    (D) about equally in males and females

59. There is no oxidation-reduction in a reac-tion involving

    (A) single replacement
    (B) double replacement
    (C) simple decomposition
    (D) direct combination of elements

60. When $BaCl_2$ was added to a salt solution, there was formed a white precipitate insoluble in hydrochloric acid. The salt solution was most likely a

    (A) carbonate
    (B) sulfite
    (C) nitrate
    (D) sulfate

61. The cellular organelle where respiratory reactions for the release of energy occurs is a

    (A) centrosome
    (B) chromosome
    (C) chromoplast
    (D) mitochondrion

62. In which cellular body are proteins synthesized?

    (A) ribosome
    (B) nucleus
    (C) chloroplast
    (D) lysosome

63. The most efficient cellular respiratory process, in terms of energy-yield per molecule of glucose, is

    (A) aerobic respiration
    (B) anaerobic respiration
    (C) fermentation
    (D) phosphorylation

64. Enzymes are necessary as catalysts for all processes except

    (A) cellular oxidation
    (B) digestion
    (C) egestion
    (D) proteolysis

65. A cellular organelle found in typical plant cells but not in typical animal cells is the

    (A) chloroplast
    (B) ribosome
    (C) mitochondrion
    (D) centrosome

66. Two processes that must occur during the life cycle of sexually reproducing organisms are

    (A) mitosis and fertilization
    (B) sporulation and meiosis
    (C) meiosis and syngamy
    (D) propagation and mitosis

67. Every cell contains

    (A) a cell membrane and cytoplasm
    (B) a cell wall and cytoplasm
    (C) a nucleus and cell wall
    (D) plastids and pigments

68. Darwin collected and presented evidence to support the theory of

    (A) propagation
    (B) evolution
    (C) conservatism
    (D) amalgamation

69. An example of an obligate intracellular parasitic microorganism is a

    (A) tapeworm
    (B) virus
    (C) bacterium
    (D) spirochaete

70. Which of the following substances is *not* transported by the blood?

    (A) oxygen
    (B) metabolic wastes
    (C) digestive enzymes
    (D) hormones

Answer Key

1.	**C**	25.	**B**	48.	**A**
2.	**A**	26.	**C**	49.	**B**
3.	**B**	27.	**C**	50.	**A**
4.	**A**	28.	**B**	51.	**D**
5.	**C**	29.	**D**	52.	**B**
6.	**B**	30.	**A**	53.	**D**
7.	**D**	31.	**C**	54.	**A**
8.	**C**	32.	**B**	55.	**A**
9.	**C**	33.	**D**	56.	**B**
10.	**D**	34.	**B**	57.	**B**
11.	**C**	35.	**D**	58.	**A**
12.	**C**	36.	**B**	59.	**B**
13.	**C**	37.	**B**	60.	**D**
14.	**B**	38.	**B**	61.	**D**
15.	**C**	39.	**C**	62.	**A**
16.	**C**	40.	**D**	63.	**A**
17.	**A**	41.	**D**	64.	**C**
18.	**A**	42.	**C**	65.	**A**
19.	**B**	43.	**A**	66.	**C**
20.	**C**	44.	**B**	67.	**A**
21.	**A**	45.	**C**	68.	**B**
22.	**D**	46.	**A**	69.	**B**
23.	**C**	47.	**A**	70.	**C**
24.	**B**				

Explanatory Answers

1. **(C)** All conditions are under genetic control; however, hereditary baldness is also under hormonal control. Baldness is expressed as a dominant characteristic in males but recessive in females, because of the hormones present. Thus, a male and female may inherit the same genes for baldness, but the expression of the genes will depend on the sex hormones.

2. **(A)** Phenolphthalein in an indicator that will not give a color reaction (remains colorless) at a pH below 8.3. The range for this indicator is pH 8.3–14. Thus, a color reaction of red will be seen at a pH of 9.2.

3. **(B)** There are only four basic kinds of tissues: epithelial, connective, muscle, and nerve. Gland cells are among the epithelial tissues that cover the internal and external surfaces of various parts of the body.

4. **(A)** The speed of sound in air varies slightly with temperature, increasing slightly as temperature increases. For convenience, the speed of sound in air is referred to as 1100 feet per second. This is an approximate value that can be used despite various conditions. 1100 feet is approximately one-fifth of a mile (one mile = 5280 feet).

5. **(C)** A member of the acetylene series is unsaturated, with a trip bond between two carbons. The formula for acetylene, for example, is $H-C \equiv C-H$; because of the triple bond between two carbons, the number of hydrogens is reduced by two. Thus, the general formula is $Cn_2H_2n - 2$.

6. **(B)** The *semicircular canals* of the inner ear are fluid-filled structures containing *receptors* (hair cells); the canals are oriented in three planes, lateral, posterior, and superior. As the body moves in a given plane, the fluid of the canal oriented in that plane is displaced, pushing against a receptor and signaling direction.

7. **(D)** Prothrombin is produced in insuffient quantities if there is a deficiency of vitamin K; prothrombin produces thrombin, which acts as an enzyme to convert fibrinogen to fibrin, the mesh that traps blood cells, forming the clot. Thus, if vitamin K is deficient, prothrombin is deficient, clotting is delayed or does not occur.

8. **(C)** Eggs and sperm are sexual reproductive cells and are haploid in chromosome number. A plant spore is an asexual reproductive cell and usually is haploid also. Pollen grains develop mitotically from microspores, and thus they are haploid. The plant embryo develops mitotically from a diploid zygote and is diploid in chromosome number.

9. **(C)** There are three morphological types, or shapes, of bacteria: spherical-shaped bacteria are called *cocci*; rod-shaped bacteria are called *bacilli*; curved or spiral-shaped bacteria are usually known as *spirilla*.

10. **(D)** The buoyancy of an object in water or air is determined by its *density* relative to the surrounding medium; thus objects less dense than the surrounding medium will float, and those more dense will sink. Salt water is denser than fresh water because of the much greater amount of dissolved substances. Therefore, a person will float more easily in salt water because there is a greater difference between the density of the person's body and that of the water.

11. **(C)** Warm-blooded animals have basically the same body and tissue organization; thus, a drug that injures one is likely to injure others. Rats are useful test animals because they are readily available, have a fairly short reproductive cycle, and are relatively inexpensive.

12. **(C)** A pH of 7 is neither acid nor base; it is neutral. If a base, such as sodium hydroxide, is added to an acid, such as nitric acid, until neutralization, the pH of the resultant solution is 7.

13. **(C)** Insulin increases the permeability of the cell membrane to glucose, thus increasing the rate of glucose uptake by the cells from the bloodstream. Adrenalin promotes an increase in cardiac activity, respiratory rate, and the breakdown of glycogen (stored in the liver) to glucose, thus raising the glucose level of the blood. With physical activity, glucose is more rapidly utilized by cells, which must remove glucose from the blood, thus reducing the blood level of glucose.

14. **(B)** The digestion and absorption of most nutrients occurs in the *duodenum*, the first portion of the small intestine. Therefore, digestive juices are most active at this site.

15. **(C)** A cold-blooded animal's body temperature will vary with environmental temperature, as contrasted to a warm-blooded animal, whose body temperature remains constant.

16. **(C)** Chromosomes contain genetic material, or carry genes; the separation of the chromosomes of each pair is involved in *meiosis*, or reduction division, in the production of sexual reproductive cells. The *gametes* (egg and sperm) will each receive one-half the chromosomes carried by the parent, or one chromosome of each pair carried by the parent. Thus, the gametes will be *haploid*. When fertilization occurs, the zygote becomes *diploid*, having received one chromosome of each pair from each parent. Therefore, each individual inherits one-half of its chromosomes and genes from its father and one-half from its mother.

17. **(A)** A *hertz* can be defined as the number of wavelengths per second. A wave or wavelength is the distance between successive values, for example, from crest to crest. The diagram shows four waves in the one-second period, or four hertz.

18. **(A)** Light consists of colors of varying wavelengths. Visible light ranges from red, with a wavelength of about 7000 angstrom units, down to violet, with a wavelength of about 4000 angstroms. Ultraviolet has shorter wavelengths (150-3900 Å) and is bactericidal; the highest bactericidal activity occurs between 2000 Å and 3000 Å.

19. **(B)** The lens is concave; therefore, it is thicker at the edges. Light rays passing through a concave lens are refracted or bent outward, so they spread apart. A light ray passing through the center of the lens is not bent.

20. **(C)** Sound travels in air at a rate of approximately 1100 feet/second; in five seconds the sound will have traveled approximately 5500 feet. Half of that distance was to reach the mountain, and half was the return of the echo. Therefore, the man is about 2750 feet from the mountain (half of 5500 feet), or about 900 yards.

21. **(A)** Visible light consists of different colors of light, producing a spectrum of red (with the longest wavelength) orange, yellow, green, blue, indigo, violet (with the shortest wavelength).

22. **(D)** White light consists of the colors or wavelengths of the visible spectrum, red, orange, yellow, green, blue, indigo, violet. An object appears to be a certain color when it is reflecting light of this wavelength, and absorbing all others. A white object is reflecting all of the colors or wavelengths at the same time.

23. **(C)** Magnetic properties of a substance are determined by atomic structure. Each electron of an atom spins on its axis as it moves in orbit, and each electron is a tiny magnet. In unmagnetized pieces of iron, steel, etc., the magnetic fields created by electrons are randomly arranged and move in all directions. If a steel knitting needle is stroked with a magnet, the small magnetic fields are attracted by the magnet to line up, with north and south poles pointing in opposite directions, thus increasing the magnetism in the steel.

24. **(B)** Persons with sickle cell anemia carry a variant hemoglobin molecule in the red blood cells, instead of the normal hemoglobin A. The production of hemoglobin is under genetic control.

25. **(B)** All elements listed are found in cells. Carbon, hydrogen, and phosphorus are three of the six major elements from which most organic molecules are built. Potassium is one of the five essential minor elements.

26. **(C)** An *ampere* (amp) is a unit for measuring the rate of flow of electricity. A *watt* is the metric unit of power; it is the power produced by 1 amp in a 1 volt circuit. Thus, the formula *watt = amp × volt*, can be used, or *amp = watt/volt*. If the problem is worked using this formula, the answer is (C), 16 amps.

27. **(C)** Photosynthesis is the process by which an organic, energy-containing compound (sugar or glucose) is produced from inorganic materials. This is a process basic to the production of organic compounds that can be used for food. Algae and other green plants exhibit photosynthesis.

28. **(B)** The presence of mammary glands for feeding young is the important characteristic of the class *Mammalia*. Birds are members of the class *Aves*; they do not nurse or suckle their young.

29. **(D)** A lichen is a composite organism consisting of a fungus and an alga living together. Some species of these plants can attach themselves to and break down rock by chemical and mechanical action. As organic remains from lichens become incorporated into and among the rock particles, a primitive kind of soil is formed in which some other plants can become established. As more organic material is produced, the soil becomes more enriched, leading to the establishment of higher plants, etc.

30. **(A)** The frog does not chew its food, and digestion of its food does not start in the mouth, as with man. Hence, salivary glands are not found in the frog. However, the endocrine system of the frog is basically like that of man, and the thyroid, pancreas, and adrenal glands are found in the frog as well as man.

31. **(C)** The center of gravity is that point on an object where all of the weight appears to be concentrated. Lowering the center of gravity will increase stability of the object. As the keel, the supporting frame along the bottom of a ship, is the lowest part of a ship, lowering its center of gravity will increase the stability of the ship.

32. **(B)** The root systems of plants help to hold soil in place, preventing erosion. Thus, removal of trees is most likely to speed up erosion.

33. **(D)** Vitamin D is not widely distributed in natural foods; it does occur, however, in cod-liver oil and in the tissues of certain fish. A provitamin or precursor to vitamin D is found in the skin and can be converted to vitamin D on exposure to sunlight. Commercial milk is "fortified" with vitamin D because this vitamin does not occur naturally in milk.

34. **(B)** The overproduction of the thyroid hormones causes a condition known as exophthalmic goiter, or Graves' disease. The thyroid may or may not be enlarged, but increased metabolic rate, protrusion of eyes (exophthalmus), increased blood pressure, increased heart rate, loss of weight, etc., are symptoms of Graves' disease. This disease may be treated by surgical removal of, or destruction of, a part of the thyroid gland.

35. **(D)** A person of blood group AB has antigen A and antigen B, but cannot produce antibodies against A or B. Therefore, such a person can receive blood from any of the four blood groups and is often called a "universal recipient."

36. **(B)** The Schick Test, developed by Bela Schick, is administered by injecting a weak solution of the diphtheria toxin cutaneously. A reddening of the site of injection indicates susceptibility to diphtheria; lack of reddening indicates immunity, indicating the presence of sufficient antitoxin to protect the person against diphtheria.

37. **(B)** *Evaporation* is the physical change of a substance from a liquid to a gas. The rate of movement of gas molecules into the air is more rapid in dry air or when the humidity is low, and decreases with increased humidity. The movement of air currents (wind) carries away the vapor above the surface of the liquid, thus increasing evaporation rate.

38. **(B)** K_2CO_3 in aqueous solution dissociates into potassium ions and carbonate ions. Water dissociates into hydrogen ions and hydroxyl ions. The carbonate ions can react with the hydrogen ions. forming bicarbonate ions (HCO_3-). The removal of hydrogen ions will yield an excess of hydroxyl ions, making the solution basic, and raising the pH. Since litmus, an indicator in the range of pH 6–8, is red in acid solution and blue in basic solution, K_2CO_3 will cause a basic reaction.

39. **(C)** Of the 17 atoms making up a molecule of $Al_2(SO_4)_3$, there are two atoms of aluminum, three atoms of sulfur, and twelve atoms of oxygen (four oxygens in each of the three sulfate ions). The weight of the oxygen is 192; the total weight of the molecule is 342. Thus, the percentage of oxygen by weight is 192/342, or 56 percent.

40. **(D)** To determine genotype of a hybrid, a pure recessive is always used in a test backcross. Any dominant trait carried by the hybrid parent will be expressed in some of the offspring; the recessive traits will also be expressed in some of the offspring, since the recessive parent cannot produce a dominant to mask it. Ratios and phenotypes will indicate the genotype of the hybrid parent.

41. **(D)** Maturing of cheese, formation of humus, and the synthesis of antibiotics can involve other kinds of organisms instead of, or in addition to, bacteria. The synthesis of vitamin K is a process performed by bacteria in the intestine and is not known to be performed by any other kind of organism.

42. **(C)** Reptiles do not possess a diaphragm but have the other structures listed.

43. **(A)** Light activates the chlorophylls, causing the emission of electrons at high energy levels. The energy-rich electron can pass through a series of catalysts; the light energy is converted to chemical energy resulting in phosphorylation, etc.

44. **(B)** The *vibrio* shape is curved, comma shaped. The bacilli, cocci, and rickettsiae are not curved.

45. **(C)** Coral is the hard skeleton of many marine coelenterates. The sea anemone is a coelenterate. The hard calcareous skeletal remains of these animals are the chief component of the coral reefs and coral islands found in tropical and subtropical seas. The sea anemone itself, however, does not produce coral.

46. **(A)** In a food chain, algae are the primary "producers," occupying the bottom level of the food chain since they produce organic materials through photosynthetic processes. Insect larvae are some of the animals that can feed on algae; fish, which prey on animals such as insect larvae, are in turn consumed by man.

47. **(A)** Grasses are usually pollinated by wind; the grass flower typically does not attract insects or birds. Since grasses are mostly land plants, water would not play a significant role in their pollination.

48. **(A)** The *ectoderm* is the outer germ layer, which gives rise to the nervous and integumentary systems of the embryo.

49. **(B)** Only green plants can produce organic materials (food) from inorganic materials (carbon dioxide and water) through the process of photosynthesis. Oxygen and a by-product are returned to the air by means of this process. Animals may consume green plants (direct dependence) or may consume animals that consume green plants (indirect dependence) for food and energy.

50. **(A)** Photosynthesis occurs only in the presence of light and the chlorophylls. This means that photosynthesis occurs only in the green parts of plants that are exposed to light. Roots generally are not green and are subterranean organs; therefore, roots generally do not exhibit photosynthetic activity.

51. **(D)** One mole (gram molecular weight) of nitrogen is 28 grams, since two nitrogen atoms form a nitrogen molecule (N_2). One mole of gas occupies a volume of 22.4 liters at standard conditions.

52. **(B)** The frequency, or number of vibrations per second, determines pitch, or tone. The greater the frequency, the higher the pitch; the lower the frequency, the lower the pitch.

53. **(D)** Nitrogen-fixing bacteria have the ability to convert gaseous, atmospheric nitrogen into nitrates that can be taken up by plants. These bacteria are associated with certain leguminous plants, such as clover, occurring in nodules on the root systems of the plants.

54. **(A)** Cells of the root tip, stem tip, and cambium are *meristematic* tissues in that they retain their ability to divide, thus producing other tissues and growth. Other tissues in plants generally are not meristematic when they mature.

55. **(A)** Although plants have tissues and organs that perform specific functions, these are not organized into organ systems such as one would find in animals, especially higher animals.

56. **(B)** Boyle's Law illustrates the relationship between the pressure and volume of a mass of gas at a fixed temperature. The law can be simply stated: at a given fixed temperature and mass of gas, pressure and volume are inversely proportional. For example, volume will increase as pressure decreases, or volume will decrease as pressure increases. Therefore, pressure × volume = a constant.

57. **(B)** Peas and beans are members of the legume family and have nitrogen-fixing bacteria in nodules on their roots. Nitrogen-fixing bacteria convert atmospheric gaseous nitrogen into nitrates, thus restoring nitrates to the soil. It is only in the form of nitrates that plants generally can obtain nitrogen from the soil.

58. **(A)** The male sex chromosome is referred to as the Y chromosome. It is inherited only by male offspring; thus, a male is XY and a female is XX, as far as inheritance of sex is concerned. Therefore, any gene located on the Y chromosome is inherited only by males since females will inherit an X from the male parent.

59. **(B)** Oxidation-reduction reactions are those in which one substance is oxidized by the loss of electrons, and another substance is reduced by the gain of electrons. In double replacement reactions, this does not occur. Ions are exchanged between reactants and do not lose or gain electrons.

60. **(D)** Barium carbonate and barium sulfate are both white precipitates. However, barium carbonate is formed on contact of barium, as in barium chloride, with CO_2, while barium sulfate is formed by precipitation with a sulfate salt, such as zinc sulfate.

61. **(D)** The mitochondrion is called the powerhouse of the cell; most of the respiratory process involving the release of energy occurs in this organelle.

62. **(A)** Proteins are synthesized on the messenger RNA molecule as it moves through the ribosomes. Transfer RNA transports specific amino acids to the appropriate site on the messenger RNA, forming a protein.

63. **(A)** More energy per molecule of glucose is derived from aerobic respiration, involving the use of gaseous molecular oxygen, than from anaerobic respiration or fermentation. Thus aerobic respiration is the most efficient. Anaerobic respiration ranks second in efficiency; fermentation, third. Phosphorylation, though involved in respiratory processes, is not itself a respiratory process.

64. **(C)** *Egestion* is the elimination of undigested wastes from the digestive tracts or cavity; enzymes are not involved in this process but are involved in the other processes named.

65. **(A)** Chloroplasts contain the chlorophylls, the green pigments, and are characteristic of green plants but not of animals.

66. **(C)** These two processes, meiosis and syngamy, enable the chromosome number to remain constant for the species. *Meiosis* reduces the chromosome number from the diploid to the haploid condition in the formation of gametes or some spores; *syngamy* (the union of gametes or gametic nuclei) restores the diploid number to the zygote or diploid nucleus.

67. **(A)** The cell wall and plastids are characteristic of plant cells but not animal cells. A nucleus may not be present in some cells, such as mature human red blood cells. But all cells have cytoplasm surrounded by a plasma or cell membrane.

68. **(B)** Charles Darwin was one of several scientists who collected and presented evidence in support of the theory of evolution. His best-known published work is entitled *The Origin of Species*.

69. **(B)** A virus does not exhibit reproduction, synthesis, and other characteristics of life outside a living host cell; thus, it is an obligate intracellular parasite.

70. **(C)** Digestive enzymes pass directly from the gland or gland cells producing them to the site of digestion. Thus, they are not transported in the bloodstream as are the other substances named.

UNIT IV READING COMPREHENSION

TECHNIQUES OF READING INTERPRETATION

Reading comprehension presents problems to many test-takers. To avoid this, make every effort to improve your ability to interpret reading passages.

First, understand that there are two aspects of success in reading interpretation:

1. *reading speed*
2. *reading understanding*

Too many individuals read with excellent comprehension but read too slowly. Remember, there is a time limit on your test. On the other hand, some people read rapidly, but, for reasons that we shall cite later, do not thoroughly understand what they are reading. Both speed of reading and comprehension of the material read are important during an exam. Let us, then, divide our discussion into two parts:

1. *increasing reading speed*
2. *improving reading comprehension*

General Advice

You were probably taught to read letter-by-letter; gradually, as you matured, you learned to read word-by-word. As an adult, however, you should be able to read a complete phrase as quickly as you once read just one letter. If you cannot do this, or if you have trouble understanding what you read, you should practice reading intensively.

There is no need to be discouraged if this is the case. Most students can increase the speed of their reading significantly with a little effort. The old idea that slow readers make up for their slowness by better comprehension of what they read has been proved untrue. Your ability to comprehend what you read should keep pace with your increase in speed. You can absorb as many ideas per page and get many more ideas per unit of reading time by applying specific techniques of reading.

It has been demonstrated that those who read best also read quickly. This is probably due to the fact that heavier concentration is required for rapid reading; and concentration is what enables a reader to grasp important ideas contained in the reading material.

A good paragraph generally has one central thought—that is, a *topic sentence*. Your main task is to locate and absorb that thought while reading the paragraph. The correct interpretation of the paragraph is based upon that thought, and not upon your personal opinions, prejudices, or preferences. If a selection consists of two or more paragraphs, its correct interpretation is based on the central idea of the entire passage. The ability to grasp the central idea of a passage can be acquired by practice—practice that will also increase the speed with which you read.

An important rule to follow in order to improve reading ability is to force yourself to increase your speed. Just as you once stopped reading letter-by-letter, now learn to stop reading word-by-word. Force yourself to read rapidly across the line of type, skimming it. Don't permit your eyes to stop for individual words; try instead to reconstruct the whole idea even if a word has been missed. Proceed quickly through the paragraph in this skimming fashion, without rereading or backtracking to a missed word.

If you find yourself failing to comprehend what you read, read the material over several times rapidly until you do understand. Do *not* slow down on rereading. At first, you may find yourself missing some of the ideas. With persistent practice, however, you will step up both your reading speed and your ability to comprehend what you read.

You may need to overcome certain handicaps or bad reading habits at once. Do not move your lips, pronounce words individually silently or aloud, or think of each word separately as you read. These habits can be overcome almost automatically if you learn to leap from phrase to phrase. You can synchronize your eye movements with your mind, both of which are a great deal nimbler than your lips.

Certain physical factors affect reading. You should always read sitting in a comfortable position, erect, with head slightly inclined. The light should be excellent, with both an indirect and a direct source available; direct light should come from behind you and slightly above your shoulder, in such a way that the type is evenly lit. Hold the reading matter at your own best reading distance and at a convenient height, so you don't stoop or squint. It goes without saying that if you need reading glasses, you should certainly use them.

Increasing Reading Speed: Causes and Cures of Slow Reading

Cause #1: Word-by-word reading. Our earliest reading, since it is done aloud, is, of necessity, word-by-word reading. Unfortunately, this method of reading sometimes becomes so firmly implanted that it persists as a bad reading habit.

Cure: Use the *eye-span method.* Look at the first part of a sentence that consists of a thought-unit. Then, look for the next thought-unit, if there is another one in the same sentence—then, look for still another thought-unit. For example, consider this sentence:

Reading maketh a full man, conference a ready man, and writing an exact man. How many ideas are there in the sentence? Three. Now, employ the eyespan method in reading this sentence.

Reading maketh a full man,
EYE SPAN 1

conference a ready man,
EYE SPAN 2

<u>and writing an exact man,</u>
EYE SPAN 3

Cause #2: Vocalizing.   Some readers move their lips or whisper while they read "silently." This practice slows down silent-reading time considerably.

Cure: You must consciously refrain from moving your lips or whispering during silent reading. Have someone watch you while you read. Are you vocalizing?

Cause #3: One-speed reading.   You should vary your reading speed according to what you are reading.

Cure: The pace of your reading should change not only from book to book, but even within a reading selection. Be flexible so that you can change speed from paragraph to paragraph, even from sentence to sentence.

Increasing Reading Comprehension

The following are good techniques to use on *any* reading interpretation question.

1. Read the selection through quickly to get the general sense.

2. Reread the selection, concentrating on the central idea.

3. Can you now pick out the *topic sentence* in each paragraph?

4. If the selection consists of more than one paragraph, determine the *central idea* of the entire selection.

5. Examine the four choices for each test item carefully yet rapidly. Eliminate immediately those choices that are far-fetched, ridiculous, irrelevant, false, or impossible.

6. Eliminate those choices that may be true but have nothing to do with the sense of the selection.

7. Check those few choices that now remain as possibilities.

8. Refer back to the original selection and determine which one of these remaining possibilities is best in view of
   a) information *stated* in the selection
   b) information *implied* in the selection

9. Be sure to consider only the facts *given or definitely implied* in the selection.

10. Be especially careful of trick expressions or catch-words, which sometimes destroy the validity of a seemingly acceptable answer. These include the expressions "under all circumstances," "at all times," "always," "under no conditions," "absolutely," "completely," and "entirely."

AVOID TRAPS

Trap #1 Sometimes the question cannot be answered on the basis of the stated facts. You may be required to make a *deduction* from the facts given.

Trap #2 Eliminate your personal opinions.

Trap #3 Search out significant details that are nestled in the paragraph. Reread the paragraph as many times as necessary (with an eye on your watch).

GET PLENTY OF PRACTICE

Read:

(a) editorial pages of various newspapers

(b) book reviews (also drama and movie reviews)

(c) magazine articles

For each selection that you read, do the following:

(a) Jot down the main idea of the article.

(b) Look up the meanings of words you don't know or aren't sure of.

A SAMPLE QUESTION

Here is a sample question followed by analysis. Try to understand the process of arriving at the correct answer.

> Too often, indeed, have scurrilous and offensive allegations by underworld figures been sufficient to blast the careers of irreproachable and incorruptible executives who, because of their efforts to serve the people honestly and faithfully, incurred the enmity of powerful political forces and lost their positions.

Judging from the contents of the preceding sentence, which conclusion might be most valid?

(A) The large majority of executives are irreproachable and incorruptible.

(B) Criminals often swear in court that honest officials are corrupt in order to save themselves.

(C) Political forces are always clashing with government executives.

(D) False statements by criminals sometimes cause honest officials the loss of their positions or the ruin of their careers.

INTERPRETATION

Statement (A) can generally be said to be a true statement, but it cannot be derived from the paragraph. Nothing is said in the paragraph about "the large majority" of executives.

Statement (B) may also be a true statement and can, to a certain extent, be derived from the paragraph. However, the phrase "in order to save themselves" is not relevant to the sense of the paragraph, and even if it were, this choice does not sum up its central thought.

Statement (C) cannot be derived from the paragraph. The catch-word "always" makes this choice entirely invalid.

Statement (D) is the best conclusion that can be drawn from the contents of the paragraph, in light of the four choices given. It is open to no exceptions and adequately sums up the central thought of the paragraph.

ANALYSIS OF THE READING COMPREHENSION TEST ITEM

Reading Comprehension test items are designed to address specific skills. They usually elicit a response that would indicate the test-taker's ability to identify directly stated details; indirectly stated details; main idea; inferences; generalizations. Other target skills may include making judgments, drawing conclusions, and determining author's purpose.

The sample reading passage below, followed by a set of six questions, will help you to analyze comprehension test items and to understand why a particular response is the correct or appropriate one. Studying the questions before reading a passage will cause you to be more alert when reading the passage, that is, you will be aware of what information in the passage will best help you answer the questions. Now read the six questions at the end of the passage and then proceed to answer them. Note that the questions are followed by explanatory notes that indicate the skill addressed and strategies to use in your approach to a particular type question.

"The Land of Frost and Fire" is no misnomer for the elliptic island republic in the North Atlantic known as Iceland. The island is so called because erupting volcanoes and steaming hot springs lie adjacent to its glaciers and ice fields. The official name of the country in Icelandic is Lydveldid Island, or the Republic of Iceland.

The "frost" is frigidly evident in the island's numerous ice fields that traverse the hoary landscape. Approximately one-eighth of the island is covered by glaciers. In the southeast, a glacier known as Vatnajokull makes an area of about 8550 square kilometers (about 3300 square miles). Iceland, just south of the Arctic Circle, has more than 120 glaciers.

Lydveldid Island's "fire" leaps from the many hot springs and spouting geysers that cloud the panorama of the seventeen-province republic. To add heat to the "fire" are some one hundred volcanoes including at least twenty-five that have erupted and been recorded in the annals of the island's autocratic history. Lava and rocks erupting from volcanoes have contoured much of the land. The central highlands reflect the barren wilderness of lava fields. Hekla in the southwest is the best-known Icelandic volcano because of its many eruptions. The years 1766, 1940, 1947, and 1980 mark its explosive appearances.

Thermal springs are also common in Iceland. The springs occur as geysers, sizzling mud lakes, and in various other forms. The most famous geyser here is Great Geysir, which is situated in southwest Iceland. The natives of this island of swift-flowing rivers boast of Geysir's spectacular and frequent eruptions occurring at irregular intervals of five to thirty-six hours. The torrid spring reportedly thrusts a column of boiling water upward to about sixty meters or two hundred feet.

Volcanic in origin, Iceland is indeed a land of contrast. Dazzling ice and jet black lava covering most of Iceland's surface attest to the appropriateness of its nickname—"Land of Frost and Fire".

1. Where are Iceland's hot springs and glaciers located?

   (A) in the central highlands
   (B) in the southwest
   (C) next to the glaciers
   (D) in the southeast

Explanatory Note: This is a directly stated detail question. When answering this type question, always consider the *wh* word with which the question begins. *Who* can be answered by the name of a person. *When* is answered by a word or phrase that tells at what time or in what sequence something happens. *Why* is answered by a word or phrase that tells the reason something happens. *What* is usually answered by the name of a thing or event. *Which* is answered by choosing the correct person, place, or thing from two or more persons, places, or things. *Where* is answered by the name of a place or a phrase that describes the location of one person or thing in relation to another (spatial relationships). Finally, *how* should be considered with these question words. *How* is answered by the way in which something is done. Question 1 is a *where* question denoting a spatial relationship. The correct answer is C. Since adjacent means next to and encompasses the location of both the glaciers and geysers this is the appropriate response. A, B, and D could be ruled out immediately because they do not describe the location of both the glaciers and the geysers.

2. An appropriate title for this passage would be

   (A) Volcanoes and Geysers
   (B) Iceland: The Island Republic
   (C) Iceland: A Land of Contrast
   (D) Thermal Springs

Explanatory Note: This is a main idea question. This type question requires the test-taker to consider what the passage is mostly about. Read the question first. Then scan the entire passage to find out what it is mostly about. A word of caution: Some answer choices are merely details from the passage. It is not difficult to choose (C) as the best title.

3. It is apparent that this passage is intended to

   (A) inform
   (B) entertain
   (C) persuade
   (D) share an experience

Explanatory Note: The skill addressed in this question is identifying author's purpose. The test-taker must determine what the author is trying to accomplish by writing this selection. What kind of response does he or she want from the reader. If the reader can say that he or she enjoyed this passage or thought it was hilarious, obviously the passage was meant to entertain. If the reader's reaction is, "Well, I think I'll try that" or "I have to agree with that," the passage was written to persuade. If the passage is a narration or a storytelling written in the first person (I, me, my, myself—all references to the writer) the passage is probably aimed at sharing an experience. If the reader's reaction is, "I didn't know that," or "I never heard of this before," there is a good chance that the author intended to inform. The correct answer for this question is A, "inform."

4. The people of Iceland's sentiments toward the presence of geysers in their native land is one of

    (A) mixed emotions
    (B) pride
    (C) dread and fear
    (D) indifference

Explantory Note: This question requires the test-taker to infer a meaning or idea. In other words, "read between the lines". In the fourth paragraph of this passage, it is mentioned that the natives "boast of Geysir's spectacular and frequent eruptions." Usually, people boast about something when they are proud of it. The correct response would therefore be, B, "pride."

5. According to this passage, Iceland's form of government at one time reflected

    (A) total rule by the state
    (B) rule by and for the people
    (C) rule by royalty
    (D) rule by dictator

Explanatory Note: This test question is an example of indirectly stated detail. In paragraph three of this passage the phrase "the annals of the island's autocratic history" appears. The adjective autocratic, though irrelevant to the main idea of the passage, and even to the sentence in which it appears, does provide an informational detail. The term autocratic suggests government by one person having unlimited power. The correct answer therefore would be, D, "rule by dictator." In completing this type question, the test-taker should scan the passage to eliminate answer choices. Eliminate answer choices that are obviously related to the main idea, and in some cases, be careful of negative words in the question (no, not, not any).

6. Iceland is a difficult place to

    (A) grow crops
    (B) raise a family
    (C) get an education
    (D) start a business

Explanatory Note: Question 6 requires that you make a judgment or draw a conclusion. Since the passage does not mention family life, education, or industry, it would be safe to eliminate choices B, C, and D. The passage also does not mention agriculture; however it does describe the land as being "barren wilderness" and "covered by glaciers." These are conditions are unsuitable for farming. Therefore, A, "farm," is an appropriate answer.

Answer Sheet
Reading Comprehension Passages
TEST 1

1. Ⓐ Ⓑ Ⓒ Ⓓ   2. Ⓐ Ⓑ Ⓒ Ⓓ   3. Ⓐ Ⓑ Ⓒ Ⓓ   4. Ⓐ Ⓑ Ⓒ Ⓓ

TEST 2

1. Ⓐ Ⓑ Ⓒ Ⓓ   3. Ⓐ Ⓑ Ⓒ Ⓓ   5. Ⓐ Ⓑ Ⓒ Ⓓ   7. Ⓐ Ⓑ Ⓒ Ⓓ
2. Ⓐ Ⓑ Ⓒ Ⓓ   4. Ⓐ Ⓑ Ⓒ Ⓓ   6. Ⓐ Ⓑ Ⓒ Ⓓ   8. Ⓐ Ⓑ Ⓒ Ⓓ

TEST 3

1. Ⓐ Ⓑ Ⓒ Ⓓ   3. Ⓐ Ⓑ Ⓒ Ⓓ   5. Ⓐ Ⓑ Ⓒ Ⓓ   7. Ⓐ Ⓑ Ⓒ Ⓓ
2. Ⓐ Ⓑ Ⓒ Ⓓ   4. Ⓐ Ⓑ Ⓒ Ⓓ   6. Ⓐ Ⓑ Ⓒ Ⓓ   8. Ⓐ Ⓑ Ⓒ Ⓓ

TEST 4

1. Ⓐ Ⓑ Ⓒ Ⓓ   4. Ⓐ Ⓑ Ⓒ Ⓓ   7. Ⓐ Ⓑ Ⓒ Ⓓ
2. Ⓐ Ⓑ Ⓒ Ⓓ   5. Ⓐ Ⓑ Ⓒ Ⓓ   8. Ⓐ Ⓑ Ⓒ Ⓓ
3. Ⓐ Ⓑ Ⓒ Ⓓ   6. Ⓐ Ⓑ Ⓒ Ⓓ   9. Ⓐ Ⓑ Ⓒ Ⓓ

TEST 5

1. Ⓐ Ⓑ Ⓒ Ⓓ   3. Ⓐ Ⓑ Ⓒ Ⓓ   5. Ⓐ Ⓑ Ⓒ Ⓓ   7. Ⓐ Ⓑ Ⓒ Ⓓ
2. Ⓐ Ⓑ Ⓒ Ⓓ   4. Ⓐ Ⓑ Ⓒ Ⓓ   6. Ⓐ Ⓑ Ⓒ Ⓓ   8. Ⓐ Ⓑ Ⓒ Ⓓ

TEST 6

1. Ⓐ Ⓑ Ⓒ Ⓓ

2. Ⓐ Ⓑ Ⓒ Ⓓ

3. Ⓐ Ⓑ Ⓒ Ⓓ

4. Ⓐ Ⓑ Ⓒ Ⓓ

5. Ⓐ Ⓑ Ⓒ Ⓓ

6. Ⓐ Ⓑ Ⓒ Ⓓ

READING COMPREHENSION TEST 1

9 Minutes   4 Questions

Directions: *Carefully read the following passage and then answer the accompanying questions, basing your answers on what is stated or implied in the passage. When you have decided which choice is best, blacken the corresponding space on your answer sheet. There is only one best answer for each question.*

The "liberated woman" is a phrase which most of us associate with the sixties and seventies. The ERA and NOW's consciousness-raising and bra-burning blitzed the media with a fury. In reality, the American woman had begun to cast off the restrictions of feminine suppression long before the seventies, by snipping the strings of her proverbial apron, if not the straps of her bra. We are referring to both the 1920s and the postwar era.

The flood of labor-saving and timesaving devices pouring from the factories freed women of much of the never-ending drudgery that had been the plight of housewives since the beginning of time.

Women also found new freedom outside the home. The vote was finally rendered to women via the Nineteenth Amendment to the Constitution, and the long awaited dream of political equality between the sexes was fulfilled. Members of what was once known as the "gentle sex" cast down their brooms, cast forth their ballots, and fled their kitchens to take part in a social freedom that catapulted their grandmothers right out of their rocking chairs. Chaperones no longer made the scene at young people's parties. Fashion editors reported "the American woman has lifted her skirt far beyond any modest limitation." The hemline was being hoisted nine inches from the ground and was heading for the knee.

The boyish look was in, and women everywhere invaded the strictly male territory known as the barbershop to have their beautiful and once-treasured tresses "bobbed." Breast implants, no way! Damsels of every social station were binding their chests to acquire that fashionable look of masculinity. In contrast to this trend in fashion, beautiful debutantes took heed to the cliche "powder and paint will make you what you ain't" and plastered their faces doll-style with rouge and lipstick.

Young ladies no longer puffed secretly into the fireplaces of their homes to conceal the damnable sin of which they were partaking. Women were smoking in public for the first time.

Extensive vicissitudes in lifestyle and values placed women in the workplace. The "roaring twenties" were characterized by women finding new opportunities for employment in the booming cities. Though they were limited to a few low-paying jobs such as retail clerking and office typing that were hastily labeled "women's work," they were making an impact on the postwar era. A feisty feminist, Margaret Sanger, led a birth-control movement and openly defended the use of contraceptives. To add insult to injury, the women of the twenties deflated many a male ego with the organization of the National Women's Party in 1923.

"You've Come A Long Way Baby" was putting it mildly in the twenties. In all probability, the women of the 1990s can anticipate recoining the phrase "... and you ain't seen nothin' yet!"

1. This passage would suggest that women of the 1920s were

    (A) docile in their attitudes regarding social change
    (B) assertive in their views on women's social and political status
    (C) willing to compromise on political issues concerning women
    (D) eager to return to life in the kitchen

2. A fitting title for this passage would be

    (A) *You've Come a Long Way Baby— Twenties Style*
    (B) *Women in the Workplace*
    (C) *Women's Political Advancements in the Twenties*
    (D) *Male Bashing in the Twenties*

3. The tone of this passage would suggest that the author is

    (A) a male chauvinist
    (B) a product of the seventies
    (C) a trendy individual
    (D) an advocate of women's lib

4. This passage reflects that the era known as the "Roaring Twenties" was characterized by

    (A) an increase in women's unemployment
    (B) marked social change
    (C) an industrial slump
    (D) an indifference to fashion and style

READING COMPREHENSION TEST 2

10 Minutes   8 Questions

Directions: *Carefully read the following passage and then answer the accompanying questions, basing your answers on what is stated or implied in the passage. When you have decided which choice is best, blacken the corresponding space on your answer sheet. There is only one best answer for each question.*

Living organisms are unique, among the known forms of matter, because they are capable of creating their own specific highly organized structure out of substances taken from far more disorganized surroundings, and can transmit this capability to their offspring. Perhaps the oldest and most profound theoretical problem in biology is the effort to explain the curious paradox that, despite its unique capability for self-duplication and inheritance, a living organism is nevertheless a mixture of substances which are separately no more possessed of these properties than are the more prosaic molecules that never occur in living cells. This question has been at the root of a long train of experiments, debates, and speculations that began in classical times and continues unbroken through the development of present-day "molecular biology."

The basic issues are simply stated. If the component parts of a cell are not themselves alive, whence come the life-properties exhibited by the whole? Apart from the untenable notion of a mystic non-material "vital force" which supposedly animates the otherwise dead substance of the cell, the debate has elicited two main positions: (a) There is, in fact, some special cellular component which possesses the fundamental attribute of self-duplication, and which is therefore a "living molecule" and the basic source of the life-properties of the cell. (b) The unique properties of life are inherently connected with the very considerable complexity of living substance and arise from interactions among its separable constituents which are not exhibited unless these components occur together in the complex whole. In this view, only the entire living cell is capable of self-duplication.

There is at this time a widespread impression that this issue has been resolved and that the cell does indeed contain a component—DNA—which, according to the theory of the "DNA code," possesses the basic attribute of life, self-duplication, and which guides the activities of all the inheritable processes of the cell.

The importance of this conclusion is self-evident, for it would answer, at last, the basic question of the origin of the unique properties of life, and, if correct, should lead to unprecedented technological control over these properties. It is appropriate, therefore, to ask what criteria are required to establish that a molecule, such as DNA, is capable of self-duplication, to examine the degree to which the available evidence meets such criteria, and to determine whether the undoubted importance of DNA in the biology of inheritance may be due to some properties other than those attributed to it by current theory.*

1. The chief conclusion to be derived from the foregoing considerations is that

   (A) self-duplication of living organisms is the result of the biochemical aspects of genetics

   (B) the origin of unique properties of life is a "vital force"

   (C) the relationships between reproduction and inheritance are mutually exclusive

   (D) self-duplication is a process of converting non-living matter to living matter

2. In this passage, the author identifies the uniqueness of living organisms by which one of the following characteristics?

   (A) Similar life forms are created from separate substances possessing the properties of life.

   (B) Similar life forms are created from separate substances that do not possess the properties of life.

   (C) New organisms are reproduced from a single substance.

   (D) New organisms are produced from non-cellular components.

3. The author's approach to the study of inheritance is

   (A) biological and chemical
   (B) ecological and biological
   (C) chemical and ecological
   (D) physical and biological

4. Which one of the following statements best describes the "DNA code" theory?

   (A) DNA acts as a catalyst in the creation of life.

   (B) DNA controls heredity but not cell reproduction.

   (C) The cell has the ability to synthesize DNA, which animates nonliving matter.

   (D) The cell contains DNA, a living molecule capable of self-duplication.

5. The basic issues regarding self-duplication presented in this passage include all of the following *except* the

   (A) role of living and nonliving matter in the creation of life.

   (B) relationships between cellular parts and the complex whole

   (C) differences between genetic processes and reproduction in living organisms

   (D) paradox between the phenomenon of self-duplication and the biochemical

---

* Reprinted with permission of *American Scientist*. From "DNA and the Chemistry of Inheritances," by Barry Commoner, *American Scientist* 52, 1964.

processes involved in the creation of life

6. The ultimate purpose of research related to heredity is to

    (A) balance the relationships between living and non-living matter

    (B) create life through artificial techniques

    (C) control inheritable processes of the cell

    (D) create unknown forms of life

7. The author's approach to the study of the DNA theory is to

    (A) apply the principles of molecular biology to the notion of "vital force"

    (B) establish criteria for judging the capabilities of DNA to self-duplicate

    (C) assume that DNA is the isolated factor of self-duplication and study genetic processes

    (D) confirm that the creation of organisms is a self-duplication process

8. The best title for this passage might be

    (A) *DNA, the Miracle of Life*

    (B) *Self-Duplication: The Mystery of Life*

    (C) *Differences Between Self-Duplication and Heredity*

    (D) *The Status of Genetic Research*

READING COMPREHENSION TEST 3

Directions: *Carefully read the following passage and then answer the accompanying questions, basing your answers on what is stated or implied in the passage. When you have decided which choice is best, blacken the corresponding space on your answer sheet. There is only one best answer for each question.*

10 Minutes   8 Questions

The term philanthropy may be defined as a spirit of goodwill toward humanity, usually expressed in activities that promote human welfare. The word gained frequent usage and popularity in the eighteenth century. This was a time when the functions of religious charities were being adopted by both the state and private individuals.

In ancient societies, such as those of Greece and Rome, there existed self-supporting kinship groups. Urbanization resulted in these groups disbanding and, in turn, this led to the indigent, and disadvantaged. Subsequently, all the principal religions, Judaism, Christianity, Buddhism, and Islam began to realize the need for financially wealthy people to aid the less fortunate, and in recognition of this need, they encouraged their affluent parishioners to donate generously to the impoverished. So it is apparent that the concept of philanthropy is as old as recorded history.

Even during the Middle Ages in Europe, an intricate network of almshouses, orphanages, and hospitals was supported by the rich and by church collections. As the modern nation-state surfaced, secular governments assumed the duties of religious authorities as the basic philanthropic agencies.

Today, philanthropy is synonymous with the disbursement of wealth by individuals and the fund-raising activities of nonprofit organizations such as United Way. One of the most famous philanthropists was the American industrialist Andrew Carnegie. He devoted his waning years to giving away the huge fortune he had acquired in the steel industry. In keeping with the principles he proposed in his essay "Gospel of Wealth," written in 1889, Carnegie turned over $300 million to society via foundations and trusts. Significant philanthropic foundations of the twentieth century were also established by Henry Ford and John D. Rockefeller.

The Rockefeller Foundation was chartered in 1913 for the permanent purpose of promoting "the well-being" of mankind throughout the world. The nonprofit organization was conceived based on a perception of a need to extend and apply knowledge in the fields of medical education, public health, medical and biological research, agriculture, the social sciences, and humanities. The Foundation gives aid through grants to qualified agencies and to the training of personnel in related fields.

John D. Rockefeller originally provided an endowment of $100 million for the Foundation. Later he increased it to more than $183 million. The policies and operation of the organization are under the jurisdiction of a self-perpetuating board of trustees who receive no remuneration. The Rockefeller Foundation and others like it are evidence that the age-old institution of philanthropy is alive and well in our society.

1. In ancient times, philanthropic activities shifted from family circles to the church because

    (A) the church could appropriate more funds

    (B) the church demanded it

    (C) there were more people in need

    (D) people moved to towns and villages

2. According to this passage a philanthropist could be considered

    (A) profoundly religious

    (B) a humanitarian

    (C) political

    (D) an industrialist

3. Andrew Carnegie's great wealth may be attributed to his

    (A) essay writing

    (B) foundations and trusts

    (C) investment and return in the steel industry

    (D) prudent attitude toward life

4. "The Gospel of Wealth" advocates that the

    (A) prosperous give back to society

    (B) rich should get richer

    (C) church assume responsibility for the impoverished

    (D) government should oversee philanthropic organizations

5. It could be concluded that the trustees of the Rockefeller Foundation are not paid because

    (A) this enables them to be objective in their decision-making

    (B) this would greatly diminish foundation funds

    (C) government legislation forbids the practice

    (D) Rockefeller did not wish to pay them

6. As delineated in this passage, the grant provisions to the Rockefeller Foundation

    (A) would permit aid to local sports programs

    (B) would affirm assistance to AIDS research

    (C) would assist other philanthropic organizations

    (D) would provide assistance to any destitute individual

7. An appropriate title for this passage would be

    (A) *The Rockefeller Foundation*
    (B) *Sharing the Wealth*
    (C) *Alms to the Poor*
    (D) *Philanthropy in Ancient Times*

8. In comparing philanthropic institutions of ancient times to those of today, one would note the

    (A) vast increase in monies allotted
    (B) presence of government intervention
    (C) expansion of services
    (D) elimination of the church role

READING COMPREHENSION TEST 4

10 Minutes   9 Questions

Directions: *Carefully read the following passage and then answer the accompanying questions, basing your answers on what is stated or implied in the passage. When you have decided which choice is best, blacken the corresponding space on your answer sheet. There is only one best answer for each question.*

As the world's population grows, the part played by man in influencing plant life becomes increasingly great. In old and densely populated countries, as in western Europe, man determines almost wholly what shall grow and what shall not. In such regions, the influence of man on plant life is in large measure a beneficial one. Laws, often centuries old, protect plants of economic value and preserve soil fertility. In newly settled countries the situation is, unfortunately, quite the reverse. The pioneer's life is too strenuous for him to think of posterity.

Some years ago Mt. Mitchell, the highest summit east of the Mississippi, was covered with a magnificent forest. A lumber company was given full rights to fell the trees. Those not cut down were crushed. The mountain was left a waste area where fire would rage and erosion complete the destruction. There was no stopping the devastating foresting of the company, for the contract had been given. Under a more enlightened civilization, this could not have happened. The denuding of Mt. Mitchell is a minor chapter in the destruction of lands in the United States; and this country is by no means the only sufferer. China, India, Egypt, and East Africa all have their thousands of square miles of wasteland, the result of man's indifference to the future.

Deforestation, grazing, and poor farming techniques are the chief causes of the destruction of land fertility. Wasteful cutting of timber is the first step. Grazing follows lumbering, often bringing about ruin. The Caribbean slopes of northern Venezuela are barren wastes, owing first to ruthless cutting of forests and then to destructive grazing. Hordes of goats roamed these slopes until only a few thorny acacias and cacti remained. Erosion completed the devastation. What is illustrated there on a small scale is the story of vast areas in China and India, countries where famines occur regularly.

Man is not wholly to blame, for nature is often merciless. In parts of India and China, plant life, even when left undisturbed by man, cannot cope with either the disastrous floods of wet seasons or the destructive winds of the dry season. Man has learned much; prudent land management has been the policy of the Chinese people since 2700 B.C., but even they have not learned enough.

When the American forestry service was in its infancy, it met with much opposition from legislators who loudly claimed that the protected land would in one season yield a crop of cabbages of more value than all the timber on it. Herein lay the fallacy, that one season's crop is all that need be thought of. Nature, through the years, adjusts crops to the soil and to the climate. Forests usually occur where precipitation exceeds evaporation. If the reverse is true, grasslands are found; and where the evaporation is still greater, desert or scrub vegetation alone survives. The phytogeographic map of a country is very similar to the climatic map based on rainfall, evaporation, and temperature. Man ignores this natural adjustment of crops and strives for one "bumper" crop in a single season; he may produce it, but "year in and year out, the yield of the grassland is certain, that of the planted fields, never."

Man is learning; he sprays his trees with insecticides and fungicides; he imports ladybugs to destroy aphids; he irrigates, fertilizes, and rotates his crops; but he is still indifferent to many of the consequences of his shortsighted policies.

In spite of the evidence from the experience of this country, the people of other countries still in the pioneer stage farm as wastefully as did our own pioneers. In the interiors of Central and South America, natives fell superb forest trees and leave them to rot in order to obtain virgin soil for cultivation. Where the land is hilly, it readily washes, and after one or two seasons it is unfit for crops. So the frontier farmer pushes back into the primeval forest, moving his hut as he goes, and fells more monarchs to lay bare another patch of ground for his plantings to support his family. Valuable timber that will require a century to replace is destroyed and the land laid waste to produce what could be supplied for a pittance.

How badly man can err in his handling of land is shown by the draining of extensive swamp areas, which to the uninformed would seem to be a very good thing to do. One of the first effects of the drainage is the lowering of the water-table, which may bring about the death of the dominant species and leave to another species the possession of the soil, even when the difference in water level is little more than an inch. Bog country will frequently yield marketable crops of cranberries and blueberries but if drained, will grow neither these nor any other economically useful plant on the fallow soil. Swamps and marshes may have their drawbacks, but man should beware of disturbing the ecosphere. When drained, wetlands may leave waste land, the surface of which can erode rapidly and be blown away in dust blizzards disastrous to both man and wild beasts.

1. The best title for this passage might be

   (A) *How to Increase Soil Productivity*
   (B) *Conservation of Natural Resources*
   (C) *Man's Effect on Soil*
   (D) *Soil Conditions and Plant Growth*

2. A policy of good management is sometimes upset by

   (A) the indifference of man
   (B) centuries-old laws
   (C) floods and winds
   (D) grazing animals

3. Areas in which the total amounts of rain and snow falling on the ground are greater than the moisture evaporated will support

   (A) forests
   (B) grasslands
   (C) scrub vegetation
   (D) no plants

4. Pioneers usually do not have a long-range view on soil problems, since they

   (A) are not protected by laws
   (B) live under adverse conditions
   (C) use poor methods of farming
   (D) must protect themselves from famine

5. *Phytogeographic* maps are those that show

   (A) areas of grassland
   (B) areas of bumper crops
   (C) areas of similar climate
   (D) areas of similar plants

6. What is meant by, "the yield of the grasslands is certain; that of the planted field, never"?

   (A) It is impossible to get more than one bumper crop from any one cultivated area.
   (B) Crops planted in former grasslands will not give good yields.

   (C) Through the indifference of man, dust blizzards have occurred in former grasslands.
   (D) If man does not interfere, plants will grow in the most suitable environment

7. The first act of prudent land management might be to

   (A) prohibit drainage of swamps
   (B) use irrigation and crop rotation in planted areas
   (C) increase use of fertilizers
   (D) prohibit excessive forest lumbering

8. The results of good land management may usually be found in

   (A) heavily populated areas
   (B) areas not given over to grazing
   (C) underdeveloped areas
   (D) ancient civilizations

9. Long-range programs of soil management are possible only in

   (A) young nations
   (B) ancient civilizations
   (C) those nations with an agricultural economy
   (D) those nations that want it

READING COMPREHENSION TEST 5

10 Minutes   8 Questions

Directions: *Carefully read the following passage and then answer the accompanying questions, basing your answers on what is stated or implied in the passage. When you have decided which choice is best, blacken the corresponding space on your answer sheet. There is only one best answer for each question.*

The pituitary gland is a small gland, about the size of an acorn or cherry, that lies at the base of the brain. It was once thought to be the "master gland" of the body, since its secretions appeared to influence the activity of all other endocrine glands. However, it is now known that other glands, especially the thyroid and adrenal glands, influence the pituitary gland.

The pituitary gland consists of two lobes: anterior and posterior. The anterior lobe secretes several different hormones. One of these, the *somatotropic* or growth hormone, regulates the growth of the skeleton. If an oversecretion of this hormone occurs during the growing years, tremendous height may be attained. This condition is called *giantism*. Circus giants, over 8 feet tall, weighing over 300 pounds and wearing size 30 shoes, are examples of this disorder. If the oversecretion occurs during adult life, the bones of the face and hands thicken, since they cannot grow in length. However, the organs and the soft tissues enlarge tremendously. This condition is known as *acromegaly*. Victims of this disorder have greatly enlarged jawbones, noses, hands and fingers.

Somatotropic hormone deficiency results in a *pituitary dwarf*, or midget. These individuals are perfectly proportioned "men in miniature." They are quite different from the thyroid dwarf in that they have normal intelligence.

Another hormone secretion of the anterior lobe of the pituitary gland, the *gonadotropic* hormone, influences the development of the reproductive organs. It also influences hormone secretion of the ovaries and testes. The gonadotropic hormone, together with the sex hormones, causes the sweeping changes that occur during adolescence, when a child becomes an adult.

Other secretions of the anterior lobe of the pituitary gland include hormones that stimulate the secretion of milk in the mammary glands (*lactogenic* hormone), the activity of the thyroid gland (*thyrotropic* hormone), and the parathyrotropic glands (*parathyrotropic* hormone).

ACTH is a secretion of the anterior lobe of the pituitary gland and stimulates the outer part, or *cortex*, of the adrenal glands. The adrenals, in turn, secrete hormones responsible for the control of certain phases of carbohydrate, fat, and protein metabolism, and the salt and water balance in the body.

The adrenal cortex also yields hormones that control the production of some kinds of white corpuscles and the structure of connective tissue. When ACTH is given to patients with leukemia, a dramatic but, unfortunately, temporary improvement occurs. Its effects in arthritis treatment are somewhat more encouraging. Good results in the treatment of asthma and other allergies with ACTH have been reported. Even though ACTH may not give permanent cures to these diseases, its use may lead the way to the discovery of their actual causes.

The posterior lobe of the pituitary gland produces two hormones: 1) *pitressin*, which helps regulate the amount of water in the blood and the blood pressure; and 2) *pitocin*, which stimulates smooth muscles. It is administered following childbirth to cause contraction of the muscles of the uterus, thus preventing blood loss.

1. A hormone is

   (A) an important gland
   (B) a kind of medicine
   (C) a chemical secretion
   (D) a kind of germ

2. Which of the following is not a secretion of the pituitary gland?

   (A) somatotropin
   (B) gonadotrophin
   (C) pitocin
   (D) adrenalin

3. Which of the following will affect the age at which a person reaches puberty?

    (A) sex hormones
    (B) somatotrophin
    (C) lactogenic hormone
    (D) none of these

4. Cretinism results in a stunted body and a dull, stupid mentality. It is caused by a defect in which gland?

    (A) pituitary
    (B) adrenal
    (C) thyroid
    (D) parathyroid

5. The circus giant of over 8 feet in height probably got too much somatotropic hormone when he was

    (A) an infant
    (B) a teenager
    (C) a young adult
    (D) an older adult

6. A cure for leukemia is

    (A) a pituitary hormone
    (B) an adrenal hormone
    (C) a cortexial hormone
    (D) none of these

7. A cow which failed to have enough lactogenic hormone would probably

    (A) fail to become pregnant
    (B) become overly fat
    (C) lose a lot of weight
    (D) not give any milk

8. A person admitted to a hospital with swollen limbs due to too much water in the joints may be suffering from

    (A) improper functioning of the adrenal gland
    (B) overactivity of the pituitary gland
    (C) underactivity of the pituitary gland
    (D) too much pitressin

READING COMPREHENSION TEST 6

8 Minutes   6 Questions

Directions: *Carefully read the following passage and then answer the accompanying questions, basing your answers on what is stated or implied in the passage. When you have decided which choice is best, blacken the corresponding space on your answer sheet. There is only one best answer for each question.*

PET (positron emission tomography) is a sort of a Geiger counter for the brain. It displays in living color which regions are active during remembering, thinking, and other mental tasks. PET scans, in other words, show the brain recalling and cogitating.

PET was developed in 1972. Currently, six American laboratories use it in research. The procedure for administering a PET scan requires the scientist to inject radioactive water into the volunteer's bloodstream. The water, though radioactive, is safe. The "hot blood" makes its way to the brain. Active regions of the brain use more blood than inactive areas, so they illuminate with radioactivity that is captured on special detectors surrounding the person's head.

Researchers use this new "window on the mind" to observe and monitor all regions of the brain. They can tune into motor functions controlled by the cerebrum, monitor the reception and processing of sensory information in the cerebral cortex (where higher thinking takes place), and observe the formation of long-term memory in the hippocampus. The scan provides information on the activity in the amygdala, a center of emotions where scent perceptions are gathered, and in the cerebellum, where balance is controlled.

Numerous studies of the brain have been conducted using PET. One study proved the brain to be "pretty nimble when it comes to switching circuits." Common nouns were shown to 11 adult volunteers. The volunteers were asked to respond with an appropriate verb. For instance, "car" might elicit "drive." This exercise resulted in four areas of the brain lighting up, including the cerebellum and part of the cortex. After 15 minutes of practice, the same nouns were used again to test the same volunteers. None of the original areas lit up. Only the brain's motor system, which controls muscles, showed activity. It appears that if the brain knows the answer cold, it does not have to think much. However, when the subjects encountered a new list of nouns, the original thinking areas lit up again. The sudden change would indicate that when a task is novel and requires conscious thought, the brain calls on resources extremely different from those required for the simple repetition of a word.

1. PET permits neuroscientists to

(A) study an individual's vocabulary skills.
(B) perform various surgical procedures on the brain.
(C) monitor the activity in the different regions of the brain.
(D) alter the function of the hippocampus.

2. The term "hot blood" refers to

(A) blood circulation in the amygdala, a center of emotions.
(B) blood injected with radioactive water.
(C) blood transfused at elevated temperatures.
(D) blood located at the base of the brain.

3. The hippocampus

(A) receives and processes sensory information.
(B) controls balance.
(C) forms long-term memories.
(D) controls motor function.

4. One experiment conducted suggests that

(A) cognition is not exactly subtle.
(B) one can essentially rearrange the brain, and in only 15 minutes.

(C) the hippocampus is not the site of visual memory.
(D) The subject's level of intelligence is directly related to the extent of brain activity observable.

5. In this reading passage, positron emission tomography is compared to

(A) a Geiger counter.
(B) previous methods used to scan the brain.
(C) a recalling/cogitating catalyst.
(D) a new type of x-ray.

6. The study described in this passage would

(A) support an argument for the brain's ability to handle learned tasks without conscious thought.
(B) dispel the idea that someone speaks without thinking.
(C) suggest that a visual image etches a channel in the cortex.
(D) prove that there is little activity in the cerebellum.

Answer Key

TEST 1

1.	B	3.	D
2.	A	4.	B

TEST 2

1.	A	5.	C
2.	B	6.	C
3.	A	7.	B
4.	D	8.	B

TEST 3

1.	D	5.	A
2.	B	6.	B
3.	C	7.	B
4.	A	8.	C

TEST 4

1.	C	6.	D
2.	C	7.	D
3.	A	8.	A
4.	B	9.	C
5.	D		

TEST 5

1.	C	5.	B
2.	D	6.	D
3.	A	7.	D
4.	C	8.	A

TEST 6

1.	C	4.	B
2.	B	5.	A
3.	C	6.	A

Part Three

PRACTICE FOR PRACTICAL NURSING SCHOOL ENTRANCE EXAMINATIONS

Introduction

Modern nursing is complex and multifaceted. Nurses practice in a variety of settings that emphasize different nursing roles. Various educational programs are available to provide opportunities for nurses to enter different careers within the same profession of nursing. Nursing has experienced many changes throughout its history, and the changes are not yet over. A major change that has occured in practical nursing history is a gradual increase in the required formal knowledge base.

Prior to the Civil War, untrained compassionate women cared for sick relatives and friends using skills that they had learned from their mothers and friends. Today's practical nurses are educationally prepared and technically skilled persons capable of rendering competent, scientific, and personal care to the sick and those in need. They care for patients in hospitals, physicians' offices, extended-care facilities, community health centers, private homes, industries, nursing homes, hospice facilities, and the armed forces. Men as well as women find this a rewarding vocation.

The practical nurse works under the supervision of the registered professional nurse, physician, or other person(s) authorized by law. The practical nurse participates in assessing the patient's physicial and mental health; records and reports; participates in implementing health care plans designed by the registered nurse or other authorized persons; reinforces teaching, and documents the patient's response to nursing care given.

The practical nurse is a graduate of a state-approved school and is licensed to practice after passing the National Council Licensure Examination for Practical Nurses (NCLEX-PN). The nursing curriculm is based on scientific theory from the natural, social, and health sciences. Basic principles of selected nursing techniques are also included. Clinical experience is provided in such areas as nursing care of mothers and infants, pediatrics, care of the mentally ill, medical and surgical nursing, and care of the aged and the chronically ill. The programs are usually one year in length but may extend to eighteen months. Licensed practical nurses have excellent employment opportunities. Supply has not kept pace with demand. Many new positions have been created by population growth and the increase in public-health consciousness. Salaries for practical nurses have increased proportionately, as they have for professional nurses; the salary of the practical nurse is usually three-fourths that of the registered professional nurse.

Since practical nursing is comprehensive, students are required to take many theoretical and practical courses to provide them with the knowledge and information essential to their vocation. A nursing examination is usually required before admission to a school of practical nursing. This section is designed to help you achieve an acceptable score on the examination.

Answer Sheet
Verbal Skills

TEST 1

1. Ⓐ Ⓑ Ⓒ Ⓓ	11. Ⓐ Ⓑ Ⓒ Ⓓ	21. Ⓐ Ⓑ Ⓒ Ⓓ	31. Ⓐ Ⓑ Ⓒ Ⓓ	41. Ⓐ Ⓑ Ⓒ Ⓓ
2. Ⓐ Ⓑ Ⓒ Ⓓ	12. Ⓐ Ⓑ Ⓒ Ⓓ	22. Ⓐ Ⓑ Ⓒ Ⓓ	32. Ⓐ Ⓑ Ⓒ Ⓓ	42. Ⓐ Ⓑ Ⓒ Ⓓ
3. Ⓐ Ⓑ Ⓒ Ⓓ	13. Ⓐ Ⓑ Ⓒ Ⓓ	23. Ⓐ Ⓑ Ⓒ Ⓓ	33. Ⓐ Ⓑ Ⓒ Ⓓ	43. Ⓐ Ⓑ Ⓒ Ⓓ
4. Ⓐ Ⓑ Ⓒ Ⓓ	14. Ⓐ Ⓑ Ⓒ Ⓓ	24. Ⓐ Ⓑ Ⓒ Ⓓ	34. Ⓐ Ⓑ Ⓒ Ⓓ	44. Ⓐ Ⓑ Ⓒ Ⓓ
5. Ⓐ Ⓑ Ⓒ Ⓓ	15. Ⓐ Ⓑ Ⓒ Ⓓ	25. Ⓐ Ⓑ Ⓒ Ⓓ	35. Ⓐ Ⓑ Ⓒ Ⓓ	45. Ⓐ Ⓑ Ⓒ Ⓓ
6. Ⓐ Ⓑ Ⓒ Ⓓ	16. Ⓐ Ⓑ Ⓒ Ⓓ	26. Ⓐ Ⓑ Ⓒ Ⓓ	36. Ⓐ Ⓑ Ⓒ Ⓓ	46. Ⓐ Ⓑ Ⓒ Ⓓ
7. Ⓐ Ⓑ Ⓒ Ⓓ	17. Ⓐ Ⓑ Ⓒ Ⓓ	27. Ⓐ Ⓑ Ⓒ Ⓓ	37. Ⓐ Ⓑ Ⓒ Ⓓ	47. Ⓐ Ⓑ Ⓒ Ⓓ
8. Ⓐ Ⓑ Ⓒ Ⓓ	18. Ⓐ Ⓑ Ⓒ Ⓓ	28. Ⓐ Ⓑ Ⓒ Ⓓ	38. Ⓐ Ⓑ Ⓒ Ⓓ	48. Ⓐ Ⓑ Ⓒ Ⓓ
9. Ⓐ Ⓑ Ⓒ Ⓓ	19. Ⓐ Ⓑ Ⓒ Ⓓ	29. Ⓐ Ⓑ Ⓒ Ⓓ	39. Ⓐ Ⓑ Ⓒ Ⓓ	49. Ⓐ Ⓑ Ⓒ Ⓓ
10. Ⓐ Ⓑ Ⓒ Ⓓ	20. Ⓐ Ⓑ Ⓒ Ⓓ	30. Ⓐ Ⓑ Ⓒ Ⓓ	40. Ⓐ Ⓑ Ⓒ Ⓓ	50. Ⓐ Ⓑ Ⓒ Ⓓ

TEST 2

1. Ⓐ Ⓑ Ⓒ Ⓓ	5. Ⓐ Ⓑ Ⓒ Ⓓ	9. Ⓐ Ⓑ Ⓒ Ⓓ	13. Ⓐ Ⓑ Ⓒ Ⓓ	17. Ⓐ Ⓑ Ⓒ Ⓓ
2. Ⓐ Ⓑ Ⓒ Ⓓ	6. Ⓐ Ⓑ Ⓒ Ⓓ	10. Ⓐ Ⓑ Ⓒ Ⓓ	14. Ⓐ Ⓑ Ⓒ Ⓓ	18. Ⓐ Ⓑ Ⓒ Ⓓ
3. Ⓐ Ⓑ Ⓒ Ⓓ	7. Ⓐ Ⓑ Ⓒ Ⓓ	11. Ⓐ Ⓑ Ⓒ Ⓓ	15. Ⓐ Ⓑ Ⓒ Ⓓ	19. Ⓐ Ⓑ Ⓒ Ⓓ
4. Ⓐ Ⓑ Ⓒ Ⓓ	8. Ⓐ Ⓑ Ⓒ Ⓓ	12. Ⓐ Ⓑ Ⓒ Ⓓ	16. Ⓐ Ⓑ Ⓒ Ⓓ	20. Ⓐ Ⓑ Ⓒ Ⓓ

TEST 3

1. Ⓐ Ⓑ Ⓒ Ⓓ   11. Ⓐ Ⓑ Ⓒ Ⓓ   21. Ⓐ Ⓑ Ⓒ Ⓓ   31. Ⓐ Ⓑ Ⓒ Ⓓ   41. Ⓐ Ⓑ Ⓒ Ⓓ

2. Ⓐ Ⓑ Ⓒ Ⓓ   12. Ⓐ Ⓑ Ⓒ Ⓓ   22. Ⓐ Ⓑ Ⓒ Ⓓ   32. Ⓐ Ⓑ Ⓒ Ⓓ   42. Ⓐ Ⓑ Ⓒ Ⓓ

3. Ⓐ Ⓑ Ⓒ Ⓓ   13. Ⓐ Ⓑ Ⓒ Ⓓ   23. Ⓐ Ⓑ Ⓒ Ⓓ   33. Ⓐ Ⓑ Ⓒ Ⓓ   43. Ⓐ Ⓑ Ⓒ Ⓓ

4. Ⓐ Ⓑ Ⓒ Ⓓ   14. Ⓐ Ⓑ Ⓒ Ⓓ   24. Ⓐ Ⓑ Ⓒ Ⓓ   34. Ⓐ Ⓑ Ⓒ Ⓓ   44. Ⓐ Ⓑ Ⓒ Ⓓ

5. Ⓐ Ⓑ Ⓒ Ⓓ   15. Ⓐ Ⓑ Ⓒ Ⓓ   25. Ⓐ Ⓑ Ⓒ Ⓓ   35. Ⓐ Ⓑ Ⓒ Ⓓ   45. Ⓐ Ⓑ Ⓒ Ⓓ

6. Ⓐ Ⓑ Ⓒ Ⓓ   16. Ⓐ Ⓑ Ⓒ Ⓓ   26. Ⓐ Ⓑ Ⓒ Ⓓ   36. Ⓐ Ⓑ Ⓒ Ⓓ   46. Ⓐ Ⓑ Ⓒ Ⓓ

7. Ⓐ Ⓑ Ⓒ Ⓓ   17. Ⓐ Ⓑ Ⓒ Ⓓ   27. Ⓐ Ⓑ Ⓒ Ⓓ   37. Ⓐ Ⓑ Ⓒ Ⓓ   47. Ⓐ Ⓑ Ⓒ Ⓓ

8. Ⓐ Ⓑ Ⓒ Ⓓ   18. Ⓐ Ⓑ Ⓒ Ⓓ   28. Ⓐ Ⓑ Ⓒ Ⓓ   38. Ⓐ Ⓑ Ⓒ Ⓓ   48. Ⓐ Ⓑ Ⓒ Ⓓ

9. Ⓐ Ⓑ Ⓒ Ⓓ   19. Ⓐ Ⓑ Ⓒ Ⓓ   29. Ⓐ Ⓑ Ⓒ Ⓓ   39. Ⓐ Ⓑ Ⓒ Ⓓ   49. Ⓐ Ⓑ Ⓒ Ⓓ

10. Ⓐ Ⓑ Ⓒ Ⓓ   20. Ⓐ Ⓑ Ⓒ Ⓓ   30. Ⓐ Ⓑ Ⓒ Ⓓ   40. Ⓐ Ⓑ Ⓒ Ⓓ   50. Ⓐ Ⓑ Ⓒ Ⓓ

TEST 4

1. Ⓐ Ⓑ Ⓒ Ⓓ   5. Ⓐ Ⓑ Ⓒ Ⓓ   9. Ⓐ Ⓑ Ⓒ Ⓓ   13. Ⓐ Ⓑ Ⓒ Ⓓ   17. Ⓐ Ⓑ Ⓒ Ⓓ

2. Ⓐ Ⓑ Ⓒ Ⓓ   6. Ⓐ Ⓑ Ⓒ Ⓓ   10. Ⓐ Ⓑ Ⓒ Ⓓ   14. Ⓐ Ⓑ Ⓒ Ⓓ   18. Ⓐ Ⓑ Ⓒ Ⓓ

3. Ⓐ Ⓑ Ⓒ Ⓓ   7. Ⓐ Ⓑ Ⓒ Ⓓ   11. Ⓐ Ⓑ Ⓒ Ⓓ   15. Ⓐ Ⓑ Ⓒ Ⓓ   19. Ⓐ Ⓑ Ⓒ Ⓓ

4. Ⓐ Ⓑ Ⓒ Ⓓ   8. Ⓐ Ⓑ Ⓒ Ⓓ   12. Ⓐ Ⓑ Ⓒ Ⓓ   16. Ⓐ Ⓑ Ⓒ Ⓓ   20. Ⓐ Ⓑ Ⓒ Ⓓ

UNIT V   VERBAL SKILLS

Please Refer to Unit I Pages 15 Through 26 for Review
Before Doing This Section.

VERBAL SKILLS ANTONYMS TEST 1

30 Minutes   50 Questions

Directions: *For each question in this test, select the word that is opposite in meaning to the capitalized word. Blacken the corresponding space on your answer sheet.*

1. GARRULOUS

    (A) talkative
    (B) reserved
    (C) unruly
    (D) fraternal

2. TRANSLUCENT

    (A) patent
    (B) transitory
    (C) transparent
    (D) opaque

3. BENEVOLENT

    (A) generous
    (B) charitable
    (C) malevolent
    (D) good

4. LETHARGIC

    (A) energetic
    (B) sluggish
    (C) apathetic
    (D) fatal

5. AMICABLE

    (A) lonely
    (B) reactionary
    (C) hostile
    (D) laconic

6. TRANQUILITY

    (A) complacency
    (B) tumult
    (C) plagiarism
    (D) prophecy

7. PROCRASTINATE

    (A) elegiac
    (B) mediate
    (C) expedite
    (D) investiture

8. QUIESCENT

    (A) restless
    (B) lethargic
    (C) mendicant
    (D) malignant

9. DELETERIOUS

    (A) fractious
    (B) pathetic
    (C) salubrious
    (D) gullible

10. COGNIZANCE

    (A) ignorance
    (B) abeyance
    (C) anecdote
    (D) idiom

287

11. CLEMENCY

    (A) mercy
    (B) indulgence
    (C) kindness
    (D) vindictiveness

12. IGNOBLE

    (A) honorable
    (B) shameful
    (C) disgraceful
    (D) humble

13. CURSORY

    (A) hasty
    (B) superficial
    (C) awful
    (D) thorough

14. ADMONISH

    (A) warn
    (B) praise
    (C) advise
    (D) reprove

15. PHLEGMATIC

    (A) energetic
    (B) dull
    (C) extraordinary
    (D) morbid

16. LAMENTABLE

    (A) laughable
    (B) generous
    (C) emotional
    (D) doleful

17. PERILOUS

    (A) vivacious
    (B) fatal
    (C) safe
    (D) hazardous

18. INIQUITOUS

    (A) unequaled
    (B) unfriendly
    (C) righteous
    (D) injurious

19. ASSIDUOUS

    (A) cooperative
    (B) indifferent
    (C) active
    (D) satisfactory

20. CORROBORATE

    (A) fascinate
    (B) corrupt
    (C) confirm
    (D) dispute

21. CONFLUENCE

    (A) convention
    (B) sympathy
    (C) divergence
    (D) concurrence

22. DASTARDLY

    (A) cowardly
    (B) bravely
    (C) friendly
    (D) sinfully

23. ABSTRUSE

    (A) understandable
    (B) hidden
    (C) absurd
    (D) religious

24. ILLUSION

    (A) delusion
    (B) conception
    (C) reality
    (D) dramatization

25. AVARICIOUS

    (A) greedy
    (B) persuasive
    (C) generous
    (D) gracious

26. COERCE

    (A) enforce
    (B) cohere
    (C) forestall
    (D) coax

27. TEMERITY

   (A) recklessness
   (B) prudence
   (C) support
   (D) sanity

28. LACONIC

   (A) verbose
   (B) concise
   (C) serene
   (D) interesting

29. CREDULOUS

   (A) exuberant
   (B) skeptical
   (C) dangerous
   (D) legible

30. INCARCERATE

   (A) immunize
   (B) anesthetize
   (C) transport
   (D) release

31. OBTUSE

   (A) oblique
   (B) obese
   (C) perpendicular
   (D) acute

32. MUNIFICENT

   (A) political
   (B) miserly
   (C) liberal
   (D) educational

33. DERANGED

   (A) unsettled
   (B) paralyzed
   (C) sane
   (D) awkward

34. LEVITY

   (A) flippancy
   (B) peace
   (C) gravity
   (D) trickery

35. EQUANIMITY

   (A) peace
   (B) inflation
   (C) agitation
   (D) tranquility

36. MARAUD

   (A) purchase
   (B) plunder
   (C) masticate
   (D) elevate

37. ENCOMIUM

   (A) immorality
   (B) praise
   (C) egotism
   (D) defamation

38. ABOMINABLE

   (A) delightful
   (B) horrible
   (C) meaningful
   (D) insane

39. ABSTEMIOUS

   (A) frugal
   (B) happy
   (C) greedy
   (D) radiant

40. ADVERTENT

   (A) attentive
   (B) inconsiderate
   (C) empathetic
   (D) abnormal

41. ENIGMATIC

   (A) perplexing
   (B) explicit
   (C) persistent
   (D) officious

42. EXECRABLE

   (A) unusual
   (B) detestable
   (C) fallible
   (D) respectable

43. IGNOMINIOUS

(A) reputable
(B) shameful
(C) intangible
(D) irascible

44. SAGACITY

(A) sorrowfulness
(B) support
(C) satisfaction
(D) stupidity

45. PROVERBIAL

(A) innovative
(B) current
(C) wise
(D) cautious

46. ANNIHILATE

(A) advertise
(B) destroy
(C) preserve
(D) announce

47. AFFABLE

(A) discourteous
(B) beloved
(C) sociable
(D) debonair

48. CAPRICIOUS

(A) logical
(B) agreeable
(C) awkward
(D) constant

49. CONTINGENT

(A) conditional
(B) independent
(C) confinable
(D) familiar

50. OFFICIOUS

(A) meddling
(B) modest
(C) emaciated
(D) authentic

Answer Key

1.	B	18.	C	35.	C
2.	D	19.	B	36.	A
3.	C	20.	D	37.	D
4.	A	21.	C	38.	A
5.	C	22.	B	39.	C
6.	B	23.	A	40.	B
7.	C	24.	C	41.	B
8.	A	25.	C	42.	D
9.	C	26.	D	43.	A
10.	A	27.	B	44.	D
11.	D	28.	A	45.	A
12.	A	29.	B	46.	C
13.	D	30.	D	47.	A
14.	B	31.	D	48.	D
15.	A	32.	B	49.	B
16.	A	33.	C	50.	B
17.	C	34.	C		

VERBAL SKILLS ANTONYMS TEST 2

10 Minutes   20 Questions

Directions: *For each question in this test, select the word that is opposite in the meaning to the capitalized word. Blacken the corresponding space on your answer sheet.*

1. DECEIT
   - (A) fraud
   - (B) truthfulness
   - (C) treachery
   - (D) imposition

2. DOCILE
   - (A) teachable
   - (B) compliant
   - (C) tame
   - (D) inflexible

3. HARMLESS
   - (A) safe
   - (B) hurtful
   - (C) innocent
   - (D) innocuous

4. MELANCHOLY
   - (A) jolly
   - (B) low-spirited
   - (C) dreamy
   - (D) sad

5. IMPETUOUS
   - (A) violent
   - (B) furious
   - (C) calm
   - (D) vehement

6. JOY
   - (A) gladness
   - (B) grief
   - (C) mirth
   - (D) delight

7. LUNACY
   - (A) sanity
   - (B) madness
   - (C) derangement
   - (D) mania

8. MOIST
   - (A) dank
   - (B) dry
   - (C) damp
   - (D) humid

9. PUERILE
   - (A) youthful
   - (B) weak
   - (C) silly
   - (D) mature

10. WEIGHT
    - (A) gravity
    - (B) heaviness
    - (C) lightness
    - (D) burden

11. SUPERFLUOUS
    - (A) necessary
    - (B) excessive
    - (C) unnecessary
    - (D) expanded

12. REFORM
    - (A) amend
    - (B) correct
    - (C) better
    - (D) corrupt

13. SCANTY
    - (A) bare
    - (B) ample
    - (C) insufficient
    - (D) meager

14. MISERY
    - (A) happiness
    - (B) woe
    - (C) privation
    - (D) penury

15. PROPER

    (A) honest
    (B) appropriate
    (C) wrong
    (D) pertinent

16. INCONGRUOUS

    (A) compatible
    (B) absurd
    (C) contrary
    (D) incoherent

17. FATIGUE

    (A) lassitude
    (B) weariness
    (C) malaise
    (D) vigor

18. HASTEN

    (A) delay
    (B) accelerate
    (C) dispatch
    (D) expedite

19. ABSORB

    (A) emit
    (B) engulf
    (C) engross
    (D) consume

20. ABUSE

    (A) ribaldry
    (B) protection
    (C) contumely
    (D) obloquy

Answer Key

1.	**B**	6.	**B**	11.	**A**	16.	**A**
2.	**D**	7.	**A**	12.	**D**	17.	**D**
3.	**B**	8.	**B**	13.	**B**	18.	**A**
4.	**A**	9.	**D**	14.	**A**	19.	**A**
5.	**C**	10.	**C**	15.	**C**	20.	**B**

VERBAL SKILLS SYNONYMS TEST 3

30 Minutes   50 Questions

Directions: *In each of the following sentences, one word is in italics. Below each sentence are words lettered A, B, C, D. For each sentence choose the word that best corresponds in meaning to the italicized word. Blacken the corresponding space on your answer sheet.*

1. Her efforts to revive the child were *futile*.

   (A) strong
   (B) clumsy
   (C) useless
   (D) sincere

2. The supply of pamphlets has been *depleted*.

   (A) exhausted
   (B) delivered
   (C) included
   (D) rejected

3. The *gist* of his speech was that we should strike.

   (A) end
   (B) essence
   (C) strength
   (D) spirit

4. The soldier was decorated for his *valor* in battle in Korea.

   (A) injury
   (B) ability
   (C) cooperation
   (D) courage

5. When Mary arrived in California, her future seemed *auspicious*.

   (A) bleak
   (B) uncertain
   (C) promising
   (D) somber

6. To our *consternation*, the child's bicycle rolled into the busy street.

   (A) dismay
   (B) amazement
   (C) incompetence
   (D) annoyance

7. *Indolence* is a habit that cannot be excused.

   (A) incompetency
   (B) snoring
   (C) carelessness
   (D) idleness

8. The political candidate made *cogent* remarks.

   (A) pleasing
   (B) convincing
   (C) flattering
   (D) slandering

9. A *prolific* writer is one who is

   (A) productive
   (B) popular
   (C) frank
   (D) effective

10. He was *meticulous* when performing his work.

    (A) careless
    (B) patient
    (C) scrupulous
    (D) nervous

11. There were *sporadic* outbreaks of food poisoning at the camp.

    (A) epidemic
    (B) widespread
    (C) serious
    (D) scattered

12. The motion passed even though there were three *dissenting* votes.

    (A) annoying
    (B) disagreeing
    (C) abstaining
    (D) approving

13. It is *traditional* for the bride to wear a white gown.

    (A) normal
    (B) customary
    (C) ordinary
    (D) gracious

14. The company has *rescinded* the order.

    (A) canceled
    (B) revised
    (C) confirmed
    (D) misinterpreted

15. Although the prisoner was released early, he was *vindictive* toward society.

    (A) prejudiced
    (B) impatient
    (C) revengeful
    (D) unreasonable

16. The *sedulous* student worked many hours in the laboratory.

    (A) eager
    (B) persistent
    (C) intelligent
    (D) inexperienced

17. The neighbors were *interrogated* by the police.

    (A) arrested
    (B) detained
    (C) investigated
    (D) questioned

18. The lifeguard *disparaged* his brave rescue of the child.

    (A) explained
    (B) belittled
    (C) demonstrated
    (D) elucidated

19. The water could not *permeate* the rubber apron.

    (A) saturate
    (B) wet
    (C) harm
    (D) discolor

20. The *docile* dog waited at the gate.

    (A) mongrel
    (B) hungry
    (C) intractable
    (D) obedient

21. The two hospitals in our town will *amalgamate* next year.

    (A) close
    (B) expand
    (C) relocate
    (D) merge

22. She wasted her money on *frivolous* things.

    (A) sweet
    (B) expensive
    (C) unimportant
    (D) cheap

23. The teacher *divulged* the test grades.

    (A) whispered
    (B) disregarded
    (C) revealed
    (D) averaged

24. *Remuneration* to the shareholders was ten percent higher than last year.

    (A) shares
    (B) payment
    (C) liquidation
    (D) speculation

25. The art dealer *scrutinized* the painting to verify its authenticity.

    (A) touched
    (B) bought
    (C) inspected
    (D) measured

26. The bridge was closed because it was *decrepit*.

    (A) slippery
    (B) weak
    (C) swaying
    (D) flooded

27. The driver *conceded* that he was at fault.

    (A) denied
    (B) explained
    (C) complained
    (D) admitted

28. The machinery in the vocational classroom was *obsolete*.

    (A) out of date
    (B) new
    (C) reliable
    (D) complicated

29. The speaker made *candid* remarks about the candidate's record.

    (A) biased
    (B) confidential
    (C) frank
    (D) insulting

30. When the hostage was released, he was speaking *incoherently*.

    (A) disconnectedly
    (B) cohesively
    (C) prolifically
    (D) sluggishly

31. The mother tried to *pacify* the child.

    (A) detain
    (B) restrain
    (C) accompany
    (D) calm

32. The head nurse on 2 West was young and *vivacious*.

    (A) kind
    (B) lively
    (C) short
    (D) talkative

33. The town was *devastated* after the earthquake.

    (A) rebuilt
    (B) deserted
    (C) destroyed
    (D) saved

34. The teacher *digressed* from her custom and didn't give any homework.

    (A) deviated
    (B) reposed
    (C) alighted
    (D) moored

35. The Colonel was a *gallant* man.

    (A) rude
    (B) fastidious
    (C) cowardly
    (D) chivalrous

36. The family gathering was a *melancholic* scene.

    (A) happy
    (B) sad
    (C) heart-warming
    (D) ardent

37. When I visited her in the nursing home, she was *querulous* and unhappy.

    (A) satisfied
    (B) cheerful
    (C) complaining
    (D) painful

38. The FBI agent kept a *vigilant* guard on the suspect.

    (A) careful
    (B) continuous
    (C) observant
    (D) reciprocal

39. The play treated current social issues *satirically*.

    (A) frankly
    (B) interminably
    (C) musically
    (D) ironically

40. She felt an *antipathy* for lizards.

    (A) aversion
    (B) fondness
    (C) interest
    (D) fear

41. The hiker had a *premonition* of danger.

    (A) vision
    (B) forewarning
    (C) recurrence
    (D) apprehension

42. The policeman *confiscated* the illegal drugs.

    (A) stored
    (B) distributed
    (C) destroyed
    (D) appropriated

43. John was asked to resign because of his *improbity*.

    (A) age
    (B) tardiness
    (C) dishonesty
    (D) absenteeism

44. There is no *tangible* evidence of damage.

    (A) concrete
    (B) theoretical
    (C) verified
    (D) scientific

45. Her *blithe* spirit made her popular.

    (A) free
    (B) cheerful
    (C) kind
    (D) insolent

46. The jury *deliberated* for eight hours.

    (A) met
    (B) convened
    (C) considered
    (D) summarized

47. He had a *sinister* motive for entering the building.

    (A) practical
    (B) wrong
    (C) important
    (D) honest

48. The requirements for admission to the school were *stringent*.

    (A) unusual
    (B) numerous
    (C) rigid
    (D) lax

49. The students refused to give up their *prerogatives*.

    (A) demands
    (B) rights
    (C) ideals
    (D) duties

50. The widow and her children were *destitute*.

    (A) impoverished
    (B) detained
    (C) loathed
    (D) ill

Answer Key

1.	**C**	18.	**B**	35.	**D**
2.	**A**	19.	**A**	36.	**B**
3.	**B**	20.	**D**	37.	**C**
4.	**D**	21.	**D**	38.	**C**
5.	**C**	22.	**C**	39.	**D**
6.	**A**	23.	**C**	40.	**A**
7.	**D**	24.	**B**	41.	**B**
8.	**B**	25.	**C**	42.	**D**
9.	**A**	26.	**B**	43.	**C**
10.	**C**	27.	**D**	44.	**A**
11.	**D**	28.	**A**	45.	**B**
12.	**B**	29.	**C**	46.	**C**
13.	**B**	30.	**A**	47.	**B**
14.	**A**	31.	**D**	48.	**C**
15.	**C**	32.	**B**	49.	**B**
16.	**B**	33.	**C**	50.	**A**
17.	**D**	34.	**A**		

VERBAL SKILLS SYNONYMS TEST 4

10 Minutes   20 Questions

Directions: *For each question in this test, select the word that corresponds in meaning to the capitalized word. Blacken the corresponding space on your answer sheet.*

1. COMPETENT

    (A) agreeable
    (B) inept
    (C) vigorous
    (D) capable

2. OMNIBUS

    (A) threatening
    (B) all-embracing
    (C) rotund
    (D) slow-moving

3. INGENUITY

    (A) deceitfulness
    (B) appeal
    (C) cleverness
    (D) innocence

4. CONCAVE

    (A) curving inward
    (B) curving outward
    (C) oval-shaped
    (D) rounded

5. CANON

    (A) barrier
    (B) noisy place
    (C) guiding principle
    (D) vigorous

6. AUSPICIOUS

    (A) questionable
    (B) well-known
    (C) free
    (D) favorable

7. VACILLATING

    (A) changable
    (B) decisive
    (C) equalizing
    (D) progressing

8. FORFEIT

    (A) exchange
    (B) relinquish
    (C) protect
    (D) withdraw

9. QUERY

    (A) question
    (B) look over carefully
    (C) follow through
    (D) act peculiarly

10. STEADFAST

    (A) gradual
    (B) strong
    (C) friendly
    (D) unwavering

11. ACCESS

    (A) too much
    (B) extra
    (C) admittance
    (D) arrival

12. PERMUTATION

    (A) alteration
    (B) permission
    (C) combination
    (D) seepage

13. SPRITZ

    (A) spray
    (B) bubble
    (C) protrude
    (D) sail

14. PERSONABLE

    (A) intimate
    (B) cheerful
    (C) attractive
    (D) superficial

15. EXPEDITE

    (A) dismiss
    (B) advise
    (C) accelerate
    (D) demolish

16. COMPULSORY

    (A) imperative
    (B) impossible
    (C) imminent
    (D) logical

17. PRACTICABLE

    (A) lenient
    (B) feasible
    (C) simple
    (D) visible

18. AGREE

    (A) inquire
    (B) acquiesce
    (C) discharge
    (D) endeavor

19. FLORID

    (A) overflowing
    (B) ruddy
    (C) seedy
    (D) flowery

20. NEARNESS

    (A) adherence
    (B) declivity
    (C) worldliness
    (D) proximity

Answer Key

1. **D**	6. **D**	11. **C**	16. **A**
2. **B**	7. **A**	12. **A**	17. **B**
3. **C**	8. **B**	13. **A**	18. **B**
4. **A**	9. **A**	14. **C**	19. **B**
5. **C**	10. **D**	15. **C**	20. **D**

SPELLING USAGE TEST 5

20 Minutes   35 Questions

Directions: *Select the letter that belongs in the blank space in the sentence.*

1. The demonstrators were _____ from the property.

    (A) band
    (B) banned

2. The nurse had to _____ the baby.

    (A) weigh
    (B) way

3. She looked on the _____ for the date of the meeting.

    (A) calendar
    (B) calender

4. The perfume had a _____ of roses.

    (A) sent
    (B) scent

5. The injury caused a _____ on her arm.

    (A) bruise
    (B) brews

6. The student received a _____ for passing the test.

    (A) complement
    (B) compliment

7. The _____ gave the faculty their assignments.

    (A) principal
    (B) principle

8. The ulcer on the patient's foot did not _____.

    (A) heel
    (B) heal

9. A tiny opening in the skin is called a _____.

    (A) pour
    (B) pore

10. The _____ after surgery caused the child to cry.

    (A) pain
    (B) pane

11. A _____ is a sour berry.

    (A) current
    (B) currant

12. It is important to _____ in order to strengthen muscles.

    (A) exercise
    (B) exorcise

13. The secretary purchased new _____ on which to type letters.

    (A) stationery
    (B) stationary

14. They wanted _____ food right away.

    (A) there
    (B) their

15. He was too _____ to climb the stairs.

    (A) week
    (B) weak

16. The _____ is a timid animal.

    (A) dear
    (B) deer

17. I want to _____ the president.

    (A) meat
    (B) meet

18. She wanted a _____ of candy.

    (A) piece
    (B) peace

19. The child did not _____ the vase.

    (A) brake
    (B) break

20. To _____ means to stop living.

    (A) dye
    (B) die

21. She wanted to purchase two _____ of milk.

    (A) quartz
    (B) quarts

22. He could not _____ his book.

    (A) find
    (B) fined

23. The _____ led to a dead-end street.

    (A) rode
    (B) road

24. The telephone was _____ .

    (A) ringing
    (B) wringing

25. The _____ was chocolate cake.

    (A) dessert
    (B) desert

26. The thief was going to _____ the money.

    (A) steel
    (B) steal

27. She placed an _____ in the local newspaper.

    (A) ad
    (B) add

28. He turned _____ because he was so afraid.

    (A) pale
    (B) pail

29. The man wanted the bank to _____ him some money.

    (A) lone
    (B) loan

30. The area around the incision was _____.

    (A) sore
    (B) soar

31. The _____ in the paragraph was not clear.

    (A) clause
    (B) claws

32. The passenger had to pay a _____ to ride the bus.

    (A) fair
    (B) fare

33. When her blood pressure dropped, she started to _____ .

    (A) feint
    (B) faint

34. He _____ a loud sound.

    (A) heard
    (B) herd

35. We will go _____ it rains or not.

    (A) weather
    (B) whether

Answer Key

1. **B**	10. **A**	19. **B**	28. **A**
2. **A**	11. **B**	20. **B**	29. **B**
3. **A**	12. **A**	21. **B**	30. **A**
4. **B**	13. **A**	22. **A**	31. **A**
5. **A**	14. **B**	23. **B**	32. **B**
6. **B**	15. **B**	24. **A**	33. **B**
7. **A**	16. **B**	25. **A**	34. **A**
8. **B**	17. **B**	26. **B**	35. **B**
9. **B**	18. **A**	27. **A**	

UNIT VI ARITHMETIC AND MATHEMATICS

Arithmetic is an important part of the study of pharmacology and the related sciences. In this section practice problems on fractions, decimals, ratio, proportion, and percent are included with a review of the appropriate processes. The problem solutions are presented after each set of exercises. If you have made errors, go back to the explanation for that kind of problem. After you have completed all practice tests, take the final test.

REVIEW OF BASIC OPERATIONS

Fractions

REDUCTION OF FRACTIONS

To reduce fractions to lowest terms, divide both the numerator and the denominator by the same number:

Example:

$$\frac{4}{8} = \frac{4 \div 4}{8 \div 4} = \frac{1}{2}$$

Practice Exercise A

Reduce the following fractions to their lowest terms.

1. $\frac{8}{16}$ = _____

2. $\frac{3}{12}$ = _____

3. $\frac{5}{10}$ = _____

4. $\frac{25}{100}$ = _____

5. $\frac{18}{72}$ = _____

6. $\frac{50}{60}$ = _____

7. $\frac{27}{54}$ = _____

8. $\frac{4}{64}$ = _____

9. $\frac{12}{144}$ = _____

10. $\frac{25}{150}$ = _____

IMPROPER FRACTIONS

To change an improper fraction to a mixed number, divide the numerator by the denominator.

Example:

$$\frac{3}{2} \quad \begin{array}{r} 1.5 \\ 2\overline{)3.0} \\ \underline{2} \\ 1.0 \end{array} = 1\frac{5}{10} = 1\frac{1}{2}$$

Practice Exercise B

Change the following improper fractions to mixed numbers.

1. $\frac{15}{4}$ = _____   6. $\frac{19}{4}$ = _____

2. $\frac{13}{6}$ = _____   7. $\frac{36}{7}$ = _____

3. $\frac{27}{5}$ = _____   8. $\frac{39}{12}$ = _____

4. $\frac{17}{3}$ = _____   9. $\frac{14}{4}$ = _____

5. $\frac{99}{10}$ = _____   10. $\frac{57}{3}$ = _____

ADDITION OF FRACTIONS

To add two or more fractions, find the lowest common denominator, divide the lowest common denominator by the original denominator, and multiply this figure by the original numerator. Then add the numerators and reduce to lowest terms.

Practice Exercise C

1. $\frac{1}{2}$
   $\frac{1}{3}$
   $\frac{1}{6}$

2. $\frac{3}{4}$
   $\frac{1}{12}$
   $\frac{2}{3}$

3. $7\frac{2}{3}$
   $3\frac{5}{24}$
   $\frac{5}{12}$

4. $1\frac{1}{4}$
   $5\frac{3}{16}$
   $2\frac{5}{12}$

5. $26\frac{3}{5}$
$14\frac{1}{6}$
$5\frac{7}{8}$

8. $7\frac{11}{12}$
$16\frac{3}{4}$
$2\frac{4}{18}$

6. $7\frac{5}{8}$
$\frac{1}{32}$
$3\frac{1}{10}$

9. $1\frac{3}{24}$
$8\frac{1}{3}$
$3\frac{5}{6}$

7. $4\frac{1}{2}$
$3\frac{1}{4}$
$9\frac{3}{8}$

10. $5\frac{5}{6}$
$7\frac{3}{8}$
$2\frac{3}{10}$

SUBTRACTION OF FRACTIONS

To subtract one fraction from another, find their lowest common denominator. If the fraction to be subtracted is larger than the one from which it is to be subtracted, a whole number (1) will have to be borrowed from the whole number in the mixed number.

Practice Exercise D

1. $\frac{5}{8}$
   $-\frac{3}{16}$

6. $\frac{17}{20}$
   $-\frac{3}{4}$

2. $7\frac{5}{12}$
   $-3\frac{1}{4}$

7. $5\frac{3}{8}$
   $-1\frac{7}{16}$

3. $\frac{1}{2}$
   $-\frac{1}{8}$

8. $\frac{2}{5}$
   $-\frac{2}{9}$

4. $3\frac{1}{8}$
   $-1\frac{3}{4}$

9. $4\frac{3}{4}$
   $-2\frac{2}{3}$

5. $\frac{7}{9}$
   $-\frac{1}{6}$

10. $11\frac{7}{8}$
    $-1\frac{3}{4}$

MULTIPLICATION OF FRACTIONS

To multiply a fraction by a fraction, multiply the numerators to obtain the new numerator and multiply denominators to obtain the new denominator. Cancellation may be done before multiplication to allow you to work with smaller numbers. *To multiply a fraction by a whole number,* multiply the numerator by the whole number. The denominator remains unchanged. In order to cancel, divide numerator and denominator by the same number. Cancellation is optional, and it allows you to work with smaller numbers. *To multiply a fraction by a mixed number,* change the mixed number to an improper fraction and proceed as in multiplying two fractions.

Practice Exercise E

1. $\frac{2}{5} \times \frac{1}{8} =$ _____

2. $\frac{2}{5} \times \frac{5}{12} =$ _____

3. $\frac{4}{21} \times \frac{7}{8} =$ _____

4. $\frac{15}{16} \times \frac{9}{10} =$ _____

5. $\frac{4}{6} \times \frac{2}{4} =$ _____

6. $3\frac{3}{8} \times \frac{27}{8} =$ _____

7. $\frac{1}{2} \times 8 =$ _____

8. $6\frac{1}{2} \times 5\frac{4}{8} =$ _____

9. $3\frac{2}{3} \times \frac{3}{4} =$ _____

10. $9 \times 3\frac{1}{3} =$ _____

DIVISION OF FRACTIONS

To divide fractions, invert the divisor and change the sign from division ($\div$) to multiplication ($\times$) and then follow the rules for multiplication. Whole numbers are written as a fraction whose denominator is 1. Mixed numbers are written as improper fractions.

Practice Exercise F

1. $2\frac{1}{5} \div 11 =$ _____

2. $\frac{1}{50} \div \frac{1}{200} =$ _____

3. $6\frac{3}{5} \div 8\frac{3}{10} =$ _____

4. $\frac{3}{4} \div \frac{1}{8} =$ _____

5. $\frac{5}{12} \div \frac{5}{60} =$ _____

6. $10\frac{1}{2} \div \frac{1}{3} =$ _____

7. $\frac{1}{60} \div \frac{1}{2} =$ _____

8. $8 \div \frac{2}{3} =$ _____

9. $\frac{1}{6} \div \frac{1}{3} =$ _____

10. $\frac{7}{8} \div \frac{3}{4} =$ _____

Decimals, Ratios and Proportions, Percent
Decimals

The decimal system is based on the number ten. All numbers to the right of the decimal point are decimal fractions whose denominator is ten or a multiple of ten. *Tenths* are directly after the decimal point, *hundredths* two places after, *thousandths* three places after, *ten-thousandths* four places, etc. Whole numbers are written to the left of the decimal point and the decimal point is read as "and."

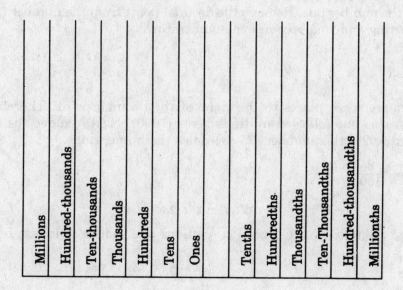

CHANGING FRACTIONS TO DECIMALS

To change fractions to decimals, divide the numerator by the denominator.

Example:

$$\frac{3}{4} = \begin{array}{r} .75 \\ 4\overline{)3.00} \\ \underline{2\ 8} \\ 20 \\ \underline{20} \end{array}$$

Answer: .75

Practice Exercise G

Change the following fractions to decimals.

1. $\frac{1}{4}$ = _____

2. $\frac{7}{8}$ = _____

3. $\frac{5}{6}$ = _____

4. $\frac{5}{125}$ = _____

5. $\dfrac{5}{16}$ = _____

6. $\dfrac{3}{25}$ = _____

7. $\dfrac{9}{20}$ = _____

8. $\dfrac{1}{75}$ = _____

9. $\dfrac{3}{8}$ = _____

10. $\dfrac{3}{10}$ = _____

CHANGING DECIMALS TO FRACTIONS

Decimals may be changed to fractions by dropping the decimal point and using the proper denominator. The number of decimal places to the right of the decimal point represents the number of zeros to be used in the denominator preceded by the number one. Remove the decimal point from the number that you are converting and this becomes the numerator.

Example:

0.025

There are three places to the right of the decimal point. Therefore, the denominator is one followed by three zeros (1000). Next, remove the decimal point from 0.025; this number (25) becomes the numerator.

$$0.025 = \dfrac{25}{1000}$$

Practice Exercise H

Change the following decimals to fractions and reduce to lowest terms.

1. 0.16 = _____

2. 0.04 = _____

3. 0.125 = _____

4. 0.06 = _____

5. 0.257 = _____

6. 0.75 = _____

7. 0.250 = _____

8. 0.525 = _____

9. 0.2 = _____

10. 4.75 = _____

ADDING DECIMALS

To add decimals, place the numbers in columns so that the decimal points are directly under each other. Then add in the same manner that you would add columns of whole numbers. Place a decimal point in your answer directly under the others.

Example:

Add 22.05 + 1.375 + 10.2.

22.05
 1.375
10.2
———
33.625

Practice Exercise I

Add the following decimals.

1. 7.2 + 3.57 + 10.8   = _____
6. 29.042 + 2.6 + 3.120   = _____

2. 48.3 + 18.25 + 4.002   = _____
7. 5.4 + 8.62 + 0.95   = _____

3. 6.3 + 0.005 + 2.67   = _____
8. 2.246 + 16.8 + 4.26   = _____

4. 25.4 + 37.06 + 41.   = _____
9. 16.1 + 1.12 + 3.525   = _____

5. 8.50 + 19.625 + 0.17   = _____
10. 30.7 + 4.05 + 20.5   = _____

SUBTRACTING DECIMALS

To subtract decimals, use the same rule as for adding decimals—place decimal points directly under one another. Then subtract in the same manner you would subtract whole numbers, placing the decimal point in your answer directly under the others.

Example:

$$
\begin{array}{r}
50.789 \\
-24.19 \\
\hline
26.599
\end{array}
$$

Practice Exercise J

Subtract the following decimals.

1. 5.67 − 3.9   = _____
6. 15 − 7.82   = _____

2. 37.2 − 25.37   = _____
7. 205.6 − 105.23   = _____

3. 17.4 − 13.262   = _____
8. 246.52 − 107.988   = _____

4. 58.94 − 27.363   = _____
9. 35.25 − 17.0   = _____

5. 2.425 − 0.675   = _____
10. 1725.5 − 50.6325   = _____

MULTIPLYING DECIMALS

To multiply decimals, multiply the numbers as if they were whole numbers. Then place the decimal point in the answer by counting from the right the number of decimal places in the multiplier and the multiplicand.

Example:

$$
\begin{array}{r}
2.56 \\
\times\ 0.6 \\
\hline
1.536
\end{array}
$$

Practice Exercise K

Multiply the following decimals.

1. 5.64×1.2 = _____

2. 4.25×12 = _____

3. 35.6×2.5 = _____

4. 4.92×9.5 = _____

5. $51. \times 0.92$ = _____

6. 28.6×8.16 = _____

7. 50.06×2.15 = _____

8. 32.2×3.15 = _____

9. 21.0×41.6 = _____

10. 8.06×3.654 = _____

DIVIDING DECIMALS

To divide decimals, the divisor must always be a whole number. If the divisor is a decimal, move the decimal to the right as many places as necessary to make the decimal a whole number. Then move the decimal point in the dividend the same number of places to the right to avoid changing the value of the quotient. The decimal point in the quotient is placed directly above the decimal point in the dividend.

Practice Exercise L

1. $100 \div 2.5$ = _____

2. $0.9 \div 0.3$ = _____

3. $38.6 \div 1.7$ = _____

4. $115 \div 1.5$ = _____

5. $5.5 \div 2.5$ = _____

6. $3.22 \div 0.46$ = _____

7. $4.65 \div 1.5$ = _____

8. $15 \div 7.5$ = _____

9. $0.042 \div 0.3$ = _____

10. $0.006 \div 0.05$ = _____

Ratios and Proportions

RATIO

Ratio is the relationship between two numbers which are separated by a colon. The ratio 1 : 8 shows the relationship between one and eight. A fraction may be written as a ratio by writing the numerator to the left of the colon and the denominator to the right of the colon. Ratios, like fractions, should be reduced to their lowest terms.

Example:

$2 : 50 = 1 : 25$

Practice Exercise M

Write the following fractions as ratios and reduce to lowest terms:

1. $\dfrac{4}{5}$ = _____

2. $\dfrac{1}{3}$ = _____

3. $\dfrac{3}{4}$ = _____

4. $\dfrac{3}{8}$ = _____

5. $\dfrac{1}{10}$ = _____

6. $\dfrac{2}{3}$ = _____

7. $\dfrac{1}{2}$ = _____

8. $\dfrac{25}{50}$ = _____

9. $\dfrac{3}{9}$ = _____

10. $\dfrac{2}{5}$ = _____

PROPORTION

A proportion states that two ratios are equal. Proportions may be expressed in two ways:

$$\frac{1}{2} = \frac{50}{100} \text{ or } 1 : 2 :: 50 : 100$$

Both are read: *One is to two as fifty is to one hundred.* The product of the means equals the product of the extremes.

Example:

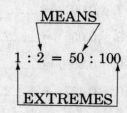

$$1 : 2 = 50 : 100$$

$$1 \times 100 = 2 \times 50$$

If one number is not known, substitute an alphabet letter and solve for the unknown number by multiplying the means and the extremes.

Example:

$$5 : y = 25 : 125$$
$$25 \times y = 5 \times 125$$
$$25y = 625$$
$$y = 25$$

Practice Exercise N

Solve for x in the following proportions.

1. $8 : 10 = x : 30$

2. $9 : 15 = x : 5$

3. $x : 80 = 3 : 12$

4. $3 : x = 8 : 24$

5. $2 : 3 = x : 63$

6. $5 : 15 = x : 60$

7. $7 : x = 4 : 28$

8. $0.2 : 8 = 25 : x$

9. $5 : 7 = x : 28$

10. $\frac{1}{10} x : 2000 = 1 : 100$

Percentages

To change a decimal to percent, multiply the decimal by 100 (move the decimal point two places to the right), and then add the percent sign.

Example:

$$0.25 = .25$$

$$= 25\%$$

Practice Exercise O

Change the following decimals to percents.

1. 0.225 = _____

2. 3.45 = _____

3. 0.7 = _____

4. 0.14 = _____

5. 4.5 = _____

6. 1.23 = _____

7. 0.001 = _____

8. 0.055 = _____

9. 0.30 = _____

10. 0.427 = _____

Roman Numerals

Roman numerals are written using letters of the alphabet. The letters used to designate arabic numbers are:

Roman	Arabic Equivalent
I	1
V	5
X	10
L	50
C	100
D	500
M	1000

Rules governing the use of Roman numerals:

Addition—Placing one or more Roman numerals after the basic numeral adds to its value.

Example:

VII = 7

The same numeral cannot be repeated more than three times in succession. If this seems necessary the rule for subtraction is used.

Example:

XXX = 30   XXXX—not allowed   XL = 40

Subtraction—Placing one or more Roman numerals in front of the basic numeral removes value from it.

Example:

IV = 4

The symbols, V, D, and L are never used in subtraction.

Practice Exercise P

Write the proper Roman numerals:

1.	8	_____	11.	25	_____
2.	15	_____	12.	100	_____
3.	50	_____	13.	37	_____
4.	4	_____	14.	7	_____
5.	23	_____	15.	18	_____
6.	44	_____	16.	526	_____
7.	93	_____	17.	94	_____
8.	36	_____	18.	39	_____
9.	56	_____	19.	62	_____
10.	19	_____	20.	1980	_____

Write the proper Arabic numbers:

1.	XXIV	_____	11.	VI	_____
2.	XVII	_____	12.	LXX	_____
3.	L	_____	13.	C	_____
4.	XL	_____	14.	XCII	_____
5.	V	_____	15.	LXIX	_____
6.	III	_____	16.	XVII	_____
7.	M	_____	17.	XXII	_____
8.	XIX	_____	18.	XI	_____
9.	XXX	_____	19.	CCIV	_____
10.	XXIX	_____	20.	MCXV	_____

Solutions to Practice Exercises

Practice Exercise A

1. $\frac{8}{16} = \frac{1}{2}$

2. $\frac{3}{12} = \frac{1}{4}$

3. $\frac{5}{10} = \frac{1}{2}$

4. $\frac{25}{100} = \frac{1}{4}$

5. $\frac{18}{72} = \frac{1}{4}$

6. $\frac{50}{60} = \frac{5}{6}$

7. $\frac{27}{54} = \frac{1}{2}$

8. $\frac{4}{64} = \frac{1}{16}$

9. $\frac{12}{144} = \frac{1}{12}$

10. $\frac{25}{150} = \frac{1}{6}$

Practice Exercise B

1. $\frac{15}{4} = 3\frac{3}{4}$

2. $\frac{13}{6} = 2\frac{1}{6}$

3. $\frac{27}{5} = 5\frac{2}{5}$

4. $\frac{17}{3} = 5\frac{2}{3}$

5. $\frac{99}{10} = 9\frac{9}{10}$

6. $\frac{19}{4} = 4\frac{3}{4}$

7. $\frac{36}{7} = 5\frac{1}{7}$

8. $\frac{39}{12} = 3\frac{3}{12} = 3\frac{1}{4}$

9. $\frac{14}{4} = 3\frac{2}{4} = 3\frac{1}{2}$

10. $\frac{57}{3} = 19$

Practice Exercise C

1. $\frac{1}{2} = \frac{3}{6}$

   $\frac{1}{3} = \frac{2}{6}$

   $\underline{\frac{1}{6} = \frac{1}{6}}$

   $\frac{6}{6} = 1$

2. $\frac{3}{4} = \frac{9}{12}$

   $\frac{1}{12} = \frac{1}{12}$

   $\underline{\frac{2}{3} = \frac{8}{12}}$

   $\frac{18}{12} = 1\frac{6}{12} = 1\frac{1}{2}$

3. $7\frac{2}{3} = 7\frac{16}{24}$

   $3\frac{5}{24} = 3\frac{5}{24}$

   $\underline{\frac{5}{12} = \frac{10}{24}}$

   $10\frac{31}{24} = 11\frac{7}{24}$

4. $1\frac{1}{4} = 1\frac{12}{48}$

   $5\frac{3}{16} = 5\frac{9}{48}$

   $\underline{2\frac{5}{12} = 2\frac{20}{48}}$

   $8\frac{41}{48}$

5. $26\frac{3}{5}$ = $26\frac{72}{120}$

$14\frac{1}{6}$ = $14\frac{20}{120}$

$5\frac{7}{8}$ = $5\frac{105}{120}$

$45\frac{197}{120}$ = $46\frac{77}{120}$

6. $7\frac{5}{8}$ = $7\frac{100}{160}$

$\frac{1}{32}$ = $\frac{5}{160}$

$3\frac{1}{10}$ = $3\frac{16}{160}$

$10\frac{121}{160}$

7. $4\frac{1}{2}$ = $4\frac{4}{8}$

$3\frac{1}{4}$ = $3\frac{2}{8}$

$9\frac{3}{8}$ = $9\frac{3}{8}$

$16\frac{9}{8}$ = $17\frac{1}{8}$

8. $7\frac{11}{12}$ = $7\frac{33}{36}$

$16\frac{3}{4}$ = $16\frac{27}{36}$

$2\frac{4}{18}$ = $2\frac{8}{36}$

$25\frac{68}{36}$ = $26\frac{32}{36}$ = $26\frac{8}{9}$

9. $1\frac{3}{24}$ = $1\frac{3}{24}$

$8\frac{1}{3}$ = $8\frac{8}{24}$

$3\frac{5}{6}$ = $3\frac{20}{24}$

$12\frac{31}{24}$ = $13\frac{7}{24}$

10. $5\frac{5}{6}$ = $5\frac{100}{120}$

$7\frac{3}{8}$ = $7\frac{45}{120}$

$2\frac{3}{10}$ = $2\frac{36}{120}$

$14\frac{181}{120}$ = $15\frac{61}{120}$

Practice Exercise D

1. $\frac{5}{8}$ = $\frac{10}{16}$

$-\frac{3}{16}$ = $\frac{3}{16}$

$\frac{7}{16}$

2. $7\frac{5}{12}$ = $7\frac{5}{12}$

$-3\frac{1}{4}$ = $3\frac{3}{12}$

$4\frac{2}{12}$ = $4\frac{1}{6}$

3. $\frac{1}{2}$ = $\frac{4}{8}$

$-\frac{1}{8}$ = $\frac{1}{8}$

$\frac{3}{8}$

4. $3\frac{1}{8}$ = $3\frac{1}{8}$ = $2\frac{9}{8}$

$-1\frac{3}{4}$ = $1\frac{6}{8}$ = $1\frac{6}{8}$

$1\frac{3}{8}$

5. $\frac{7}{9}$ = $\frac{14}{18}$

$-\frac{1}{6}$ = $\frac{3}{18}$

$\frac{11}{18}$

6. $\frac{17}{20}$ = $\frac{17}{20}$

$-\frac{3}{4}$ = $\frac{15}{20}$

$\frac{2}{20}$ = $\frac{1}{10}$

7. $5\frac{3}{8}$ = $5\frac{6}{16}$ = $4\frac{22}{16}$

$-1\frac{7}{16}$ = $-1\frac{7}{16}$ = $-1\frac{7}{16}$

$3\frac{15}{16}$

8. $\frac{2}{5}$ = $\frac{18}{45}$

$-\frac{2}{9}$ = $-\frac{10}{45}$

$\frac{8}{45}$

9. $4\frac{3}{4}$ $=$ $4\frac{9}{12}$

$-\;2\frac{2}{3}$ $=-2\frac{8}{12}$

$\overline{}$

$2\frac{1}{12}$

10. $11\frac{7}{8}$ $=$ $11\frac{7}{8}$

$-\;\frac{3}{4}$ $=-\;1\frac{6}{8}$

$\overline{}$

$10\frac{1}{8}$

Practice Exercise E

1. $\frac{\overset{1}{\cancel{2}}}{5} \times \frac{1}{\underset{4}{\cancel{8}}} = \frac{1}{20}$

2. $\frac{\overset{1}{\cancel{2}}}{\underset{1}{\cancel{8}}} \times \frac{\overset{1}{\cancel{8}}}{\underset{6}{\cancel{12}}} = \frac{1}{6}$

3. $\frac{\overset{1}{\cancel{4}}}{\underset{3}{\cancel{21}}} \times \frac{\overset{1}{\cancel{7}}}{\underset{2}{\cancel{8}}} = \frac{1}{6}$

4. $\frac{\overset{3}{\cancel{15}}}{16} \times \frac{9}{\underset{2}{\cancel{10}}} = \frac{27}{32}$

5. $\frac{\overset{1}{\cancel{4}}}{\underset{3}{\cancel{8}}} \times \frac{\overset{1}{\cancel{2}}}{\underset{1}{\cancel{4}}} = \frac{1}{3}$

6. $3\frac{3}{8} \times \frac{27}{8} = \frac{27}{8} \times \frac{27}{8} = \frac{729}{64}$

$= 11\frac{25}{64}$

7. $\frac{1}{2} \times 8 = \frac{1}{\underset{1}{\cancel{2}}} \times \frac{\overset{4}{\cancel{8}}}{1} = 4$

8. $6\frac{1}{2} \times 5\frac{4}{8} = \frac{13}{2} \times \frac{\overset{11}{\cancel{44}}}{\underset{2}{\cancel{8}}} = \frac{143}{4}$

$= 35\frac{3}{4}$

9. $3\frac{2}{3} \times \frac{3}{4} = \frac{11}{\underset{1}{\cancel{3}}} \times \frac{\overset{1}{\cancel{3}}}{4} = \frac{11}{4}$

$= 2\frac{3}{4}$

10. $9 \times 3\frac{1}{3} = \frac{\overset{3}{\cancel{9}}}{1} \times \frac{10}{\underset{1}{\cancel{3}}} = 30$

Practice Exercise F

1. $2\frac{1}{5} + 11 = \frac{11}{5} + \frac{11}{1}$

$= \frac{\overset{1}{\cancel{11}}}{5} \times \frac{1}{\underset{1}{\cancel{11}}} = \frac{1}{5}$

2. $\frac{1}{50} \div \frac{1}{200} = \frac{1}{\underset{1}{\cancel{50}}} \times \frac{\overset{4}{\cancel{200}}}{1}$

$= \frac{4}{1} = 4$

3. $6\frac{3}{5} + 8\frac{3}{10} = \frac{33}{5} + \frac{83}{10}$

$= \frac{33}{\underset{1}{\cancel{5}}} \times \frac{\overset{2}{\cancel{10}}}{83} = \frac{66}{83}$

4. $\frac{3}{4} \div \frac{1}{8} = \frac{3}{\underset{1}{\cancel{4}}} \times \frac{\overset{2}{\cancel{8}}}{1}$

$= \frac{6}{1} = 6$

5. $\dfrac{5}{12} \div \dfrac{5}{60} = \dfrac{\overset{1}{\cancel{5}}}{\underset{1}{\cancel{12}}} \times \dfrac{\overset{5}{\cancel{60}}}{\underset{1}{\cancel{5}}} = \dfrac{5}{1}$

$= 5$

6. $10\tfrac{1}{2} \div \dfrac{1}{3} = \dfrac{21}{2} \times \dfrac{3}{1} = \dfrac{63}{2}$
$= 31\tfrac{1}{2}$

7. $\dfrac{1}{60} \div \dfrac{1}{2} = \dfrac{1}{\underset{30}{\cancel{60}}} \times \dfrac{\cancel{2}}{1} = \dfrac{1}{30}$

8. $8 \div \dfrac{2}{3} = \dfrac{\overset{4}{\cancel{8}}}{1} \times \dfrac{3}{\underset{1}{\cancel{2}}} = \dfrac{12}{1}$
$= 12$

9. $\dfrac{1}{6} \div \dfrac{1}{3} = \dfrac{1}{\underset{2}{\cancel{6}}} \times \dfrac{\cancel{3}}{1} = \dfrac{1}{2}$

10. $\dfrac{7}{8} \div \dfrac{3}{4} = \dfrac{7}{\underset{2}{\cancel{8}}} \times \dfrac{\cancel{4}}{3} = \dfrac{7}{6}$
$= 1\tfrac{1}{6}$

Practice Exercise G

1. $\dfrac{1}{4} =$
$$\begin{array}{r} .25 \\ 4\overline{)1.00} \end{array}$$
Answer: 0.25

2. $\dfrac{7}{8} =$
$$\begin{array}{r} .87 \\ 8\overline{)7.00} \\ 6\,4 \\ \hline 60 \\ 56 \\ \hline 4 \end{array}$$
Answer: 0.87

3. $\dfrac{5}{6} =$
$$\begin{array}{r} .83 \\ 6\overline{)5.00} \\ 4\,8 \\ \hline 20 \\ 18 \end{array}$$
Answer: 0.83

4. $\dfrac{5}{125} =$
$$\begin{array}{r} .04 \\ 125\overline{)5.00} \\ 5\,00 \\ \hline 00 \end{array}$$
Answer: 0.04

5. $\dfrac{5}{16} =$
$$\begin{array}{r} .31 \\ 16\overline{)5.00} \\ 4\,8 \\ \hline 20 \\ 16 \\ \hline 4 \end{array}$$
Answer: 0.31

6. $\dfrac{3}{25} =$
$$\begin{array}{r} .12 \\ 25\overline{)3.00} \\ 2\,5 \\ \hline 50 \\ 50 \\ \hline \end{array}$$
Answer: 0.12

7. $\dfrac{9}{20} =$
$$\begin{array}{r} .45 \\ 20\overline{)9.00} \\ 8\,0 \\ \hline 1\,00 \\ 1\,00 \end{array}$$
Answer: 0.45

8. $\dfrac{1}{75} =$
$$\begin{array}{r} .013 \\ 75\overline{)1.000} \\ 75 \\ \hline 250 \\ 225 \\ \hline 25 \end{array}$$
Answer: 0.013

9. $\dfrac{3}{8} =$
$$\begin{array}{r} .37 \\ 8\overline{)3.00} \\ 2\,4 \\ \hline 60 \\ 56 \\ \hline 4 \end{array}$$
Answer: 0.37

10. $\dfrac{3}{10} =$
$$\begin{array}{r} .30 \\ 10\overline{)3.00} \\ 3\,0 \\ \hline 00 \end{array}$$
Answer: 0.3

Practice Exercise H

1. $0.16 = \dfrac{16}{100} = \dfrac{4}{25}$

2. $0.04 = \dfrac{4}{100} = \dfrac{1}{25}$

3. $0.125 = \dfrac{125}{1000} = \dfrac{1}{8}$

4. $0.06 = \dfrac{6}{100} = \dfrac{3}{50}$

5. $0.257 = \dfrac{257}{1000}$

6. $0.75 = \dfrac{75}{100} = \dfrac{3}{4}$

7. $0.250 = \dfrac{250}{1000} = \dfrac{1}{4}$

8. $0.525 = \dfrac{525}{1000} = \dfrac{21}{40}$

9. $0.2 = \dfrac{2}{10} = \dfrac{1}{5}$

10. $4.75 = 4\frac{75}{100} = 4\frac{3}{4}$

Practice Exercise I

1.
```
    7.2
    3.57
+  10.8
   21.57
```

2.
```
   48.3
   18.25
+   4.002
   70.552
```

3.
```
    6.3
    0.005
+   2.67
    8.975
```

4.
```
   25.4
   37.06
+  41.0
  103.46
```

5.
```
    8.50
   19.625
+   0.17
   28.295
```

6.
```
   29.042
    2.6
+   3.12
   34.762
```

7.
```
    5.4
    8.62
+   0.95
   14.97
```

8.
```
    2.246
   16.8
+   4.26
   23.306
```

9.
```
   16.1
    1.12
+   3.525
   20.745
```

10.
```
   30.7
    4.05
+  20.5
   55.25
```

Practice Exercise J

1.
```
    5.67
 -  3.90
 _____
    1.77
```

6.
```
   15.00
 -  7.82
 _____
    7.18
```

2.
```
   37.20
 - 25.37
 _____
   11.83
```

7.
```
  205.60
 -105.23
 _____
  100.37
```

3.
```
   17.400
 - 13.262
 _____
    4.138
```

8.
```
  246.520
 -107.988
 _____
  138.532
```

4.
```
   58.940
 - 27.363
 _____
   31.577
```

9.
```
   35.25
 - 17.00
 _____
   18.25
```

5.
```
    2.425
 -  0.675
 _____
    1.750
```

10.
```
 1725.5000
 -  50.6325
 _____
 1674.8675
```

Practice Exercise K

1.
```
    5.64
 ×  1.2
 _____
    1128
     564
 _____
   6.768
```

4.
```
    4.92
 ×  9.5
 _____
    2460
    4428
 _____
  46.740
```

2.
```
    4.25
 ×   12
 _____
     850
     425
 _____
   51.00
```

5.
```
      51
 ×   .92
 _____
     102
     459
 _____
   46.92
```

3.
```
    35.6
 ×  2.5
 _____
    1780
     712
 _____
   89.00
```

6.
```
    28.6
 ×  8.16
 _____
    1716
     286
    2288
 _____
 233.376
```

7.
```
      50.06
    ×  2.15
    ───────
      25030
       5006
      10012
    ───────
    107.6290
```

8.
```
      32.2
    × 3.15
    ──────
      1610
       322
       966
    ──────
    101.430
```

9.
```
       21.0
    ×  41.6
    ───────
       1260
        210
        840
    ───────
     873.60
```

10.
```
       8.06
    × 3.654
    ───────
       3224
       4030
       4836
       2418
    ────────
    29.45124
```

Practice Exercise L

1.
```
           40.
    2,5)100,0
```
Answer: 40

2.
```
          3.
    3)9
```
Answer: 3

3.
```
          22.7
    1,7)38,60
        34
        ──
        46
        34
        ───
        120
        119
```
Answer: 22.7

4.
```
            76.66
    1,5)115,000
        105
        ───
        100
         90
        ───
        100
         90
        ───
        100
```
Answer: 76.66

5.
```
          2.2
    2,5)5,50
        5 0
        ───
         50
         50
```
Answer: 2.2

6.
```
           7.
    ,46)3.22
        3 22
        ────
           0
```
Answer: 7

7.
```
          3.1
    1,5)4,65
        4.5
        ───
         15
         15
```
Answer: 3.1

8.
```
          2.
    7,5)15,0
        15 0
        ────
           0
```
Answer: 2

9.
$$.3 \overline{).042}$$

Answer: 0.14

10.
$$.05 \overline{).0060}$$

Answer: 0.12

Practice Exercise M

1. $\frac{4}{5} = 4 : 5$

2. $\frac{1}{3} = 1 : 3$

3. $\frac{3}{4} = 3 : 4$

4. $\frac{3}{8} = 3 : 8$

5. $\frac{1}{10} = 1 : 10$

6. $\frac{2}{3} = 2 : 3$

7. $\frac{1}{2} = 1 : 2$

8. $\frac{25}{50} = 25 : 50 = 1 : 2$

9. $\frac{3}{9} = 3 : 9 = 1 : 3$

10. $\frac{2}{5} = 2 : 5$

Practice Exercise N

1. $8 : 10 = x : 30$
   $10x = 240$
   $x = 24$

2. $9 : 15 = x : 5$
   $15x = 45$
   $x = 3$

3. $x : 80 = 3 : 12$
   $12x = 240$
   $x = 20$

4. $3 : x = 8 : 24$
   $8x = 72$
   $x = 9$

5. $2 : 3 = x : 63$
   $3x = 126$
   $x = 42$

6. $5 : 15 = x : 60$
   $15x = 300$
   $x = 20$

7. $7 : x = 4 : 28$
   $4x = 196$
   $x = 49$

8. $0.2 : 8 = 25 : x$
   $0.2x = 200$
   $x = 1000$

9. $5 : 7 = x : 28$
   $7x = 140$
   $x = 20$

10. $\frac{1}{10} x : 2000 = 1 : 100$
    $10x = 2000$
    $x = 200$

Practice Exercise O

1. 0.225 = 22.5%

2. 3.45 = 345%

3. 0.7 = 70%

4. 0.14 = 14%

5. 4.5 = 450%

6. 1.23 = 123%

7. 0.001 = 0.1%

8. 0.055 = 5.5%

9. 0.30 = 30%

10. 0.427 = 42.7%

Practice Exercise P

Roman Numerals:

1. VIII
2. XV
3. L
4. IV
5. XXIII
6. XLIV
7. XCIII
8. XXXVI
9. LVI
10. XIX

11. XXV
12. C
13. XXXVII
14. VII
15. XVIII
16. DXXVI
17. XCIV
18. XXXIX
19. LXII
20. MCMLXXX

Arabic Numbers:

1. 24
2. 17
3. 50
4. 40
5. 5
6. 3
7. 1000
8. 19
9. 30
10. 29

11. 6
12. 70
13. 100
14. 92
15. 69
16. 17
17. 22
18. 11
19. 204
20. 1115

ARITHMETIC TEST 1

30 Questions   30 Minutes

Directions: *Work out each problem and fill in your answer in the space provided.*

Reduce to lowest terms:

1. $\dfrac{3}{6}$ = _____

2. $\dfrac{10}{12}$ = _____

3. $\dfrac{40}{1000}$ = _____

4. $\dfrac{15}{50}$ = _____

5. $\dfrac{75}{90}$ = _____

Change to improper fractions:

6. $2\frac{3}{5}$ = _____

7. $10\frac{3}{5}$ = _____

8. $6\frac{5}{6}$ = _____

9. $17\frac{1}{2}$ = _____

10. $9\frac{1}{3}$ = _____

Add:

11. $\dfrac{2}{3}$
$\dfrac{1}{4}$
$\dfrac{5}{6}$

12. $\dfrac{5}{9}$
$\dfrac{3}{8}$
$\dfrac{1}{4}$

13. $\dfrac{4}{5}$
$\dfrac{3}{8}$
$\dfrac{1}{20}$

14. $17\frac{2}{3}$
$\dfrac{8}{9}$
$2\frac{1}{12}$

15. $1\frac{9}{10}$
$8\frac{4}{5}$
$9\frac{2}{3}$

Subtract:

16. $\dfrac{7}{8}$
$-\dfrac{1}{3}$

17. $\dfrac{11}{18}$
$-\dfrac{2}{9}$

18. $7\frac{1}{3}$
$-\ 2\frac{3}{4}$

19. $2\frac{5}{6}$

      $-\ \frac{8}{9}$

20. $17\frac{1}{3}$

      $-\ 8\frac{5}{15}$

Multiply:

21. $\frac{1}{5} \times \frac{25}{50} =$ _____

22. $\frac{1}{3} \times \frac{3}{4} =$ _____

23. $\frac{7}{10} \times \frac{5}{6} =$ _____

24. $15 \times 2\frac{1}{3} =$ _____

25. $\frac{2}{3} \times \frac{9}{16} =$ _____

Divide:

26. $\frac{1}{2} \div \frac{1}{50} =$ _____

27. $\frac{1}{2} \div 6 =$ _____

28. $2\frac{1}{4} \div 3\frac{1}{2} =$ _____

29. $2\frac{4}{5} \div 7 =$ _____

30. $\frac{1}{2} \div \frac{1}{50} =$ _____

Answer Key

1. $\frac{1}{2}$

2. $\frac{5}{6}$

3. $\frac{1}{25}$

4. $\frac{3}{10}$

5. $\frac{5}{6}$

6. $\frac{13}{5}$

7. $\frac{53}{5}$

8. $\frac{41}{6}$

9. $\frac{35}{2}$

10. $\frac{28}{3}$

11. $1\frac{3}{4}$

12. $1\frac{13}{72}$

13. $1\frac{9}{40}$

14. $20\frac{11}{36}$

15. $20\frac{11}{30}$

16. $\frac{13}{24}$

17. $\frac{7}{18}$

18. $4\frac{7}{12}$

19. $1\frac{17}{18}$

20. 9

21. $\frac{1}{10}$

22. $\frac{1}{4}$

23. $\frac{7}{12}$

24. 35

25. $\frac{3}{8}$

26. 25

27. $\frac{1}{12}$

28. $\frac{9}{14}$

29. $\frac{2}{5}$

30. 25

Solutions to Arithmetic Test 1

1. $\dfrac{3}{6} = \dfrac{1}{2}$

2. $\dfrac{10}{12} = \dfrac{5}{6}$

3. $\dfrac{40}{1000} = \dfrac{1}{25}$

4. $\dfrac{15}{50} = \dfrac{3}{10}$

5. $\dfrac{75}{90} = \dfrac{5}{6}$

6. $2\frac{3}{5} = \dfrac{13}{5}$

7. $10\frac{3}{5} = \dfrac{53}{5}$

8. $6\frac{5}{6} = \dfrac{41}{6}$

9. $17\frac{1}{2} = \dfrac{35}{2}$

10. $9\frac{1}{3} = \dfrac{28}{3}$

11. $\dfrac{2}{3} = \dfrac{8}{12}$

$\dfrac{1}{4} = \dfrac{3}{12}$

$\dfrac{5}{6} = \dfrac{10}{12}$

$\quad\dfrac{21}{12} = 1\frac{9}{12} = 1\frac{3}{4}$

12. $\dfrac{5}{9} = \dfrac{40}{72}$

$\dfrac{3}{8} = \dfrac{27}{72}$

$\dfrac{1}{4} = \dfrac{18}{72}$

$\quad\dfrac{85}{72} = 1\frac{13}{72}$

13. $\dfrac{4}{5} = \dfrac{32}{40}$

$\dfrac{3}{8} = \dfrac{15}{40}$

$\dfrac{1}{20} = \dfrac{2}{40}$

$\quad\dfrac{49}{40} = 1\frac{9}{40}$

14. $17\frac{2}{3} = 17\frac{24}{36}$

$\frac{5}{9} = \frac{20}{36}$

$2\frac{1}{12} = 2\frac{3}{36}$

$\quad 19\frac{47}{36} = 20\frac{11}{36}$

15. $1\frac{9}{10} = 1\frac{27}{30}$

$8\frac{4}{5} = 8\frac{24}{30}$

$9\frac{2}{3} = 9\frac{20}{30}$

$\quad 18\frac{71}{30} = 20\frac{11}{30}$

16. $\dfrac{7}{8} = \dfrac{21}{24}$

$-\dfrac{1}{3} = \dfrac{8}{24}$

$\quad\dfrac{13}{24}$

17. $\dfrac{11}{18} = \dfrac{11}{18}$

$-\dfrac{2}{9} = \dfrac{4}{18}$

$\quad\dfrac{7}{18}$

18. $7\frac{1}{3} = 7\frac{4}{12} = 6\frac{11}{12}$

$-2\frac{3}{4} = 2\frac{9}{12} = 2\frac{9}{12}$

$\phantom{-2\frac{3}{4} = 2\frac{9}{12} = }4\frac{7}{12}$

19. $2\frac{5}{6} = 2\frac{15}{18} = 1\frac{33}{18}$

$-\frac{8}{9} = \frac{16}{18} = \frac{16}{18}$

$\phantom{-2\frac{5}{6} = 2\frac{15}{18} = }1\frac{17}{18}$

20. $17\frac{1}{3} = 17\frac{5}{15}$

$-\ \ 8\frac{5}{15} = 8\frac{5}{15}$

$= 9$

21. $\dfrac{1}{5} \times \dfrac{\cancel{25}^{1}}{\cancel{50}_{2}} = \dfrac{1}{10}$

22. $\dfrac{1}{\cancel{8}_{1}} \times \dfrac{\cancel{8}^{1}}{4} = \dfrac{1}{4}$

23. $\dfrac{7}{\cancel{10}_{2}} \times \dfrac{\cancel{5}^{1}}{6} = \dfrac{7}{12}$

24. $15 \times 2\frac{1}{3} = \cancel{15}^{5} \times \dfrac{7}{\cancel{3}_{1}}$

$= \dfrac{35}{1}$

25. $\dfrac{\cancel{2}^{1}}{\cancel{3}_{1}} \times \dfrac{\cancel{9}^{3}}{\cancel{16}_{8}} = \dfrac{3}{8}$

26. $\dfrac{1}{2} \div \dfrac{1}{50} = \dfrac{1}{\cancel{2}_{1}} \times \dfrac{\cancel{50}^{25}}{1} = \dfrac{25}{1} = 25$

27. $\dfrac{1}{2} \div 6 = \dfrac{1}{2} \times \dfrac{1}{6} = \dfrac{1}{12}$

28. $2\frac{1}{4} \div 3\frac{1}{2} = \dfrac{9}{4} \div \dfrac{7}{2} = \dfrac{9}{\cancel{4}_{2}} \times \dfrac{\cancel{2}^{1}}{7} = \dfrac{9}{14}$

29. $2\frac{4}{5} \div 7 = \dfrac{14}{5} \div \dfrac{7}{1} = \dfrac{\cancel{14}^{2}}{5} \times \dfrac{1}{\cancel{7}_{1}} = \dfrac{2}{5}$

30. $\dfrac{1}{2} \div \dfrac{1}{50} = \dfrac{1}{\cancel{2}_{1}} \times \dfrac{\cancel{50}^{25}}{1} = \dfrac{25}{1} = 25$

Answer Sheet
Arithmetic

TEST 2

1. Ⓐ Ⓑ Ⓒ Ⓓ   5. Ⓐ Ⓑ Ⓒ Ⓓ   9. Ⓐ Ⓑ Ⓒ Ⓓ   13. Ⓐ Ⓑ Ⓒ Ⓓ   17. Ⓐ Ⓑ Ⓒ Ⓓ

2. Ⓐ Ⓑ Ⓒ Ⓓ   6. Ⓐ Ⓑ Ⓒ Ⓓ   10. Ⓐ Ⓑ Ⓒ Ⓓ   14. Ⓐ Ⓑ Ⓒ Ⓓ   18. Ⓐ Ⓑ Ⓒ Ⓓ

3. Ⓐ Ⓑ Ⓒ Ⓓ   7. Ⓐ Ⓑ Ⓒ Ⓓ   11. Ⓐ Ⓑ Ⓒ Ⓓ   15. Ⓐ Ⓑ Ⓒ Ⓓ   19. Ⓐ Ⓑ Ⓒ Ⓓ

4. Ⓐ Ⓑ Ⓒ Ⓓ   8. Ⓐ Ⓑ Ⓒ Ⓓ   12. Ⓐ Ⓑ Ⓒ Ⓓ   16. Ⓐ Ⓑ Ⓒ Ⓓ   20. Ⓐ Ⓑ Ⓒ Ⓓ

FINAL ARITHMETIC TEST

1. Ⓐ Ⓑ Ⓒ Ⓓ   5. Ⓐ Ⓑ Ⓒ Ⓓ   9. Ⓐ Ⓑ Ⓒ Ⓓ   13. Ⓐ Ⓑ Ⓒ Ⓓ   17. Ⓐ Ⓑ Ⓒ Ⓓ

2. Ⓐ Ⓑ Ⓒ Ⓓ   6. Ⓐ Ⓑ Ⓒ Ⓓ   10. Ⓐ Ⓑ Ⓒ Ⓓ   14. Ⓐ Ⓑ Ⓒ Ⓓ   18. Ⓐ Ⓑ Ⓒ Ⓓ

3. Ⓐ Ⓑ Ⓒ Ⓓ   7. Ⓐ Ⓑ Ⓒ Ⓓ   11. Ⓐ Ⓑ Ⓒ Ⓓ   15. Ⓐ Ⓑ Ⓒ Ⓓ   19. Ⓐ Ⓑ Ⓒ Ⓓ

4. Ⓐ Ⓑ Ⓒ Ⓓ   8. Ⓐ Ⓑ Ⓒ Ⓓ   12. Ⓐ Ⓑ Ⓒ Ⓓ   16. Ⓐ Ⓑ Ⓒ Ⓓ   20. Ⓐ Ⓑ Ⓒ Ⓓ

ARITHMETIC TEST 2

20 Minutes   20 Questions

Directions: *Read each question carefully, then decide which choice is the best. Blacken the corresponding space on your answer sheet.*

1. $23 + 4.67 + 19.2 + 0.365 =$

    (A) 1047.0
    (B) 47.235
    (C) 1172.4
    (D) 46.235

2. $2.37 \times 0.6 =$

    (A) 14.22
    (B) 1.282
    (C) 1.422
    (D) 12.82

3. The freshman nursing class consists of 40 students. Seven-eighths of the class are women. How many women are in the class?

    (A) 35
    (B) 38
    (C) 21
    (D) 24

4. What percentage of 20 is 12?

    (A) 12 percent
    (B) 60 percent
    (C) 14 percent
    (D) 8 percent

5. What is the value of x in the proportion 1 : 5 :: x : 1500?

    (A) 5
    (B) $\frac{1}{3}$
    (C) 750,000
    (D) 300

6. Three percent of the 900 students in a school went on a trip. How many students remained in school?

    (A) 27
    (B) 30
    (C) 873
    (D) 773

 7. The fraction $\frac{7}{16}$ expressed as a decimal is

    (A) .1120
    (B) .2286
    (C) .4850
    (D) .4375

8. If 30 is divided by .06, the result is

    (A) 5
    (B) 50
    (C) 500
    (D) 5000

9. The sum of 637.894, 8352.16, 4.8673, and 301.5 is, most nearly,

    (A) 8989.5
    (B) 9021.35
    (C) 9294.9
    (D) 9296.4

10. The sum of $82.79, $103.06, and $697.85 is

    (A) $883.70
    (B) $1628
    (C) $791
    (D) $873

11. One percent of $23,000 is

    (A) $23
    (B) $2.30
    (C) $230
    (D) $2300

12. If one and one-half pounds of candy are required to fill an Easter basket, how many baskets can be filled with ten and one-half pounds of candy?

    (A) 7.5
    (B) 2.5
    (C) $5\frac{1}{2}$
    (D) 7

13. If one tee shirt costs $5.60, how many tee shirts can be bought for $61.60?

   (A) $8\frac{1}{2}$
   (B) 10
   (C) 9
   (D) 11

14. The decimal 410.07 less 38.49 equals

   (A) 372.58
   (B) 371.58
   (C) 381.58
   (D) 382.68

15. The fraction $\frac{3}{10}$ written as a decimal is

   (A) 0.3
   (B) 0.03
   (C) 0.003
   (D) 0.0003

16. The decimal 12.5 written as a fraction is

   (A) $\frac{1}{25}$
   (B) $12\frac{1}{2}$
   (C) $1\frac{1}{2}$
   (D) $\frac{125}{100}$

17. The product of 8.3 × 80 is

   (A) 6.64
   (B) 66.4
   (C) 664
   (D) 6640

18. The fraction equal to 0.0625 is

   (A) $\frac{1}{16}$
   (B) $\frac{1}{15}$
   (C) $\frac{1}{14}$
   (D) $\frac{1}{13}$

19. The number 0.03125 equals

   (A) $\frac{3}{64}$
   (B) $\frac{1}{16}$
   (C) $\frac{1}{64}$
   (D) $\frac{1}{32}$

20. The quantity 21.70 divided by 1.75 equals

   (A) 124
   (B) 12.4
   (C) 1.24
   (D) .124

Answer Key

1.	**B**	11.	**C**
2.	**C**	12.	**D**
3.	**A**	13.	**D**
4.	**B**	14.	**B**
5.	**D**	15.	**A**
6.	**C**	16.	**B**
7.	**D**	17.	**C**
8.	**C**	18.	**A**
9.	**D**	19.	**D**
10.	**A**	20.	**B**

Solutions for Arithmetic Test 2

1. (B)
$$
\begin{array}{r}
23.0 \\
4.67 \\
19.2 \\
\underline{0.365} \\
47.235
\end{array}
$$

2. (C)
$$
\begin{array}{r}
2.37 \\
\underline{\times\ 0.6} \\
1.422
\end{array}
$$

3. (A) $\dfrac{7}{\cancel{8}} - \dfrac{\cancel{40}^{\ 5}}{1} = 35$
$$1$$

4. (B) $\dfrac{12}{20} = \dfrac{3}{5} = .6 = 60\%$

$$5x = 355$$
$$x = 60\%$$

5. (D) $1:5 :: x:1500$
$$5x = 1500$$
$$x = 300$$

6. (C)
$$
\begin{array}{rr}
900 & 900 \\
\underline{\times\ .03} & \underline{-\ \ 27} \\
27.00 & 873
\end{array}
$$

7. (D) $\dfrac{7}{16} = $
$$
\begin{array}{r}
.4375 \\
16\overline{)7.0000} \\
\underline{6\,4} \\
60 \\
\underline{48} \\
120 \\
\underline{112} \\
80 \\
\underline{80}
\end{array}
$$

8. (C)
$$
\begin{array}{r}
500. \\
.06\overline{)30,00} \\
\underline{30} \\
00
\end{array}
$$

9. (D)
$$
\begin{array}{r}
637.894 \\
8352.16 \\
4.8673 \\
\underline{301.5} \\
9296.4213
\end{array}
$$

10. (A)
$$
\begin{array}{r}
\$\ 82.79 \\
103.06 \\
\underline{697.85} \\
\$883.70
\end{array}
$$

11. (C)
$$
\begin{array}{r}
\$23,000 \\
\underline{\times\ \ \ 0.01} \\
\$230.00
\end{array}
$$

12. **(D)** $\dfrac{1.5}{1} = \dfrac{10.5}{x}$

$1.5x = 10.5$

$x = 7$

13. **(D)**

$$5.60\overline{)61.60}$$
$$56\ 0$$
$$5\ 60$$

11.

14. **(B)**   410.07
− 38.49
———
371.58

15. **(A)** $\frac{3}{10} = 0.3$

16. **(B)** $12.5 = 12\frac{5}{10} = 12\frac{1}{2}$

17. **(C)**   8.3
× 80
———
00
664
———
664.0

18. **(A)** $.0625 = \dfrac{625}{10,000} = \frac{1}{16}$

19. **(D)** $0.03125 = \dfrac{3125}{100,000} = \frac{1}{32}$

20. **(B)**

$$1.75\overline{)21.70.0}$$

12.4
17.5
4.20
3.50
700
700

FINAL ARITHMETIC AND MATHEMATICS TEST

30 Minutes   20 Questions

Directions: *Work out each of the following problems. Blacken the corresponding space on your answer sheet.*

1. Add $\frac{1}{4}$, $\frac{3}{8}$, and $\frac{7}{16}$
   - (A) $\frac{11}{16}$
   - (B) $1\frac{1}{16}$
   - (C) $\frac{11}{28}$
   - (D) $\frac{18}{16}$

2. Multiply 25.5 by 0.326.
   - (A) 83.13
   - (B) 25.826
   - (C) 0.2805
   - (D) 8.313

3. Subtract 25.246 from 307.401.
   - (A) 282.155
   - (B) 54.941
   - (C) 549.41
   - (D) 28.2155

4. $14.75 + 15.1256 + 0.07 =$
   - (A) 299.46
   - (B) 36.8756
   - (C) 29.946
   - (D) 268.756

5. Divide 36.36 by 0.0606.
   - (A) .06
   - (B) 0.6
   - (C) 60
   - (D) 600

6. Write the fraction $\frac{1}{8}$ as a ratio.
   - (A) 8 : 1
   - (B) 0.18
   - (C) 1 : 8
   - (D) 0.125

7. Solve for x in $2 : 8 = 11 : x$
   - (A) 44
   - (B) $2\frac{3}{4}$
   - (C) $\frac{11}{16}$
   - (D) 4.4

8. Change 85 percent to a fraction and reduce to lowest terms.
   - (A) $\frac{85}{100}$
   - (B) $\frac{17}{20}$
   - (C) $\frac{100}{85}$
   - (D) $\frac{20}{17}$

9. Change 0.12 to a percent.
   - (A) 0.12 percent
   - (B) 0.0012 percent
   - (C) .12 percent
   - (D) 12 percent

10. Subtract $\frac{1}{8}$ from $\frac{1}{6}$.
    - (A) $\frac{2}{8}$
    - (B) $\frac{3}{24}$
    - (C) $\frac{1}{24}$
    - (D) $\frac{1}{12}$

11. How many grains of codeine are there in one and one-half tablets of one-eighth grain each?
    - (A) $\frac{2}{8}$
    - (B) $\frac{3}{16}$
    - (C) $\frac{3}{8}$
    - (D) $\frac{5}{8}$

12. Mary drank eight ounces of milk from a quart containing 32 ounces of milk. What part of the quart had she consumed?
    - (A) $\frac{1}{4}$
    - (B) $\frac{1}{8}$
    - (C) $\frac{1}{3}$
    - (D) $\frac{1}{2}$

13. There are 75 nursing students in the freshman class and 15 are men. What is the ratio of women students to men students?

(A) $\frac{1}{4}$
(B) $\frac{1}{5}$
(C) $\frac{4}{1}$
(D) $\frac{5}{1}$

14. If a recipe calls for five ounces of sugar for every 15 ounces of flour, what part of the mixture will be sugar?

(A) $\frac{1}{2}$
(B) $\frac{1}{5}$
(C) $\frac{1}{3}$
(D) $\frac{1}{4}$

15. If a suit is on sale for $120.00, and the original cost was $150.00, what percentage would you save by buying it on sale?

(A) 40 percent
(B) 30 percent
(C) 10 percent
(D) 20 percent

16. A seamstress bought two and two-thirds yards of wool material and one and three-fourths yards of crepe material. How many yards of material did she buy?

(A) $4\frac{5}{12}$
(B) $4\frac{2}{3}$
(C) $5\frac{1}{4}$
(D) $4\frac{1}{3}$

17. A sack contained ten pounds of potatoes. Mrs. Brown used one and three-fourths pounds for french fries yesterday and two and one-third pounds for a casserole today. How many pounds of potatoes does she have left?

(A) $5\frac{1}{2}$
(B) $5\frac{11}{12}$
(C) $6\frac{2}{3}$
(D) $6\frac{11}{12}$

18. How many ounces is three-eighths of a pound if a pound equals 16 ounces?

(A) 6 ounces
(B) 12 ounces
(C) 8 ounces
(D) 10 ounces

19. If John receives two-fifths of $10.00, how much does he receive?

(A) $2.00
(B) $4.00
(C) $5.00
(D) $3.00

20. If there are 3000 registered voters in Center City and three-fifths of them are Democrats, how many Democrats are there in Center City?

(A) 500
(B) 600
(C) 1800
(D) 1500

Answer Key

1.	B	11.	B
2.	D	12.	A
3.	A	13.	C
4.	C	14.	D
5.	D	15.	D
6.	C	16.	A
7.	A	17.	B
8.	B	18.	A
9.	D	19.	B
10.	C	20.	C

Solutions for Arithmetic Test 2

1. **(B)**

$$\frac{1}{4} = \frac{4}{16}$$
$$\frac{3}{8} = \frac{6}{16}$$
$$\frac{7}{16} = \frac{7}{16}$$
$$\overline{\qquad \frac{17}{16}} = 1\frac{1}{16}$$

2. **(D)**

$$
\begin{array}{r}
25.5 \\
\times \; .326 \\
\hline
1530 \\
510 \\
765 \quad \\
\hline
8.3130
\end{array}
$$

3. **(A)**

$$
\begin{array}{r}
307.401 \\
- \; 25.246 \\
\hline
282.155
\end{array}
$$

4. **(C)**

$$
\begin{array}{r}
14.75 \\
15.1256 \\
0.07 \quad \\
\hline
29.9456 = 29.946
\end{array}
$$

5. **(D)**

$$
0.0606)\overline{36.3600}\;(600.
$$
$$
\underline{36.36}
$$
$$
00
$$

6. **(C)** $\frac{1}{8} = 1 : 8$

7. **(A)** $2 : 8 = 11 : x$
$$2x = 88$$
$$x = 44$$

8. **(B)** $85\% = 0.85 = \dfrac{85}{100} = \dfrac{17}{20}$

9. **(D)** $0.12 = 12\%$

10. **(C)**

$$\frac{1}{6} = \frac{4}{24}$$
$$- \frac{1}{8} = \frac{3}{24}$$
$$\overline{\qquad \frac{1}{24}}$$

11. **(B)** $1\frac{1}{2} \times \dfrac{1}{8} = \dfrac{3}{2} \times \dfrac{1}{8} = \dfrac{3}{16}$

12. **(A)** $\dfrac{8}{32} = \dfrac{1}{4}$

13. **(C)** $\dfrac{60 \text{ women}}{15 \text{ men}} = \dfrac{4}{1}$

14. **(D)** $\dfrac{5 \text{ oz. sugar}}{20 \text{ oz. total mixture}} = \dfrac{1}{4}$

15. **(D)** $\dfrac{30}{150} = 150)\overline{30.00}\;(.20 = 20\%$
$$\underline{30\;0}$$
$$00$$

16. **(A)** $2\frac{2}{3} = 2\frac{8}{12}$
$$1\frac{3}{4} = 1\frac{9}{12}$$
$$\overline{\qquad 3\frac{17}{12}} = 4\frac{5}{12}$$

17. **(B)** $1\frac{3}{4} = 1\frac{9}{12}$

$+\ 2\frac{1}{3} = 2\frac{4}{12}$

$3\frac{13}{12} = 4\frac{1}{12}$

$10\ \ \text{lbs}$

$-\ 4\frac{1}{12}\ \text{lbs}$

$5\frac{11}{12}\ \text{lbs}$

18. **(A)** $\dfrac{3}{\underset{1}{\cancel{8}}} \times \dfrac{\overset{2}{\cancel{16}}}{1} = 6$ ounces

19. **(B)** $\dfrac{2}{\underset{1}{\cancel{5}}} \times \dfrac{\overset{2}{\cancel{10}}}{1} = \$4.00$

20. **(C)** $\dfrac{3}{\underset{1}{\cancel{5}}} \times \dfrac{\overset{600}{\cancel{3000}}}{1} = 1800$ Democrats

Answer Sheet
Health and Science

TEST 1

1. Ⓐ Ⓑ Ⓒ Ⓓ	9. Ⓐ Ⓑ Ⓒ Ⓓ	17. Ⓐ Ⓑ Ⓒ Ⓓ	25. Ⓐ Ⓑ Ⓒ Ⓓ	33. Ⓐ Ⓑ Ⓒ Ⓓ
2. Ⓐ Ⓑ Ⓒ Ⓓ	10. Ⓐ Ⓑ Ⓒ Ⓓ	18. Ⓐ Ⓑ Ⓒ Ⓓ	26. Ⓐ Ⓑ Ⓒ Ⓓ	34. Ⓐ Ⓑ Ⓒ Ⓓ
3. Ⓐ Ⓑ Ⓒ Ⓓ	11. Ⓐ Ⓑ Ⓒ Ⓓ	19. Ⓐ Ⓑ Ⓒ Ⓓ	27. Ⓐ Ⓑ Ⓒ Ⓓ	35. Ⓐ Ⓑ Ⓒ Ⓓ
4. Ⓐ Ⓑ Ⓒ Ⓓ	12. Ⓐ Ⓑ Ⓒ Ⓓ	20. Ⓐ Ⓑ Ⓒ Ⓓ	28. Ⓐ Ⓑ Ⓒ Ⓓ	36. Ⓐ Ⓑ Ⓒ Ⓓ
5. Ⓐ Ⓑ Ⓒ Ⓓ	13. Ⓐ Ⓑ Ⓒ Ⓓ	21. Ⓐ Ⓑ Ⓒ Ⓓ	29. Ⓐ Ⓑ Ⓒ Ⓓ	37. Ⓐ Ⓑ Ⓒ Ⓓ
6. Ⓐ Ⓑ Ⓒ Ⓓ	14. Ⓐ Ⓑ Ⓒ Ⓓ	22. Ⓐ Ⓑ Ⓒ Ⓓ	30. Ⓐ Ⓑ Ⓒ Ⓓ	38. Ⓐ Ⓑ Ⓒ Ⓓ
7. Ⓐ Ⓑ Ⓒ Ⓓ	15. Ⓐ Ⓑ Ⓒ Ⓓ	23. Ⓐ Ⓑ Ⓒ Ⓓ	31. Ⓐ Ⓑ Ⓒ Ⓓ	39. Ⓐ Ⓑ Ⓒ Ⓓ
8. Ⓐ Ⓑ Ⓒ Ⓓ	16. Ⓐ Ⓑ Ⓒ Ⓓ	24. Ⓐ Ⓑ Ⓒ Ⓓ	32. Ⓐ Ⓑ Ⓒ Ⓓ	40. Ⓐ Ⓑ Ⓒ Ⓓ

TEST 2

1. Ⓐ Ⓑ Ⓒ Ⓓ	7. Ⓐ Ⓑ Ⓒ Ⓓ	13. Ⓐ Ⓑ Ⓒ Ⓓ	19. Ⓐ Ⓑ Ⓒ Ⓓ	25. Ⓐ Ⓑ Ⓒ Ⓓ
2. Ⓐ Ⓑ Ⓒ Ⓓ	8. Ⓐ Ⓑ Ⓒ Ⓓ	14. Ⓐ Ⓑ Ⓒ Ⓓ	20. Ⓐ Ⓑ Ⓒ Ⓓ	26. Ⓐ Ⓑ Ⓒ Ⓓ
3. Ⓐ Ⓑ Ⓒ Ⓓ	9. Ⓐ Ⓑ Ⓒ Ⓓ	15. Ⓐ Ⓑ Ⓒ Ⓓ	21. Ⓐ Ⓑ Ⓒ Ⓓ	27. Ⓐ Ⓑ Ⓒ Ⓓ
4. Ⓐ Ⓑ Ⓒ Ⓓ	10. Ⓐ Ⓑ Ⓒ Ⓓ	16. Ⓐ Ⓑ Ⓒ Ⓓ	22. Ⓐ Ⓑ Ⓒ Ⓓ	28. Ⓐ Ⓑ Ⓒ Ⓓ
5. Ⓐ Ⓑ Ⓒ Ⓓ	11. Ⓐ Ⓑ Ⓒ Ⓓ	17. Ⓐ Ⓑ Ⓒ Ⓓ	23. Ⓐ Ⓑ Ⓒ Ⓓ	29. Ⓐ Ⓑ Ⓒ Ⓓ
6. Ⓐ Ⓑ Ⓒ Ⓓ	12. Ⓐ Ⓑ Ⓒ Ⓓ	18. Ⓐ Ⓑ Ⓒ Ⓓ	24. Ⓐ Ⓑ Ⓒ Ⓓ	30. Ⓐ Ⓑ Ⓒ Ⓓ

TEST 3

1. Ⓐ Ⓑ Ⓒ Ⓓ	7. Ⓐ Ⓑ Ⓒ Ⓓ	13. Ⓐ Ⓑ Ⓒ Ⓓ	19. Ⓐ Ⓑ Ⓒ Ⓓ	25. Ⓐ Ⓑ Ⓒ Ⓓ
2. Ⓐ Ⓑ Ⓒ Ⓓ	8. Ⓐ Ⓑ Ⓒ Ⓓ	14. Ⓐ Ⓑ Ⓒ Ⓓ	20. Ⓐ Ⓑ Ⓒ Ⓓ	26. Ⓐ Ⓑ Ⓒ Ⓓ
3. Ⓐ Ⓑ Ⓒ Ⓓ	9. Ⓐ Ⓑ Ⓒ Ⓓ	15. Ⓐ Ⓑ Ⓒ Ⓓ	21. Ⓐ Ⓑ Ⓒ Ⓓ	27. Ⓐ Ⓑ Ⓒ Ⓓ
4. Ⓐ Ⓑ Ⓒ Ⓓ	10. Ⓐ Ⓑ Ⓒ Ⓓ	16. Ⓐ Ⓑ Ⓒ Ⓓ	22. Ⓐ Ⓑ Ⓒ Ⓓ	28. Ⓐ Ⓑ Ⓒ Ⓓ
5. Ⓐ Ⓑ Ⓒ Ⓓ	11. Ⓐ Ⓑ Ⓒ Ⓓ	17. Ⓐ Ⓑ Ⓒ Ⓓ	23. Ⓐ Ⓑ Ⓒ Ⓓ	29. Ⓐ Ⓑ Ⓒ Ⓓ
6. Ⓐ Ⓑ Ⓒ Ⓓ	12. Ⓐ Ⓑ Ⓒ Ⓓ	18. Ⓐ Ⓑ Ⓒ Ⓓ	24. Ⓐ Ⓑ Ⓒ Ⓓ	30. Ⓐ Ⓑ Ⓒ Ⓓ

UNIT VII
HEALTH AND SCIENCE

The Practical Nurse needs a comprehensive knowledge of the basic concepts of the biological and physical sciences in order to understand normal body structure and functions and to recognize deviations from the normal. In order for the practical nurse to function as a competent health care provider, basic principles of chemistry, physics, microbiology, and pathology must be included in the nursing curriculum. The questions in this section include facts and principles related to:

1. knowledge of the body structure
2. understanding of how the body functions
3. knowledge of principles of nutrition
4. knowledge of factors affecting health

HEALTH AND SCIENCE GLOSSARY

The purpose of this glossary is to acquaint the reader with some of the common terms that are used in body structure and functions.

A

abductor	A muscle that draws a part of the body away from the median line or normal position.
acetabulum	The socket of the hip bone.
adductor	A muscle that pulls a part of the body toward the median line.
adrenal glands	The two small glands that are on the upper part of the kidneys.
adrenalin	A hormone produced by the adrenal glands; a drug containing this hormone used to raise blood pressure.
alimentary canal	The passageway in the body extending from the mouth to the anus.
alveolus	An air cell of a lung; a tooth socket.
anatomy	The science of the structure of plants and animals.
aorta	The main artery of the body.
artery	A blood vessel carrying blood away from the heart to all parts of the body.
atrium	A chamber of the heart.
atrophy	A wasting away or failure of an organ to grow.
auditory	A term referring to the sense of hearing.
axilla	The armpit.

B

backbone	The column of bones (vertebrae) along the center of the back.
bile	A substance produced by the liver and stored in the gallbladder.
brachial	A term referring to the upper part of the forelimb of the vertebrae.

bronchus	Either of the two main branches or tubes extending from the trachea (windpipe).
bursa	A sac or cavity, especially between joints.

C

cardiac	Of or near the heart.
caudal	Near the tail.
cell	The basic unit of protoplasm.
cephalic	Of the head, skull, or cranium.
clavicle	The collarbone.
clonus	A series of muscle spasms.
colon	That part of the large intestine extending from the cecum to the rectum.
conjunctivitis	The mucous membrane lining the inner surface of the eyelids and covering the front part of the eyeball.
cornea	The transparent outer coating of the eyeball.
cranium	The skull; especially that part containing the brain.
cutaneous	Of or on the skin; affecting the skin.

D

dactyl	A finger or toe.
dermis	The layer of skin just below the epidermis.
digit	A finger or toe.
duct	A tube through which secretions or excretions pass through the body.
duodenum	The first section of the small intestine, below the stomach.

E

enamel	The hard, white coating of the crowns of teeth.
endothelium	A membrane that lines the heart, blood vessels, and lymphatic vessels.

epidermis	The outermost layer of the skin.
esophagus	The passage for food from the pharynx to the stomach; gullet.
eviscerate	To remove the entrails from; disembowel.
extensor	A muscle that straightens some part of the body.

F

fascia	A thin layer of connective tissue.
femur	The thighbone.
fibrin	A protein formed in the clotting of blood.
flexor	A muscle that bends a part of the body.
foramen	A small opening.

G

ganglion	A mass of nerve cells serving as a center from which nerve impulses are transmitted.
gastric	In or near the stomach.
genitals	The sexual organs.
glottis	The opening between the vocal cords in the larynx.
gullet	The esophagus.

H

hemoglobin	The red coloring matter of the red blood cells.
humerus	The bone of the upper arm or forelimb, extending from the shoulder to the elbow.
hyoid	A u-shaped bone at the base of the tongue.
hypophysis	The pituitary gland.

I

ileum	The lowest part of the small intestine.
ilium	The uppermost part of the three sections of the hipbone.

insulin	A secretion of the pancreas that helps the body use sugar.
intestines	The lower part of the alimentary canal, extending from the stomach to the anus.

J

jejunum	The middle part of the small intestine.
jugular	Two large veins in the neck carrying blood from the head to the heart.

K

kidney	Either of a pair of organs that separate water and products from the blood and excrete them as urine through the bladder.

L

lacrimal	Of, for, or producing tears.
larynx	A structure serving as an organ of the voice.
ligament	A band of tough tissue connecting bones or holding organs in place.
lumbar	Pertaining to the small of the back.
lymph	A clear, yellowish fluid found in the lymphatic system of the body.
lymphatic system	A system of vessels and nodes that leads from the tissue spaces to large veins entering the heart.

M

mastication	The act of chewing.
maxilla	The upper jawbone.
membrane	A thin, soft layer of tissue that covers or lines an organ or part.
meninges	The three membranes that enclose the brain and spinal cord.
meningitis	Inflammation of the meninges.
metacarpals	The bones in the hand between the wrist and the fingers.
metatarsals	The bones in the foot between the ankle and toes.

mucus	The slimy secretion that moistens and protects the mucous membrane.
mucous membrane	A membrane lining cavities leading to the outside of the body, such as to the mouth, anus, etc.

N

neural	Pertaining to the nerves or the nervous system.
nutrition	The series or processes by which an organism takes in and assimilates food for promoting growth and repairing tissues.

O

occiput	The back of the skull or head.
ocular	Pertaining to the eye.
olfactory	A term referring to the sense of smell.
ophthalmic	Of or connected with the eyes.
optic nerve	The nerve running from the brain to the eye.
orbit	The eye socket.
osteology	The study of bones.

P

pancreas	The gland that secretes insulin and other digestive juices.
parathyroid	Four small glands embedded in the thyroid gland; their secretions increase the calcium content in the blood.
pathogenic	Disease-producing.
pepsin	An enzyme secreted in the stomach, aiding in the digestion of proteins.
pharynx	The cavity extending from the mouth and nasal passages to the larynx and esophagus; throat.
placenta	The structure through which the fetus is nourished.
protoplasm	The essential living matter of animal and plant cells.

protozoa   A one-celled microscopic animal.

pubis   The bone that makes up the front part of the pelvis.

Q

quadruped   A mammal or animal with four feet.

quadrant   A term referring to four or part of four.

R

radius   The bone of the forearm on the same side as the thumb.

rectum   The lowest segment of the large intestine, ending at the anus.

retina   The innermost coating of the back part of the eyeball.

riboflavin   A factor of the vitamin B complex, found in milk, eggs, liver, fruits, leafy vegetables, etc.

S

scapula   The shoulder blade.

semen   The fluid secreted by the male reproductive organs containing sperm.

sphincter   A round muscle that can open or close a natural opening in the body by expanding and contracting.

sternum   The breastbone.

striated   Streaked with fine lines.

T

tarsals   The bones of the ankle.

tendons   The connective tissue that joins muscles to bones.

thrombin   A substance that aids in the clotting of blood.

thyroid gland   A large ductless gland near the trachea that produces thyroxine, which regulates metabolism.

tibia   The inner bone of the leg below the knee; shinbone.

trachea   The windpipe; the tube that conveys air from the larynx to the bronchi.

U

ulna   The bone of the forearm on the side opposite the thumb.

urea   A soluble, crystalline solid, found in urine.

urine   A yellowish fluid in mammals, containing urea and other waste products.

V

vagina   In female mammals, the canal leading from the vulva to the uterus.

vermiform appendix   A small saclike appendage of the large intestine.

viscera   The internal organs of the body, such as the heart, lungs, stomach, etc.

vomer   A bone forming part of the nasal septum.

Z

zoology   The branch of biology dealing with the classification of animals and the study of animal life.

HEALTH AND SCIENCE TEST 1

35 Minutes   40 Questions

Directions: *Each question or incomplete statement below is followed by four suggested answers or completions, lettered A, B, C, D. For each question select the best of the four choices and blacken the corresponding space on your answer sheet.*

1. Muscles whose functions are to close off body openings are

   (A) flexors
   (B) sphincters
   (C) extensors
   (D) adductors

2. Bile aids in the digestion of

   (A) amino acids
   (B) fats
   (C) starches
   (D) carbohydrates

3. Urea is removed from the blood as it goes through the

   (A) bladder
   (B) pancreas
   (C) spleen
   (D) kidney

4. The blood group of a universal recipient is

   (A) AB
   (B) B
   (C) O
   (D) A

5. The stimulant in coffee is

   (A) tannic acid
   (B) theobromine
   (C) theophylline
   (D) caffeine

6. Which of the following foods is the most economical source of proteins?

   (A) dried milk
   (B) green leafy vegetables
   (C) meats
   (D) eggs

7. Connective tissue that attaches muscles to the bones is called

   (A) tendons
   (B) ligaments
   (C) cartilage
   (D) osseous

8. The hormone produced by the testes is

   (A) progesterone
   (B) estrogen
   (C) testosterone
   (D) aldosterone

9. The elbow joint is an example of

   (A) ball-and-socket joint
   (B) hinge joint
   (C) pivot joint
   (D) saddle joint

10. The movement that propels food down the digestive tract is called

    (A) pyloraspasm
    (B) rugae
    (C) mastication
    (D) peristalsis

11. In mumps, the gland affected is the

    (A) parathyroid
    (B) pituitary
    (C) parotid
    (D) pineal

12. The negative charged particle found within the atom is the

    (A) proton
    (B) electron
    (C) nucleus
    (D) neutron

353

13. The exchange of nutrients and waste products occurs in the

   (A) venules
   (B) capillaries
   (C) arterioles
   (D) arteries

14. Hemoglobin is found in

   (A) basophils
   (B) neutrophils
   (C) monocytes
   (D) erythrocytes

15. Organic substances made up of several amino acids bound together are

   (A) carbohydrates
   (B) fats
   (C) proteins
   (D) fatty acids

16. The exchange of carbon dioxide and oxygen in the lungs occurs in the

   (A) venules
   (B) alveoli
   (C) bronchi
   (D) bronchioles

17. The pacemaker of the heart is the

   (A) Bundle of His
   (B) AV node
   (C) purkinje fibers
   (D) SA node

18. Mitral stenosis involves the

   (A) aortic valve
   (B) pulmonary valve
   (C) bicuspid valve
   (D) tricuspid valve

19. The smallest known microorganisms are

   (A) bacteria
   (B) viruses
   (C) fungi
   (D) protozoa

20. All arteries carry oxygenated blood *except*

   (A) pulmonary
   (B) coronary
   (C) popliteal
   (D) aorta

21. Electrolyte balance is maintained primarily by the action of the

   (A) testes
   (B) kidney
   (C) bladder
   (D) liver

22. The mineral that is necessary for the proper functioning of the thyroid gland is

   (A) sodium
   (B) iodine
   (C) calcium
   (D) iron

23. Vitamin C prevents

   (A) beriberi
   (B) rickets
   (C) pellagra
   (D) scurvy

24. The function of leukocytes is to

   (A) carry oxygen
   (B) engulf bacteria
   (C) carry food
   (D) regulate metabolism

25. Insulin is produced in the

   (A) pituitary gland
   (B) ilium
   (C) islets of Langerhans
   (D) pineal gland

26. The end product of protein metabolism is

   (A) amino acids
   (B) glucose
   (C) glycogen
   (D) ptyalin

27. Carbohydrates are absorbed into the blood as

    (A) glycogen
    (B) amino acids
    (C) glucose
    (D) fatty acids

28. When one muscle of a pair contracts, the opposing must

    (A) also contract
    (B) relax
    (C) produce more energy
    (D) remain in the same position

29. The respiratory center is located in the part of the brain known as the

    (A) thalamus
    (B) cerebrum
    (C) pons
    (D) medulla oblongata

30. Rays pass through various parts of the eye in a process of bending which is called

    (A) refraction
    (B) reflexion
    (C) retraction
    (D) retroversion

31. The part of the eye commonly called the "window" is

    (A) retina
    (B) cornea
    (C) lens
    (D) pupil

32. A calorie is a form of

    (A) light
    (B) heat
    (C) darkness
    (D) sound

33. The vitamin known as the "sunshine" vitamin is

    (A) vitamin E
    (B) vitamin B
    (C) vitamin K
    (D) vitamin D

34. The process by which the body changes food into substances that can be readily used by the body is

    (A) digestion
    (B) deglutition
    (C) micturition
    (D) absorption

35. The thyroid gland cannot function properly without

    (A) chloride
    (B) iodine
    (C) phosphorous
    (D) iron

36. The vitamin that is necessary for coagulation of the blood is

    (A) vitamin K
    (B) vitamin C
    (C) vitamin A
    (D) vitamin E

37. Another name for vitamin B_1 is

    (A) niacin
    (B) thiamin
    (C) riboflavin
    (D) pyridoxine

38. Food is moved through the alimentary canal by wave-like motions called

    (A) excretions
    (B) mastication
    (C) contractions
    (D) peristalsis

39. The femur is a bone located in the

    (A) forearm
    (B) upper arm
    (C) thigh
    (D) lower leg

40. The liquid portion of the blood is called

    (A) serum
    (B) gamma globulin
    (C) plasma
    (D) lymph

Answer Key

1.	B	21.	B
2.	B	22.	B
3.	D	23.	D
4.	A	24.	B
5.	D	25.	C
6.	A	26.	A
7.	A	27.	C
8.	C	28.	B
9.	B	29.	D
10.	D	30.	A
11.	C	31.	B
12.	B	32.	B
13.	B	33.	D
14.	D	34.	A
15.	C	35.	B
16.	B	36.	A
17.	D	37.	B
18.	C	38.	D
19.	B	39.	C
20.	A	40.	C

Explanatory Answers

1. **(B)** Sphincters are circular muscles that will contract when stimulated, closing an opening.

2. **(B)** Bile is released into the duodenum and breaks down the undigested fats into small droplets.

3. **(D)** Urea is filtered from the blood by the kidneys and excreted in urine.

4. **(A)** Group AB blood contains both group A and B antigens and neither A nor B antibodies; therefore, it cannot clump any donor red cells containing A and B antigens.

5. **(D)** Caffeine is a stimulant found in coffee.

6. **(A)** Dried milk is an inexpensive but a good source of protein.

7. **(A)** Tendons are connective tissue made of dense fibers in the shape of a cord and have great strength.

8. **(C)** Testosterone is the hormone that regulates male sex characteristics.

9. **(B)** Hinge joints allow movement in two directions only.

10. **(D)** Peristalsis is the progressive, wavelike movement that occurs involuntarily to force food forward.

11. **(C)** The parotid gland is a large salivary gland and is affected by mumps.

12. **(B)** The electron is the unit of negative electricity.

13. **(B)** Capillaries connect arterioles with venules and function as exchange vessels.

14. **(D)** Erythrocytes (red blood cells) contain hemoglobin.

15. **(C)** Proteins are nutrients essential for growth and repair of tissue.

16. **(B)** The diffusion of gas occurs across the thin, squamous epithelium lining of the alveoli.

17. **(D)** The SA node, located in the right atrium, starts each heart beat.

18. **(C)** The mitral valve located between the left atrium and left ventricle of the heart is also called the bicuspid valve.

19. **(B)** Viruses are so small that they can be seen only through special electron microscopes.

20. **(A)** The pulmonary artery carries deoxygenated blood from the heart.

21. **(B)** When water intake is excessive, the kidneys excrete generous amounts of urine; if water intake is lost, they produce less urine; the process is regulated by hormones.

22. **(B)** Iodine makes up about 65 percent of thyroxine, a hormone secreted by the thyroid gland.

23. **(D)** Scurvy is a disease caused by a deficiency of vitamin C.

24. **(B)** Leukocytes (white blood cells) engulf bacteria when there is an infection in the body.

25. **(C)** The islets of Langerhans are located in the pancreas and produce insulin.

26. **(A)** Gastric and intestinal enzymes gradually break down the protein molecule into its separate amino acids.

27. **(C)** Glucose is the end product of carbohydrate digestion.

28. **(B)** When one muscle contracts, the opposing muscle must relax; in this way movements are coordinated and normal function is carried out.

29. **(D)** The medulla oblongata is located between the pons and the spinal cord, and the vital centers are located in it.

30. **(A)** Rays pass through a series of transparent colorless eye parts. On the way, they undergo a process of bending called refraction which makes it possible for light from a large area to focus on the retina.

31. **(B)** The cornea is referred to frequently as the "window" of the eye.

32. **(B)** A calorie is the unit of measure of heat—the amount of heat required to raise the temperature of one kilogram of water by $1°C$.

33. **(D)** Vitamin D is referred to as the "sunshine" vitamin because it is formed in the body by the action of the sunshine on the cholesterol products in the skin.

34. **(A)** Digestion is the process whereby the enzymes in the body change food into simple substances that can be readily used by the body.

35. **(B)** The thyroid gland needs iodine for the formation of thyroxine.

36. **(A)** Vitamin K helps the liver to produce substances necessary for the clotting of blood.

37. **(B)** Thiamine is another name for vitamin B_1.

38. **(D)** Peristalsis is a wave-like progression of muscular contractions that moves food through the alimentary canal.

39. **(C)** The thigh bone is the femur. It is the longest and strongest bone in the body.

40. **(C)** Plasma is the liquid portion of the blood in which corpuscles are suspended.

HEALTH AND SCIENCE TEST 2

25 Minutes   30 Questions

Directions: *For each question in this test, choose the answer that you consider correct or most nearly correct. Blacken the appropriate space on your answer sheet.*

1. The force of the blood exerted against the wall of the blood vessel is called

   (A) pulse deficit
   (B) apical pulse
   (C) blood pressure
   (D) pulse pressure

2. The relative amount of moisture in the air is the

   (A) evaporation factor
   (B) temperature
   (C) dew
   (D) humidity

3. A laboratory sample is called

   (A) collection
   (B) agar
   (C) specimen
   (D) symptom

4. Defecation means

   (A) swallowing
   (B) eliminating solid waste
   (C) irrigating the colon
   (D) relieving flatus

5. An object completely free of all microorganisms is

   (A) sterile
   (B) clean
   (C) septic
   (D) contaminated

6. Carbon dioxide is a

   (A) respiratory depressant
   (B) circulatory stimulant
   (C) respiratory stimulant
   (D) circulatory depressant

7. The presence of protein in the urine is called

   (A) polyuria
   (B) anuria
   (C) albuminuria
   (D) hematuria

8. The substance basic to life is

   (A) carbohydrates
   (B) proteins
   (C) starches
   (D) fats

9. In diseases of the gallbladder, which of the following nutrients is limited?

   (A) starches
   (B) proteins
   (C) fats
   (D) carbohydrates

10. Water soluble vitamins include

    (A) vitamin A
    (B) vitamin C
    (C) vitamin D
    (D) vitamin K

11. Diets in the United States are most often deficient in

    (A) iron and calcium
    (B) calcium and potassium
    (C) iodine and sodium
    (D) phosphorous and iron

12. Tetany may be corrected by increasing the amount of

    (A) iron
    (B) iodine
    (C) calcium
    (D) thiamine

13. Which helps conserve body heat?

    (A) increased sweat production
    (B) increased respiratory activity
    (C) dilation of the capillaries of the skin
    (D) constriction of the capillaries of the skin

14. Milk is not a "perfect food" because it lacks

    (A) iron
    (B) calcium
    (C) phosphorous
    (D) carbohydrates

15. The body obtains most of its nitrogen from

    (A) carbohydrates
    (B) proteins
    (C) fats
    (D) cellulose

16. An ion is

    (A) one molecule of water
    (B) one particle of hydrogen
    (C) the same as a neutron
    (D) an atom with an electric charge

17. The basic unit of the living organism is

    (A) the brain
    (B) the cell
    (C) a tissue
    (D) the nervous system

18. The diffusion of water through a semipermeable membrane is known as

    (A) anabolism
    (B) synthesis
    (C) mitosis
    (D) osmosis

19. A physician who specializes in diseases of the heart is known as a

    (A) dermatologist
    (B) cardiologist
    (C) pediatrician
    (D) neurologist

20. A fracture that occurs without breaking through the skin is called

    (A) complex
    (B) compound
    (C) greenstick
    (D) comminuted

21. Smoking and pollution have a deadly effect upon the lungs and pulmonary function. These are classified as

    (A) environmental factors
    (B) biological factors
    (C) sociological factors
    (D) physiological factors

22. In the digestive process, almost all of the water is reabsorbed by the

    (A) sigmoid
    (B) cecum
    (C) colon
    (D) rectum

23. In what structure does fertilization normally occur?

    (A) vagina
    (B) cervix
    (C) ovary
    (D) fallopian tube

24. The process in which carbon dioxide and water is combined under the influence of light in green plants is called

    (A) respiration
    (B) fermentation
    (C) assimilation
    (D) photosynthesis

25. The most abundant gas in the atmosphere is

    (A) oxygen
    (B) nitrogen
    (C) carbon dioxide
    (D) chlorine

26. A protein substance that initiates and accelerates a chemical reaction is called a(n)

   (A) gene
   (B) enzyme
   (C) hormone
   (D) base

27. Amino acids that cannot be manufactured by the body are called

   (A) essential amino acids
   (B) synthetic amino acids
   (C) basic amino acids
   (D) dependent amino acids

28. The instrument used to measure air pressure is called a

   (A) thermometer
   (B) hydrometer
   (C) barometer
   (D) sphygmomanometer

29. An elevation above normal body temperature is called

   (A) hypothermia
   (B) pyrexia
   (C) intermittent
   (D) remittent

30. The instrument used to examine the ears is called the

   (A) ophthalmoscope
   (B) stethoscope
   (C) cystoscope
   (D) otoscope

Answer Key

1.	C	16.	D
2.	D	17.	B
3.	C	18.	D
4.	B	19.	B
5.	A	20.	C
6.	C	21.	A
7.	C	22.	C
8.	B	23.	D
9.	C	24.	D
10.	C	25.	B
11.	A	26.	B
12.	C	27.	A
13.	D	28.	C
14.	A	29.	B
15.	B	30.	D

Explanatory Answers

1. **(C)** Blood pressure is the force of the blood exerted against the wall of the blood vessel.

2. **(D)** Relative humidity refers to the amount of moisture in the air in relation to the temperature.

3. **(C)** Specimen is a laboratory sample used to help the physician make a diagnosis.

4. **(B)** Defecation means the act of having a bowel movement or removing solid waste materials from the body.

5. **(A)** Sterile means that an object is completely free of all microorganisms. Steam under pressure (autoclave) will give complete sterilization.

6. **(C)** Carbon dioxide stimulates the respiratory center in the brain (medulla oblongata).

7. **(C)** Protein substance in the urine is called albuminuria. It results from the failure of the kidneys to filter.

8. **(B)** Protein is the body's vital building material that makes up the basic structure of all cells.

9. **(C)** The gallbladder stores and concentrates bile which is used to break down fats into droplets and aids in the absorption of fatty acids and glyceral. Therefore, fats are restricted when there are diseases of the gallbladder.

10. **(C)** Water-soluble vitamins include vitamin C and vitamin B complex.

11. **(A)** Calcium and iron are the minerals most often deficient in the American diet.

12. **(C)** Tetany, which is due to lack of calcium, may be corrected by increasing milk or milk products, which are rich in calcium salts. Drugs containing high amounts of calcium may be given intravenously in emergencies.

13. **(D)** Restricting skin blood flow reduces heat radiation to the from the blood environment.

14. **(A)** Milk contains only about 0.1 milligrams of iron per cup. The recommended daily amount is 15–18 milligrams.

15. **(B)** Food proteins supply our bodies with nitrogen to replace that lost in urine, feces, and perspiration.

16. **(D)** The electrical charge results when a neutral atom or group of atoms loses or gains one or more electrons during chemical reactions.

17. **(B)** The cell is the unit of structure and function of all living things. The simplest organisms consist of one cell only.

18. **(D)** Osmosis is the diffusion of water through a semipermeable membrane from a region of greater concentration of water to a region of lesser concentration.

19. **(B)** From the word *cardiology*, meaning the study of the heart's physiology and pathology.

20. **(C)** Greenstick fractures are incomplete fractures with a longitudinal split of the shaft. They usually occur in long bones of children.

21. **(A)** Environmental factors are the relationships of living things to their surroundings.

22. **(C)** The fluid-like residue of digestion found in the colon contains valuable water, which is absorbed into the blood stream.

23. **(D)** After ovulation the egg travels into the fallopian tube. If sperms are present, the union of the sperm and the egg (fertilization) takes place in the fallopian tube.

24. **(D)** Photosynthesis is the process by which certain living plant cells combine carbon dioxide and water, in the presence of chlorophyll and light energy, to form carbohydrates and release oxygen as a waste product.

25. **(B)** The atmosphere is composed of about 78 percent nitrogen.

26. **(B)** Enzymes are protein substances that act as biochemical catalysts. They affect the rate at which a specific reaction occurs.

27. **(A)** Essential amino acids are those that cannot be manufactured by the body and, therefore, must be included in the daily diet.

28. **(C)** The barometer is an instrument used to measure air pressure. It is used in forecasting weather.

29. **(B)** An elevation of body temperature above normal is referred to as fever or pyrexia.

30. **(D)** The otoscope is a lighted instrument used to examine the ear canal, eustachian tube, eardrum, and the middle ear.

HEALTH and SCIENCE TEST 3

25 Minutes   30 Questions

Directions: *For each question in this test, choose the answer that you consider correct. Blacken the appropriate space on your answer sheet.*

1. The body's continual response to changes in the external and internal environment is called

   (A) homeostasis
   (B) diffusion
   (C) osmosis
   (D) filtration

2. The ability of a cell to reproduce is called

   (A) osmosis
   (B) crenation
   (C) lyse
   (D) mitosis

3. The immunity that occurs when a person is given a substance containing antibodies or antitoxins is called

   (A) active
   (B) autoimmune
   (C) passive
   (D) permanent

4. The part of the cell necessary for reproduction is the

   (A) cytoplasm
   (B) nucleus
   (C) protoplasm
   (D) cytoplasmic membrane

5. The hormone that regulates the metabolic rate of the body cells is

   (A) oxytocin
   (B) aldosterone
   (C) thyroxin
   (D) cortisone

6. The sudoriferous glands

   (A) secrete sebum
   (B) secrete perspiration
   (C) secrete hormones
   (D) secrete synovial fluid

7. Tanning of the skin is due to

   (A) keratin
   (B) sebum
   (C) sweat
   (D) melanin

8. The ovaries produce the hormones

   (A) estrogen and testosterone
   (B) progesterone and testosterone
   (C) estrogen and progesterone
   (D) progesterone and prolactin

9. The tissue that forms a protective covering for the body and lines the intestinal and respiratory tract is called the

   (A) periosteum
   (B) pericardium
   (C) ephithelium
   (D) connective tissue

10. The hip joint is an example of a

    (A) ball and socket joint
    (B) hinge joint
    (C) pivot joint
    (D) saddle joint

11. The endocrine gland that prepares the body for the "fight or flight" response is the

    (A) adrenal cortex
    (B) adrenal medulla
    (C) pituitary
    (D) thyroid

12. Tears drain into the nose through the

    (A) ciliary body
    (B) lacrimal gland
    (C) eustachian tube
    (D) nasolacrimal duct

13. Respiration and heart rate are controlled by the

    (A) cerebellum
    (B) cerebrum
    (C) medulla
    (D) pons

14. The main function of the large intestine is to

    (A) absorb digested food
    (B) absorb water from waste materials
    (C) produce digestive enzymes
    (D) secrete digestive enzymes

15. The hormone produced by the adrenal glands is

    (A) progesterone
    (B) estrogen
    (C) testosterone
    (D) aldosterone

16. The sloughing off of the endometrium is called

    (A) menarche
    (B) menopause
    (C) menstruation
    (D) myometritis

17. The dorsal cavity has two subdivisions, namely

    (A) thoracic and abdominopelvic
    (B) cranial and spinal
    (C) thoracic and spinal
    (D) medial and lateral

18. The chamber of the heart that receives venous blood from body tissue is the

    (A) right atrium
    (B) left atrium
    (C) right ventricle
    (D) left ventricle

19. The major work of the heart is completed by the

    (A) right ventricle
    (B) left ventricle
    (C) right atrium
    (D) left atrium

20. The shape of the eyeball is maintained by the

    (A) acqueous humor
    (B) vitreous humor
    (C) eye muscles
    (D) eyelid

21. The inner lining of the heart is the

    (A) endocardium
    (B) myocardium
    (C) pericardium
    (D) pleura

22. The muscular structure that forms the floor of the pelvis is the

    (A) peritoneum
    (B) perineum
    (C) mons pubis
    (D) rectus abdominis

23. The large, round portion at the upper and lateral portion of the femur most often involved in hip fractures is the

    (A) acetabulum
    (B) acromiom
    (C) greater trochanter
    (D) tricuspid valve

24. One of the large muscles that is used in climbing stairs and that forms most of the buttocks is the

    (A) gluteus maximus
    (B) gluteus medius
    (C) vastus lateralis
    (D) vastus medialis

25. The basic unit of function of the kidney is the

    (A) medulla
    (B) hilus
    (C) nephron
    (D) cortex

26. Normal urine has the following characteristics *except*

    (A) clear, amber liquid
    (B) nitrogenous waste products
    (C) being slightly aromatic
    (D) high specific gravity

27. The hormone that regulates blood composition and blood volume by acting on the kidney is

    (A) antidiuretic (ADH)
    (B) aldosterone
    (C) parathormone
    (D) oxytocin

28. Composition of urine normally includes

    (A) creatinine, urea, water
    (B) creatinine, ammonia, sugar
    (C) nitrogen wastes, sugar, hormones
    (D) nitrogen wastes, water, pus cells

29. An injury to the left motor area of the cerebrum would cause paralysis of

    (A) the right side of the body
    (B) the left side of the body
    (C) both arms and legs
    (D) both arms

30. Electrolyte balance is maintained chiefly by the action of the

    (A) bladder
    (B) kidney
    (C) islets of Langerhans
    (D) gonads

Answer Key

1. **A**
2. **D**
3. **C**
4. **B**
5. **C**
6. **B**
7. **D**
8. **C**
9. **C**
10. **A**

11. **B**
12. **D**
13. **C**
14. **B**
15. **D**
16. **C**
17. **B**
18. **A**
19. **B**
20. **B**

21. **A**
22. **B**
23. **C**
24. **A**
25. **C**
26. **D**
27. **B**
28. **A**
29. **A**
30. **B**

Explanatory Answers

1. **(A)** The body is constantly stabilizing and equalizing its environment to prevent any sudden or severe changes.

2. **(D)** The DNA molecules in the nucleus of a cell duplicate themselves and the cell divides, forming two cells.

3. **(C)** In acquiring passive immunity the body of the recipient plays an active part in response to an antigen.

4. **(B)** The functional unit is suspended near the center of the cell and has the property of division.

5. **(C)** Produced by the thyroid gland, thyroxin controls the rate at which glucose is burned and converts it to heat and energy.

6. **(B)** Sweat glands are distributed in the skin and produce perspiration, primarily water.

7. **(D)** Melanin, a brown pigment, increases when exposed to sun.

8. **(C)** Estrogen and progesterone promote development of female sex characteristics and regulate menstruation.

9. **(C)** Epithelial tissue has many forms—flat and irregular, square, long and narrow—that are arranged in single or many layers to form a protective covering and lining.

10. **(A)** The ball-shaped head of the femur fits into the concave socket of the hipbone and allows for a wide range of motion.

11. **(B)** Adrenaline is released from the adrenal medulla to prepare the body for emergency situations.

12. **(D)** A small opening into the nose at the inner corner of the eye allows the fluid to drain through.

13. **(C)** Many gray-matter areas that form the cranial nerves are located in the medulla and are involved in the control of vital activities.

14. **(B)** As peristalsis moves content along, water is absorbed through the walls into the circulation, and the remaining cellulose passes on to the rectum.

15. **(D)** Aldosterone is the hormone released from the adrenal cortex that helps regulate sodium and potassium balance.

16. **(C)** The shedding of the lining of the uterus occurs if the egg has not been fertilized by the sperm.

17. **(B)** Dorsal pertains to the back; the cranial and spinal cavities contain the brain and the spinal cord.

18. **(A)** Deoxygenated blood returns from the body tissues via the superior and inferior vena cava into the right atrium.

19. **(B)** The left ventricle has the major responsibility for pumping blood into the aorta to be dispersed throughout the body.

20. **(B)** The jellylike substance prevents the eyeball from collapsing inward.

21. **(A)** The endocardium is a smooth lining, which helps blood flow smoothly through the heart.

22. **(B)** The perineum is the external region between the vulva and anus in the female or between the scrotum and anus in the male and forms the pelvic floor.

23. **(C)** The greater trochanter is the ball-like head that articulates with the hipbone.

24. **(A)** The gluteus maximus is part of the hips and buttocks.

25. **(C)** Nephrons are responsible for the processes of filtration, absorption, and secretion.

26. **(D)** Normal urine has a low specific gravity.

27. **(B)** Aldosterone is released by the adrenal cortex in response to decreased blood volume, decreased blood sodium ions, or increased potassium ions.

28. **(A)** Water plus creatinine and urea, which are nitrogenous wastes, are normal substances in urine.

29. **(A)** The left motor control center in the brain controls the right side of the body because of the crossing of the nerve tracts within the brain.

30. **(B)** When the water intake is excessive, the kidneys excrete generous amounts of urine; if the water intake is lost, they produce less urine. The process is regulated by hormones.

Answer Sheet
Reading

TEST 1

1 Ⓐ Ⓑ Ⓒ Ⓓ

2 Ⓐ Ⓑ Ⓒ Ⓓ

3 Ⓐ Ⓑ Ⓒ Ⓓ

4 Ⓐ Ⓑ Ⓒ Ⓓ

5 Ⓐ Ⓑ Ⓒ Ⓓ

TEST 2

1 Ⓐ Ⓑ Ⓒ Ⓓ

2 Ⓐ Ⓑ Ⓒ Ⓓ

3 Ⓐ Ⓑ Ⓒ Ⓓ

4 Ⓐ Ⓑ Ⓒ Ⓓ

5 Ⓐ Ⓑ Ⓒ Ⓓ

TEST 3

1 Ⓐ Ⓑ Ⓒ Ⓓ

2 Ⓐ Ⓑ Ⓒ Ⓓ

3 Ⓐ Ⓑ Ⓒ Ⓓ

4 Ⓐ Ⓑ Ⓒ Ⓓ

TEST 4

1 Ⓐ Ⓑ Ⓒ Ⓓ

2 Ⓐ Ⓑ Ⓒ Ⓓ

3 Ⓐ Ⓑ Ⓒ Ⓓ

4 Ⓐ Ⓑ Ⓒ Ⓓ

5 Ⓐ Ⓑ Ⓒ Ⓓ

TEST 5

1 Ⓐ Ⓑ Ⓒ Ⓓ

2 Ⓐ Ⓑ Ⓒ Ⓓ

3 Ⓐ Ⓑ Ⓒ Ⓓ

TEST 6

1 Ⓐ Ⓑ Ⓒ Ⓓ

2 Ⓐ Ⓑ Ⓒ Ⓓ

3 Ⓐ Ⓑ Ⓒ Ⓓ

4 Ⓐ Ⓑ Ⓒ Ⓓ

TEST 7

1 Ⓐ Ⓑ Ⓒ Ⓓ

2 Ⓐ Ⓑ Ⓒ Ⓓ

3 Ⓐ Ⓑ Ⓒ Ⓓ

TEST 8

1 Ⓐ Ⓑ Ⓒ Ⓓ

2 Ⓐ Ⓑ Ⓒ Ⓓ

3 Ⓐ Ⓑ Ⓒ Ⓓ

UNIT VIII   READING

Please Review Unit IV, Pages 259 Through 265
Before Completing This Section

READING COMPREHENSION TEST 1

6 Minutes   5 Questions

Directions: *Following the passage below, you will find a number of incomplete statements about the passage. Select the word or expression that most satisfactorily completes each statement. Blacken the corresponding space on your answer sheet.*

A nearby flow of water is a very convenient place to dispose of waste materials, and people have been doing this for many years. If the right chemicals are dumped into the water, it can be beneficial. Lakes tend to follow a course from being deep, clear, nutrient-poor lakes to becoming shallow and more productive nutrient-rich lakes. This is the natural course of most lakes, and the addition of chemicals such as phosphates and nitrates can actually accelerate this process. To a certain extent, this is good, and it has been done intentionally in some cases; but when carried to extremes, it can lead to a man-made natural disaster. The water produces so much algae that most other forms of life cannot exist, and the lake chokes to death. In most cases, factories and sewage drains have carried this addition of chemicals too far.

Another consequence of dumping waste material into waterways, especially lakes, occurs when the waste contains metals, such as copper. Some metals literally cover the lake bottom and kill off all the bottom-dwelling organisms. Since many of these organisms are responsible for the decomposition of organic material on the bottom, the removal of these animals results in a great deal of the organic material remaining undecomposed, and this decreases the nutrient content of the environment.

The dumping of waste materials from combustion into the air is quite obvious every time you look at the skyline of any major industrial area: Dumping poisonous materials into the environment has resulted in the destruction of many of our oxygen-producing plants and has driven many animals from our immediate environment. Another result that strikes perhaps closer to home is the increase in lung disease attributed to air pollution. Moreover, the propellants from aerosol cans cause problems by deteriorating the ozone layer of the atmosphere. This depletion allows greater amounts of ultraviolet radiation to reach the surface of the earth. This higher level of radiation reputedly causes an increase in skin cancer.

Both air and water pollution are a retaliation by nature to man's abuse. We assume that the dumping of wastes into the environment is a one-way process, and we do not count on any repercussions. But the cost of dumping garbage into the environment is slowly coming back to haunt us. Whether it be by the return of mercury and DDT to us in our food, or the destruction of shields in the atmosphere that protect us from being burned by the sun's radiation, we will pay for our assaults on the environment.

1. The title that best expresses the main idea of this section is

   (A) *Save Our Lakes*
   (B) *Man's Responsibility Toward Nature*
   (C) *Air Pollution*
   (D) *How Pollution Causes Cancer*

2. According to this passage, one of the negative results of dumping waste chemicals into lakes is the

   (A) increased growth of algae, which kills other organisms
   (B) discoloration of water
   (C) limitation of recreational activities
   (D) increased temperature in the water

3. Two causes of air pollution are

   (A) smoke and copper
   (B) aerosol cans and recycling of waste materials

   (C) decomposition of organisms and de-oxygenation of plants
   (D) dumping of waste materials and use of aerosol cans

4. The author's attitude toward environmental protection is

   (A) complacency
   (B) pro-conservation
   (C) indifference
   (D) apathetic

5. The author's reference to the driving of animals from our immediate environment implies

   (A) migration
   (B) extinction
   (C) destruction
   (D) poaching

READING COMPREHENSION TEST 2

6 Minutes   5 Questions

Directions: *Following the passage below you will find a number of incomplete statements about the passage. Select the word or expression that most satisfactorily completes each statement. Blacken the corresponding space on your answer sheet.*

Some of you still enjoy fairy tales, but you are probably not as deeply absorbed in them as you were a few years ago. It is an interesting part of growing up to keep adding to our enthusiasms, never wholly discarding what we outgrow, but tying on new pieces of muslin to the tail of our kite. The age of fairy tales belongs to a period when we are interested chiefly in the world of unreality. Goblins, wizards, dwarfs—all those creatures of the imagination—seem to children so much more engaging than the people and things in the everyday world.

Adults find pleasure in remembering their childhood fantasies. But other interests have displaced those early flights of fancy. In fairy tales, of course, all one needs for success or happiness is a fairy godmother. Then everything turns out all right for the hero or heroine. But, as we grow older, these imaginary victories, which once satisfied us, lose their power of enchantment. We want real success and real happiness. It is this growing interest in a real world, in contrast to the fanciful world of fairy lore, that marks the first great advance in reading taste. An interest in *The Adventures of Alice in Wonderland* is likely to give way to an interest in more practical, "real" adventure. The fascination of "Jack the Giant Killer" is lost to a keen interest in Commander Byrd and his Antarctic exploration, for example. The world of real people, real problems, real victories, real facts—these are the reading interests of a mind growing up.

1. The title that best expresses the main idea of this selection is

    (A) *Fairy Tales*
    (B) *Growing Up in Reading Taste*
    (C) *Real Happiness*
    (D) *Our Interest in Goblins*

2. "Tying new pieces of muslin to the tail of our kite" means

    (A) adding new interests to our lives
    (B) finding new excuses
    (C) forgetting the past
    (D) making up stories

3. According to the selection, grown people remember their childhood fantasies with

    (A) difficulty

    (B) enchantment
    (C) enthusiasm
    (D) pleasure

4. The author states that in a fairy tale, all one needs for success or happiness is a

    (A) wizard
    (B) hero
    (C) fairy godmother
    (D) heroine

5. According to the author, "realistic" stories appeal chiefly to a person who is

    (A) childish
    (B) undeveloped
    (C) successful and happy
    (D) becoming mature

READING COMPREHENSION TEST 3

5 Minutes   4 Questions

Directions: *Following the passage below, you will find a number of incomplete statements about the passage. Select the word or expression that most satisfactorily completes each statement. Blacken the corresponding space on your answer sheet.*

Early in the nineteenth century, American youth in the eastern states were playing a game somewhat akin to the English game of rounders that contained all the elements of modern baseball. It was neither scientifically planned nor skillfully played, but it furnished considerable excitement. The playing field was a square, sixty feet on a side, with a goal or base at each of its four corners. In the center of the square was stationed the pitcher. A catcher and an indefinite number of fielders completed the team supporting the pitcher. Usually there were from eight to twenty players on a side, but none of them were stationed at the bases, for the batter was out on balls caught on the fly or on the first bound, and the base runner was out if he was hit by a thrown ball while off a base. The bat was generally nothing more than a stout paddle with a blade two inches thick, while the ball was apt to be an impromptu affair composed of a bullet, a piece of cork, or a metal slug, wound around tightly with wool yarn and string. Under the name of "town ball," this game with simple equipment and few rules steadily increased in popularity during the first half of the century.

1. The title below that best expresses the main theme or subject of this selection is

    (A) *Baseball Rules*
    (B) *A Player's Skill*
    (C) *An English Game*
    (D) *An Early Form of Baseball*

2. The game described in this selection required

    (A) eight fielders
    (B) no set number of fielders
    (C) one fielder near each base
    (D) an even number of fielders

3. The author suggests that the game he is describing

    (A) required extensive training
    (B) required trained, skilled players
    (C) was more scientific than modern baseball
    (D) was less complicated than modern baseball

4. The author informs us that this game was popular because

    (A) only skilled persons could play
    (B) anyone could play, since there were few rules and the equipment was simple
    (C) this game was reserved for the town's elite
    (D) American youth in the early nineteenth century had no other form of recreation

READING COMPREHENSION TEST 4

6 Minutes   5 Questions

Directions: *Following the passage below, you will find one or more incomplete statements about the passage. Select the word or expression that most satisfactorily completes each statement. Blacken the corresponding space on your answer sheet.*

How can we know that the birds we see in the South in the winter are the same ones that come north in the spring? John J. Audubon, a bird lover, wondered about this. Every year he watched a pair of little phoebes nesting in the same place. He wondered if they were the same birds and so decided to put tiny silver bands on their legs. The next spring back came the birds with the bands to build their nests on the walls of farm buildings in the neighborhood. The phoebe, it was learned, wintered wherever it was warm enough to find flies. In summer, phoebes could be seen from Georgia to Canada; in winter, anywhere from Georgia to Florida and Mexico. The phoebe was the first kind of bird to be banded, and Mr. Audubon was the first birdbander. Today there are thousands of birdbanders all over America, people who band all kinds of birds.

The government of the United States has a special birdbanding department that makes all the birdbands. The bands do not hurt the birds because they are made of aluminum and are very light. They come in different sizes for different-sized birds. Each band has a special number and the words, "Notify Fish and Wildlife Service, Washington, DC." Anyone who finds a dead bird with a band on one of its legs is asked to send the band to Washington with a note telling where and when the bird was found. In this way naturalists add to their knowledge of the habits and needs of birds.

1. The title below that best expresses the main theme or subject of this selection is

   (A) *The Migration of Birds*
   (B) *The Work of John Audubon*
   (C) *The Habits and Needs of Birds*
   (D) *Studying Bird Life through Bird-banding*

2. According to the selection, Audubon proved his theory that

   (A) birds prefer a diet of flies
   (B) birds return to the same nesting place each spring
   (C) silver is the best material for bird-bands
   (D) phoebes are the most interesting birds to study

3. Audubon's purpose in banding the phoebes was to

   (A) satisfy his curiosity
   (B) notify the government
   (C) start a birdbanding department
   (D) gain fame as the first birdbander

4. The migration habits of phoebes depend upon

   (A) nesting places
   (B) the help of bird lovers
   (C) the available food supply
   (D) the number of young birds

5. Which statement is *true* according to the selection?

   (A) Residents of Georgia may expect to see phoebes all year long.
   (B) The weight of a band causes a bird considerable discomfort.
   (C) The government offers a reward for information about dead birds.
   (D) Phoebes are more plentiful in the East than any other kind of bird.

READING COMPREHENSION TEST 5

6 Minutes   3 Questions

Directions: *Following the passage below, you will find a number of incomplete statements about the passage. Select the word or expression that most satisfactorily completes each statement. Blacken the corresponding space on your answer sheet.*

A pair-bonded relationship, and more specifically monogamous marriage, is the "norm" for American society today. Society brings all of its weight to bear to push everyone into this mold who can feasibly fit into it. The reasons people use to justify their "deviation" from this behavior are numerous, but the most prevalent is that marriage stifles individuals and either stunts or totally prevents further individual growth of the partners. When one asks why a relationship that is supposed to be mutually fulfilling can stifle a person, five general but interrelated reasons are given most frequently. First, one central relationship for social identity and emotional support is both confining and unrealistic. Second, the security and interdependence of marriage hinders learning, experimentation, and independence; in other words, it leads to boredom. Third, an exclusive relationship breeds a sense of isolation from other people. Fourth, an exclusive relationship cuts down on the number of friends for both partners, since friends now have to be appealing to both partners. Finally, an exclusive dependency on one's mate cannot satisfy all the needs encountered in self-development.

The underlying factor in all of the above explanations is the inherent need in man for highly integrated social relationships. The very fact that we can live in areas where the living quarters are as closely stacked as the cells in a beehive attests to that fact. Man needs many and diverse interactions if he is to reach his full personal development. This is just part of the social nature of man. Exclusive relationships such as marriage, it seems, may not allow for diverse enough interactions, especially in the areas of sex and dating. The basic principles of the relationship are restrictive in nature, and it is in an attempt to avoid these restrictions on personal interactions that many people are choosing to remain single.

Singlehood provides the individual with the opportunity to continue his or her personal growth without the stifling aspects of marriage. On the other hand, marriage provides a sense of security and a ready framework for emotional and sexual feelings. Both states have good and bad aspects, and neither can be said to be right for everyone. It is only fitting, though, that singlehood should be accepted as a viable and "normal" alternative to marriage for those who do not want to marry at the present time, remarry, or marry at all. If this is allowed, it might provide a way of cutting the increasing divorce rate in this country, since people who feel they do not want to get married or are not suited for the commitments of marriage would not feel pressured by society into adopting a life-style that for them is doomed to failure.

1. An appropriate title for the above passage is

   (A) *Reducing the Divorce Rate*
   (B) *Singlehood—An Alternative to Marriage*
   (C) *Living Together*
   (D) *Monogamy*

2. According to the passage,

   (A) marriage can stifle diverse social interactions
   (B) everyone should marry at least once
   (C) marriage is the only normal relationship
   (D) married couples are lonely people

3. The author implies that

   (A) society accepts singlehood equally with marriage
   (B) married couples are usually independent of each other
   (C) society helps increase the divorce rate by accepting only marriage as "normal"
   (D) two can live as cheaply as one

READING COMPREHENSION TEST 6

6 Minutes   4 Questions

Directions: *Following the passage below, you will find a number of incomplete statements about the passage. Select the word or expression that most satisfactorily completes each statement. Blacken the corresponding space on your answer sheet.*

Some analysts consider the process of automation a second industrial revolution with the same potential for social upheaval that marked the birth of the factory a century and a half ago. Others insist it is just another step in industry's progress toward greater efficiency, no different in its basic attributes from any of the other technological advances that have helped raise American wages, employment, and living standards.

Congressional investigators, puzzled about what action the government should take, have been told by union leaders that automation threatens to produce mass unemployment and by business executives that it will bring unparalleled prosperity.

Engineers say that push-button factories may eventually permit a work schedule in which the weekend will be longer than the week. Educators see this leisure encouraging a scholastic renaissance in which cultural attainments will become the yardstick of social recognition for worker and boss alike. Gloomier observers fear the trend toward "inhuman production" will end by making men obsolete.

1. The title below that best expresses the ideas of this passage is

    (A) *Robots at Work*
    (B) *Industry a Century Ago and Today*
    (C) *Machines versus Mankind*
    (D) *Speculations on Automation*

2. The passage states that automation has

    (A) greatly raised our standard of living
    (B) caused great social changes
    (C) made us a more cultured nation
    (D) already been brought to the attention of Congress

3. According to the passage, it is true that

    (A) the government favors automation
    (B) industry has made great advances in the past one hundred and fifty years
    (C) engineers oppose automation
    (D) labor and management are agreed on the potential of automation

4. This passage is developed principally by means of

    (A) chronology
    (B) examples
    (C) contrast
    (D) definition

READING COMPREHENSION
TESTS 7 and 8

6 Minutes   6 Questions

Directions: *Carefully read Passage 7, answer the three following items on your answer sheet, and proceed immediately to Passage 8. The two reading passages and six items are timed for six minutes.*

TEST 7

The moon is the nearest of all our celestial neighbors, at a distance from the earth of about a quarter-of-a-million miles. It is a globe 2,000 miles in diameter, with mountains, plains, cliffs, deserts—a very rugged landscape indeed, but decidedly distasteful to a sailor because there is no ocean at all! Nor is there a river, lake, or pond, for that matter. It never rains; there is no water and no atmosphere. It is a hard concept to teach and to believe, but all the evidence points to the fact that the beautiful silvery moon, sublime and serene as it appears, is only a barren desert utterly devoid of any life as we know it. The moon suffers from great extremes of temperature and is exposed to a constant barrage of meteorites and debris that easily reaches the surface without hindrance, because there is no atmosphere to slow it down or consume it in friction-generated heat.

1. The title that best expresses the main idea of this selection is:

   (A) *Meteorites*
   (B) *Life on the Moon*
   (C) *A Sailor on the Moon*
   (D) *Conditions on the Moon*

2. Which would most likely be found on the moon?

   (A) shrubs
   (B) insects

   (C) rocks
   (D) tides

3. Which statement is *true* according to this selection?

   (A) The moon is drawing closer to us.
   (B) The appearance of the moon is deceiving.
   (C) Sailors say that they dislike the moon.
   (D) The moon sends off frequent showers of meteorites.

TEST 8

The nursing profession is in the midst of controversy that stems from an American Nurses' Association position paper advocating two levels of nursing— professional nursing and technical nursing. If adopted, this proposal would require a BSN degree for entrance into practice at the professional level and an AD degree for entry at the technical level. Many nurses think that the professional nurse-technical nurse proposal will serve only to divide nurses rather than unite them. They believe that the nurse's greatest responsibility to society is to administer good nursing care. Some nurses fear that nursing education may become overloaded with academic theory and lose the valuable clinical experience needed in an applied science. Polls show that the majority of nurses want to unite all levels of nursing while providing a diversity of programs at all levels—LPN, AD, diploma, and BSN.

1. The best title for this passage might be

   (A) *University Based Nursing Programs versus Hospital Based Nursing Programs*
   (B) *The Professional Status of Nurses*
   (C) *The Professional Nurse-Technical Nurse Controversy*
   (D) *Restructuring the American Nurses' Association*

2. The American Nurses' Association position paper implies that

   (A) nurses with college degrees will give better nursing care
   (B) there is not a nursing shortage

   (C) LPNs should work only in the home
   (D) career mobility has no place in nursing

3. The author suggests that

   (A) most nursing educators oppose the ANA position paper.
   (B) degree nursing programs provide less clinical experience than hospital-based programs.
   (C) it is not necessary for technical nurses to understand scientific principles.
   (D) professional nurses should be paid more than technical nurses.

Answer Key

Passage 1
1. **B**
2. **A**
3. **D**
4. **B**
5. **A**

Passage 2
1. **B**
2. **A**
3. **D**
4. **C**
5. **D**

Passage 3
1. **D**
2. **B**
3. **D**
4. **B**

Passage 4
1. **D**
2. **B**
3. **A**
4. **C**
5. **A**

Passage 5
1. **B**
2. **A**
3. **C**

Passage 6
1. **D**
2. **B**
3. **B**
4. **C**

Passage 7
1. **D**
2. **C**
3. **B**

Passage 8
1. **C**
2. **A**
3. **B**

Answer Sheet
Final Reading
Comprehension Examination

1. Ⓐ Ⓑ Ⓒ Ⓓ   6. Ⓐ Ⓑ Ⓒ Ⓓ   11. Ⓐ Ⓑ Ⓒ Ⓓ   16. Ⓐ Ⓑ Ⓒ Ⓓ   21. Ⓐ Ⓑ Ⓒ Ⓓ

2. Ⓐ Ⓑ Ⓒ Ⓓ   7. Ⓐ Ⓑ Ⓒ Ⓓ   12. Ⓐ Ⓑ Ⓒ Ⓓ   17. Ⓐ Ⓑ Ⓒ Ⓓ   22. Ⓐ Ⓑ Ⓒ Ⓓ

3. Ⓐ Ⓑ Ⓒ Ⓓ   8. Ⓐ Ⓑ Ⓒ Ⓓ   13. Ⓐ Ⓑ Ⓒ Ⓓ   18. Ⓐ Ⓑ Ⓒ Ⓓ   23. Ⓐ Ⓑ Ⓒ Ⓓ

4. Ⓐ Ⓑ Ⓒ Ⓓ   9. Ⓐ Ⓑ Ⓒ Ⓓ   14. Ⓐ Ⓑ Ⓒ Ⓓ   19. Ⓐ Ⓑ Ⓒ Ⓓ   24. Ⓐ Ⓑ Ⓒ Ⓓ

5. Ⓐ Ⓑ Ⓒ Ⓓ   10. Ⓐ Ⓑ Ⓒ Ⓓ   15. Ⓐ Ⓑ Ⓒ Ⓓ   20. Ⓐ Ⓑ Ⓒ Ⓓ   25. Ⓐ Ⓑ Ⓒ Ⓓ

FINAL READING
COMPREHENSION TEST

40 Minutes   25 Questions

Directions: *Following each of the passages below, you will find a number of incomplete statements about the passage. Select the word or expression that most satisfactorily completes each statement. Blacken the corresponding space on your answer sheet.*

The art of quilting was practiced in China and then in Europe centuries before American colonial women began making quilts. Although they began making them simply to keep warm, making a quilt soon became a means of artistic expression.

The "crazy quilt" was made from whatever scraps were left from other sewing projects. No scrap of cloth was discarded, since these women spent many hours spinning, weaving, and dyeing their cloth. Sometimes as many as one hundred scraps were used in one quilt. If a spot on a quilt became worn, it was patched.

Later, blocks, triangles, and diamond shapes of various colors were used—sewed on a large piece of white cloth. Sometimes their edges were embroidered with contrasting-colored thread. Some traditional patterns were known by the same name in all the colonies—for example, a pattern with a historical or political theme, the Confederate Rose.

In the seventeenth and eighteenth centuries, quilts were considered treasured heirlooms and were handed down from one generation to the next. Quilting bees were held, farmers' wives coming from miles around to quilt and socialize.

Even today quilting is a popular craft in some parts of the country. Patterns are exchanged via magazine ads, and quilting parties are held in community centers and senior citizens' buildings.

1. The best title for the article above is

   (A) *Quilting Parties*
   (B) *The Crazy Quilt*
   (C) *A History of Quilting*
   (D) *How To Make a Quilt*

2. Quilting was first done in

   (A) Europe
   (B) China
   (C) American colonies
   (D) quilting parties

3. A "crazy quilt" is

   (A) made of many scraps of different shapes and colors

   (B) a bright-red quilt sewed with contrasting-colored thread
   (C) longer than it is wide
   (D) made of triangles, blocks, and diamonds

4. According to the above passage,

   (A) quilting is an art of the past, no longer popular today
   (B) patterns were exchanged throughout the American colonies
   (C) quilts were made to be sold at a profit during the seventeenth century
   (D) colonists bought material to make quilts

Many patterns of nursing care are being used today. In the *functional* method of organizing care, each nursing employee is assigned specific duties to be carried out on all the patients in a given unit. For example, a nurse's aide might to assigned to take all the patients' temperatures and the practical nurse to take all the patients' blood pressures. When *team nursing* is used, a professional nurse acts as the leader and assigns the team members (other professional nurses, practical nurses, aides, and orderlies) to patients according to their capabilities. In *primary nursing*, the nurse is responsible for planning and caring for patients until they leave the hospital. One of the advantages of this pattern is that the nurse is able to give more individualized care. *Progressive* patient care groups the patients according to degree of illness, including the patients on the following units—intensive care, intermediate care, self care, long-term care, and home care. When the *specialized* care pattern is used, the patients are grouped according to their age or diagnoses, for example, orthopedics, pediatrics, obstetrics, or geriatrics. Nursing-care patterns are constantly being modified in an effort to improve the quality of care.

5. An appropriate title for the above passage is

   (A) *How Nurses Care for Their Patients*
   (B) *Advantages and Disadvantages of Nursing-Care Patterns*
   (C) *Nursing-Care Patterns*
   (D) *The Modification of Nursing Care Patterns*

6. When team nursing is practiced, the person who plans for and delgates care is the

   (A) head nurse
   (B) primary nurse
   (C) supervisor
   (D) team leader

7. The nursing-care pattern that assigns specific tasks, such as administration of medicine, to individual nurses is called

   (A) total patient care
   (B) functional
   (C) progressive patient care
   (D) primary nursing

8. Placing critically ill patients in the intensive care unit is an example of

   (A) progressive patient care
   (B) functional nursing
   (C) team nursing
   (D) primary nursing

Dinosaurs were huge, cold-blooded animals related to reptiles that at one time ruled the world. They lived millions of years ago and were extinct 60 million years before man came upon the earth. They lived on land and sea. Some were 40 feet long. One of the best known was the brontosaurus, so big that the earth thundered when it walked. That is why it is called the "thunder lizard." It weighed about 80,000 pounds and was about 70 feet long. Its very small head contained a brain that weighed less than a pound. It possessed very little intelligence, acting mostly by instinct. In spite of its huge size, it was virtually defenseless; a constant prey for carnivorous dinosaurs. Brontosaurus stayed near the water so that it could escape into deep water when in danger.

9. A good title for this passage is

   (A) *Prehistoric Times*
   (B) *Hunting for Fossils*
   (C) *About Dinosaurs*
   (D) *Carnivorous Dinosaurs*

10. Dinosaurs were

   (A) warm-blooded
   (B) cold-blooded
   (C) intelligent
   (D) made extinct by man

11. The brontosaurus

    (A) was a sea serpent
    (B) was quite defenseless against carni-
        vores

    (C) had horns that grew out of its neck
    (D) had no teeth

For generations, historians and boat lovers have been trying to learn more about the ship that brought the Pilgrims to America. The task is a difficult one, because *Mayflower* was such a common name for ships in early seventeenth-century England that there were at least 20 of them when the Pilgrims left for the New World.

An exact duplicate of the *Mayflower* has been built in England and given to the people of the Unites States as a symbol of the goodwill and common ancestry linking Britons and Americans. The Pilgrims' *Mayflower* apparently was built originally as a fishing vessel. It seems to have been 90 feet long by 22 feet wide, displacing 180 tons of water. The duplicate measures 90 feet long by 26 feet, displaces 183 tons, and has a crew of 21, as did the original vessel. The new *Mayflower* has no motor but travels faster than the old boat.

What happened to the historical boat? So far as can be determined, the *Mayflower* went back to less colorful jobs and, not too many years later, was scrapped. What happened to the beams, masts, and planking is questionable. In the English city of Abington, there is a Congregational church containing two heavy wooden pillars. Some say these pillars are masts from the *Mayflower*. A barn in the English town of Jordans seemed to be built of old ship timbers. Marine experts say these timbers are impregnated with salt and, if put together, would form a vessel 90 feet by 22 feet. The man who owned the farm when the peculiar barn was built was a relative of the man who appraised the *Mayflower* when it was scrapped.

So the original *Mayflower* may still be doing service ashore while her duplicate sails the seas again.

12. The title that best expresses the main theme or subject of this selection is

    (A) *The Fate of the Mayflower*
    (B) *A Symbol of Goodwill*
    (C) *The Scrapping of the* Mayflower
    (D) *The* Mayflower—*Old and New*

13. A long search was made for the Pilgrims' boat because it

    (A) contained valuable materials
    (B) might still do sea service
    (C) has historical importance
    (D) would link Great Britain and America

14. It has been difficult to discover what happened to the original *Mayflower* because

    (A) it has become impregnated with salt

    (B) it was such a small vessel
    (C) the search was begun too late
    (D) many ships bore the same name

15. The British recently had a duplicate of the *Mayflower* built because

    (A) the original could not be located
    (B) they wanted to make a gesture of friendship
    (C) parts of the original could be used
    (D) historians recommended such a step

16. Compared with the original *Mayflower*, the modern duplicate

    (A) is longer
    (B) displaces less water
    (C) carries a larger crew
    (D) is somewhat wider

17. When the author says that the original boat "may still be doing service ashore," he means that

    (A) it may be whole and entire somewhere

    (B) present-day buildings may include parts of it

    (C) it may be in a boat-lover's private collection

    (D) its memory creates good will

Spring comes without trumpets to the city. The asphalt is a wilderness that does not quicken overnight; winds blow gritty with cinders instead of merry with the smells of earth and fertilizer. Women wear their gardens on their hats. But spring is a season in the city too, and it has its own harbingers, constant as daffodils. Shop windows change their colors; people walk more slowly on the streets; what one can see of the sky has a bluer tone; and matinee tickets go a-begging. But gayer than any of these are the carousels, which are already, in sheltered places, beginning to turn with the sound of springtime itself. Carousels are the earliest and the truest and the oldest of all the urban signs

18. The title below that best expresses the ideas in this passage is

    (A) *There Are All Kinds of Spring*
    (B) *The Coming of Urban Spring*
    (C) *Spring in City and Country*
    (D) *Trumpet of Spring*

19. In the passage, the word "harbingers" means

    (A) storms
    (B) noises
    (C) truths
    (D) forerunners

20. One of the signs that spring is arriving in the city is that

    (A) the city is silent
    (B) almost everyone wear daffodils
    (C) theatergoing becomes less popular
    (D) it is more difficult to see the sky

21. Which of the following describes the author of this passage?

    (A) observant
    (B) indifferent
    (C) confused
    (D) unimaginative

We all know people who would welcome a new American car to their garage, but one cannot expect to find a sports-car man among them. He cannot be enticed into such a circus float without feeling soiled. He resents the wanton use of chromium as much as he shudders at the tail fins, the grotesquely convoluted bumpers, and other "dishonest" lines. He blanches at the enormous bustle, which adds weight and useless space, drags on ramps and curbstones, and complicates the process of parking even in the car's own garage.

The attitude of the owner of a Detroit product is reflected in efforts of manufacturers to "take the drive out of driving." The sports-car addict regards this stand as outrageous. His interest in a car, he is forever telling himself and other captive listeners, lies in the fun of driving it, in "sensing its alertness on the road" and in "pampering it like a thoroughbred."

22. Of the titles below, the one that best expresses the ideas of this passage is

(A) *The Car of the Future*
(B) *Driving Foreign Cars*
(C) *The American Interest in New Cars*
(D) *The Sports-car Enthusiast*

23. According to the passage, the driver of a sports car prefers a car that

(A) is simple in design
(B) has no bumpers
(C) is economical in gas consumption
(D) is chrome plated

24. The passage implies that sports cars are very

(A) colorful
(B) showy
(C) maneuverable
(D) roomy

25. The passage suggests that sports-car owners

(A) regard economy as secondary in buying a car
(B) secretly admire Detroit products
(C) believe garages should be made longer
(D) are opposed to push-button driving

Answer Key

1.	**C**	10.	**B**	18.	**B**
2.	**B**	11.	**B**	19.	**D**
3.	**A**	12.	**D**	20.	**C**
4.	**B**	13.	**C**	21.	**A**
5.	**C**	14.	**D**	22.	**D**
6.	**D**	15.	**B**	23.	**A**
7.	**B**	16.	**D**	24.	**C**
8.	**A**	17.	**B**	25.	**D**
9.	**C**				

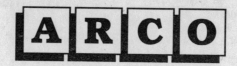

BOOKS FOR COLLEGE-BOUND STUDENTS

COLLEGE ENTRANCE

ACT: American College Testing Program
ACT Cram Course
ACT English Workbook
ACT Math Workbook
ACT SuperCourse
AP American History
AP Biology
AP Chemistry
AP Computer Science
AP English Composition and Literature
AP European History
AP Mathematics
College Board Achievement Test
  in Mathematics: Level I
College Board Achievement Test
  in Mathematics: Level II
College Board Achievement Test in Spanish
College Board Achievement Tests SuperCourse
Nursing School Entrance Examinations
PCAT: Pharmacy College Admissions Test
Preparation for the SAT: Scholastic Assessment Test
SAT Cram Course
SAT Math Workbook
SAT SuperCourse
SAT Verbal Workbook
SAT-II Writing
TOEFL: Test of English as a Foreign Language
TOEFL Grammar Workbook
TOEFL Reading and Vocabulary Workbook
TOEFL Skills for Top Scores
TOEFL SuperCourse

COLLEGE GUIDES

The American Film Institute Guide to College Courses
  in Film and Television
College Applications and Essays

College Financial Aid
College Survival
Lovejoy's College Guide
The Performing Arts Major's College Guide
The Right College
The Transfer Student's Guide

STUDY AIDS

Associated Press Guide to News Writing
Consumer and Business Mathematics
College Time Tracker
Essential English Composition for College-Bound
  Students
Essential Math for College-Bound Students
Essential Vocabulary for College-Bound
  Students
High School Time Tracker
How to Develop and Write a Research Paper
How to Read and Interpret Poetry
How to Read and Write about Drama
How to Read and Write about Fiction
How to Solve Algebra Word Problems
How to Write Book Reports
How to Write Poetry
How to Write Short Stories
How to Write Themes and Essays
How to Write a Thesis
1001 Ideas for Science Projects
Reading Lists for College-Bound Students
10,000 Ideas for Term Papers, Projects, Reports,
  and Speeches
Triple Your Reading Speed
Webster's New World™ Power Vocabulary
Webster's New World™ Student Writing
  Handbook

AVAILABLE AT BOOKSTORES EVERYWHERE

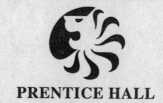

PRENTICE HALL

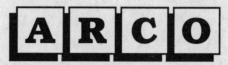

ARCO

BOOKS FOR GRADUATE SCHOOL AND BEYOND

ARCO'S SUPERCOURSES

GMAT SuperCourse
GRE SuperCourse
LSAT SuperCourse
MCAT SuperCourse
TOEFL SuperCourse

TOEFL

TOEFL: Test of English as a Foreign Language
TOEFL Grammar Workbook
TOEFL Reading and Vocabulary Workbook
TOEFL Skills for Top Scores

ARCO'S CRAM COURSES

GMAT Cram Course
GRE Cram Course
LSAT Cram Course

TEACHER CERTIFICATION

CBEST: California Educational Basic Skills Test
NTE: National Teacher Examinations
PPST: Pre-Professional Skills Tests
Teacher Certification Tests

HEALTH PROFESSIONS

Allied Health Professions
Nursing School Entrance Examinations
PCAT: Pharmacy College Admission Test

GRADUATE SCHOOL GUIDES

The Best Law Schools
Getting into Law School: Strategies for the 90's
Getting into Medical School: Strategies for the 90's
The Grad Student's Guide to Getting Published

GRADUATE & PROFESSIONAL SCHOOL ENTRANCE

GMAT: Graduate Management Admission Test
GRE: Graduate Record Examination
GRE • GMAT Math Review
Graduate Record Examination in Computer Science
Graduate Record Examination in Engineering
Graduate Record Examination in Psychology
GRE • LSAT Logic Workbook
LSAT: Law School Admission Test
MAT: Miller Analogies Test
MCAT Sample Exams

AVAILABLE AT BOOKSTORES EVERYWHERE

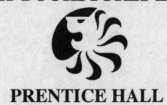

PRENTICE HALL

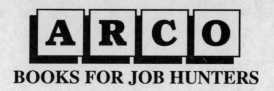

ARCO
BOOKS FOR JOB HUNTERS

CAREERS / STUDY GUIDES

Airline Pilot
Allied Health Professions
Automobile Technician Certification Tests
Federal Jobs for College Graduates
Federal Jobs in Law Enforcement
Getting Started in Film
How to Pass Clerical Employment Tests
How You Really Get Hired
Law Enforcement Exams Handbook
Make Your Job Interview a Success
Mechanical Aptitude and Spatial Relations Tests
Mid-Career Job Hunting
100 Best Careers for the Year 2000
Passport to Overseas Employment
Postal Exams Handbook
Real Estate License Examinations
Refrigeration License Examinations
Travel Agent

RESUME GUIDES

The Complete Resume Guide
Resumes for Better Jobs
Resumes That Get Jobs
Your Resume: Key to a Better Job

AVAILABLE AT BOOKSTORES EVERYWHERE

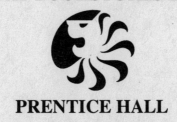

PRENTICE HALL

CANCELLED